PENNSYLVANIA COLLEGE OF TECHNOLOGY LIBRARY
5 0608 01181827 4

D1568430

White Matter Dementia

White Matter Dementia

Christopher M. Filley
University of Colorado School of Medicine
Denver Veterans Affairs Medical Center

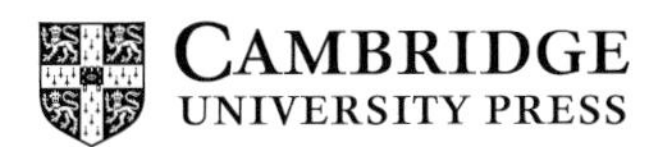

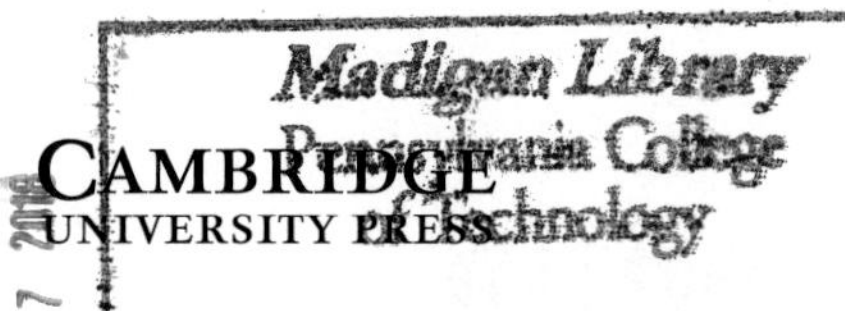

CAMBRIDGE
UNIVERSITY PRESS

University Printing House, Cambridge CB2 8BS, United Kingdom

Cambridge University Press is part of the University of Cambridge.

It furthers the University's mission by disseminating knowledge in the pursuit of education, learning and research at the highest international levels of excellence.

www.cambridge.org
Information on this title: www.cambridge.org/9781107035416

First published 2016

Printed in the United Kingdom by Clays, St Ives plc

A catalogue record for this publication is available from the British Library

Library of Congress Cataloguing in Publication data
Filley, Christopher M., 1951– , author.
White matter dementia / Christopher M. Filley.
Cambridge ; New York : Cambridge University Press, 2016. | Includes bibliographical references and index.
LCCN 2015051480 | ISBN 9781107035416 (hardback)
| MESH: Dementia – physiopathology | White Matter – physiopathology | Dementia – diagnosis
LCC RC521 | NLM WM 220 | DDC 616.8/3–dc23
LC record available at http://lccn.loc.gov/2015051480

ISBN 978-1-107-03541-6 Hardback

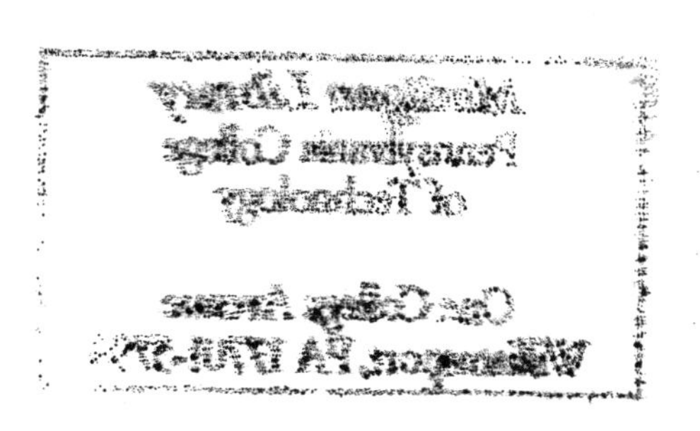

To all the patients who have contributed to my understanding of the brain in the course of their suffering

Contents

Foreword ix
Preface xi

1 **Brain–behavior relationships: a reconsideration** 1
2 **The essential contributions of neuroimaging** 9
3 **White matter neurobiology** 17
4 **A neuroanatomic overview of dementia** 27
5 **Expanding the concept of dementia** 35
6 **White matter disorders** 42
7 **White matter dementia** 95
8 **Mild cognitive dysfunction: a precursor syndrome** 118
9 **Diagnosis** 127
10 **Prognosis** 135
11 **Treatment** 142
12 **White matter and cognition: research perspectives** 153
13 **Therapeutic innovations** 162
14 **Alzheimer's Disease and white matter** 172
15 **Chronic traumatic encephalopathy and white matter** 185
16 **Beyond corticocentrism** 195

Index 203

Foreword

For years, the scientific community has focused on the influence of gray matter on cognition at the expense of white matter. In the past 30 years, advances in imaging tools have allowed us to delineate the relative contributions of white and gray matter in higher cortical function. In 1988 Chris Filley introduced the term "white matter dementia" when it became clear that white matter loss could produce cognitive decline and, when sufficiently severe, dementia.

Dr. Filley has thoughtfully considered the role of white matter in health and disease for more than 30 years, and *White Matter Dementia* is the constellation of his thinking on this critically important topic. "Corticocentrism," a term used by Dr. Filley to emphasize the lack of interest in white matter, sets the stage for this book, which provides a thorough and highly innovative review of white matter and cognition. His extensive experience with patients has shaped the scholarly approach to a topic on which he has performed his own pioneering research. This book takes the reader on a journey through white matter disorders and white matter dementia to diagnosis, prognosis, treatment, and a look at what's coming. This is a huge range of material with the fresh perspective of an experienced behavioral neurologist.

Dr. Filley describes a broad spectrum of disorders ranging from Alzheimer's Disease to traumatic brain injury and chronic traumatic encephalopathy, drug-induced white matter injury, vascular dementia, primary leukoencephalopathies, and a wide range of neuropsychiatric disorders. The early clinical manifestations of white matter dysfunction are detailed, and Dr. Filley guides the reader to a practical approach to the evaluation of white matter manifestations of brain disease. Augmented by scholarly discussions of white matter anatomy, both macroscopic and microscopic, the biological features of oligodendroglia, and gray and white matter connections and circuitry, *White Matter Dementia* is an intriguing read. The behavioral neurology of white matter is the unifying thread of this impressive and unique book.

I am proud to endorse this book and think it serves an incredibly valuable educational need. It will be an important part of any complete neurology library. We're inching closer to viable treatments for neurodegenerative diseases, and we need to have a complete picture get us across the finish line. This book brings us one step closer to the day when clinicians will be able to recognize the clinical manifestations of white matter disease, understand the biological cause, and provide effective treatments for the patient.

Bruce L. Miller, MD
A.W. and Mary Margaret Clausen Distinguished Professor in Neurology
Director, Memory and Aging Center
Joint Appointment in Psychiatry
UC San Francisco School of Medicine

Preface

My interest in the white matter of the brain as it contributes to human behavior dates back more than 30 years. In medical school during the late 1970s, I was taught that white matter had little or nothing to do with cognition, but even at that stage of my education I was not persuaded. Only as I completed residency and fellowship training, however, did I gain critical insight into this question, and joining the faculty of the University of Colorado in 1984 offered many opportunities to explore the topic in earnest. Since then, the journey in pursuit of white matter–behavior relationships has proven endlessly fascinating.

As a behavioral neurologist regularly called upon to evaluate people with cognitive loss or dementia, I naturally think in great detail about the neuroanatomic basis of cognition. Beginning with the principle that all mental operations are products of the brain, and recognizing that the brain is a highly evolved organ with almost overwhelming structural and functional complexity, is it possible to delineate neuroanatomic categories that can meaningfully shed light on cognitive dysfunction? The cerebral cortex has a long and cherished history in human neuroscience as the primary locus of higher function, and is rightly the topic of intensive study in this respect. Less well appreciated but still recognized in the architecture of cognition is the subcortical gray matter, which attracts attention as a parallel substrate of cognitive function. Between these two general gray matter areas, as every student of neuroscience knows, lies the white matter, which until recently received the least attention of all.

In this book, I have attempted to apply the idea that white matter plays a key role in cognition to the important clinical problem of dementia. The result is the concept of white matter dementia, a theoretical construct intended to help organize thinking with regard to the neural foundations of human cognition. Introduced in 1988, the syndrome of white matter dementia has served to contextualize a wide variety of observations that have been made with modern neuroimaging, offering a framework for understanding how the connectivity of the brain complements the operations of gray matter. This book reviews the original formulation of the idea, its refinement and clarification, its current position relative to trends in neuroscience (including connectomics and systems biology), and its promise for stimulating further investigation.

I am particularly indebted to Nick Dunton at Cambridge University Press for approaching me with the idea of writing this book. Many other individuals have informed, encouraged, advised, and corrected me along the long course of completing this work, and their contributions have been invaluable: C. Alan Anderson, James P. Kelly, David B. Arciniegas, Elizabeth Kozora, C. Munro Cullum, B. K. Kleinschmidt-DeMasters, Bruce L. Miller, Herbert H. Schaumburg, Jeremy D. Schmahmann, John Hart Jr., Erin D. Bigler, Marco Catani, Michael P. Alexander, Mario F. Mendez, Bruce H. Price, Allan H. Ropper, Josette G. Harris, Jose M. Lafosse, Erin D. Bigler, Jim Grigsby, Jack H. Simon, Mark S. Brown, Steven P. Ringel, John R. Corboy, Mark C. Spitz, Daniel I. Kaufer, Deborah A. Hall, Brian D. Hoyt, Michael R. Greher, Thomas R. Wodushek, Christopher Domen, Brianne M. Bettcher, Neill R. Graff-Radford, Ronald C. Petersen, Brian D. Berman, Bruce R. Ransom, Mark P. Goldberg, Melissa E. Murray, Bernard Michel, Francois Boller, Gorazd B. Stokin, Wendy B. Macklin, John R. Sladek, Leroy Hood, and R. Douglas Fields. Kristie Fields provided secretarial support, and Kenneth L. Tyler helped make possible the academic environment in which the ideas in this book could take shape and find expression. I am grateful to all.

Brain–behavior relationships: a reconsideration

In 1906, the esteemed anatomist Santiago Ramón y Cajal shared the Nobel Prize in Medicine or Physiology with Camillo Golgi, another well-known anatomist of the time. In his acceptance speech for the award, Ramón y Cajal defended what has come to be known as the neuron doctrine – the idea that all neurons of the central nervous system (CNS) are linked but not physically connected – while in his address Golgi defended his reticular theory – the notion that all CNS neurons are fused as one within a diffuse network (Bock, 2013). This vigorous debate was eventually resolved by growing evidence at the time and much subsequent work that incontrovertibly confirmed the neuron doctrine, establishing a fundamental tenet of neuroscience (Kandel et al., 2013). The neuron doctrine has exerted enormous influence in structuring thinking about how the brain subserves behavior by focusing attention squarely on the roughly 100 billion nerve cells of the human brain. In the quest to discover more precision about the relationship between the brain and behavior, however, many more details of CNS neurons become important, including their location, microstructure, physiology, pharmacology, and, most recently, their position within widespread distributed neural networks mediating cognition and emotion. All of these aspects of neural structure and function are critical not only for understanding the brain and its operations, but also for the care of millions of people around the world with devastating neurologic disorders.

Behavioral neurology is commonly described as the study of higher cortical function, a characterization held so firmly by many neuroscientists that a "corticocentric" explanation for the varieties of human behavior is often adopted without question (Parvizi, 2009). Everyday experience indicates that the vast majority of physicians and scientists, and the general public, would doubtless endorse the assumption that a person's intelligence is primarily a function of the amount of gray matter in that individual's brain. Among all the gray matter regions of the brain, however, the cerebral cortex holds a special place in neuroscientific thinking, compelling an almost reflexive allegiance to this thin mantle of tightly arrayed neuronal cell bodies, dendrites, and synapses. As much as the cortex deserves its reputation as critical for the higher functions, however, a wealth of evidence also supports the notion that brain–behavior relationships extend beyond those that can be developed with respect to the cerebral cortex (Geschwind, 1965; Schmahmann et al., 2008; Parvizi, 2009; Filley, 2012). Whereas the importance of the cortical mantle in elaborating human behavior is firmly established, the contributions of neurons and their projections in noncortical regions – the subcortical gray matter and the white matter – cannot be neglected.

As more clinical and experimental data are gathered, it is increasingly evident that a more nuanced view of the neural underpinnings of behavior is needed, and the regions below the cerebral cortex are entirely appropriate areas of study. Experienced neurologists recognize the potential for damage to these regions to produce significant neurobehavioral dysfunction, but the long-standing preeminence of the cortical gray matter in the neuroscience of behavior has to some extent hampered investigation of the full range and subtlety of brain–behavior relationships. This limitation is nowhere more evident than in the study of dementia.

The conventional emphasis on gray matter

The growing problem of Alzheimer's Disease (AD) overshadows the entire field of dementia, and indeed attracts well-deserved attention as a medical and societal menace that extends far beyond the confines of neuroscience. The widely accepted neuropathology of AD, memorized by medical students as featuring the familiar neuritic plaques and neurofibrillary tangles, naturally directs attention to the cerebral cortex in the investigation of etiopathogenesis, clinical phenomenology, and treatment (Querfurth and LaFerla, 2010). At the same time, the prominence of thinking about higher cortical function – regularly taught in many medical and graduate schools as the province of behavioral neurology – further draws investigators toward the cerebral cortex in an almost irresistible fashion. But many other dementias result from neuropathology in regions other than the cortex, and the understanding of dementia cannot be complete without inclusion of these disorders. Indeed, it can be plausibly stated that the field has been held back by the somewhat uncritical acceptance of the cortex as the only important mediator of cognition, a view that to some extent impedes innovative thinking about the phenomenology and etiopathogenesis of dementia syndromes.

The long-standing emphasis on cortical gray matter as the source of higher functions has its roots in the nineteenth century, when advances in neurology and neuroscience fostered the development of a hierarchical conceptualization of the brain (Parvizi, 2009). According to this view, the brain is composed of "lower" structures in caudal regions that subserve involuntary behaviors, with "higher" structures added rostrally in the course of evolution as humans acquired more voluntary control over instinctual behavior. At the summit of the brain's evolved structural hierarchy is the cerebral cortex, particularly the frontal lobes, which is thought to endow humans with distinctive cognitive capacities. An early impetus to corticentrism was manifest in the work of Franz Joseph Gall (1758–1828) and his collaborator Johann Kaspar Spurzheim (1776–1832), whose misguided ventures into phrenology nevertheless focused attention on the cerebral cortex as the substrate of the higher functions (Gall and Spurzheim, 1810–1818). A corticocentric focus was then prominently advanced by the English neurologist John Hughlings-Jackson (1835–1911), who maintained that higher brain centers operated for the purpose of governing lower ones (Parvizi, 2009). Hughlings-Jackson's seminal studies of epilepsy also stimulated interest in the cortex, as it was clear that a diversity of neurobehavioral experiences were associated with certain kinds of seizures. Sigmund Freud (1856–1939), who began his career as a neurologist and was an admirer of Hughlings-Jackson, followed later in a similar manner with his proposal of the id, ego, and superego forming the structure of personality; these categories, like all psychic processes, would presumably be found someday to correspond to specific areas of the brain (Parvizi, 2009). All of these ideas proved highly influential, and whereas much has been learned since the days of Gall, Hughlings-Jackson, and Freud, the hierarchical view of the brain and cognition continues to inform much contemporary thinking in neuroscience.

With the coming of the twentieth century, brain–behavior relationships were largely ignored as Freudian psychoanalysis and holistic psychology held sway for some 50 years. Still, Alzheimer's discovery of plaques and tangles in the cerebral cortex of his demented patient Auguste Deter (Alzheimer, 1907) helped keep alive the focus on the cerebral cortex. In subsequent years, as brain–behavior relationships began to attract neuroscientific interest once again, the influential neuropsychologist Alexander Luria further supported the bias toward the cerebral cortex by studying Russian soldiers who had sustained penetrating head injuries in World War II. This work culminated in the publication of his masterwork *Higher Cortical Functions in Man* (1966), a book that highlighted the term still commonly used to describe the interests of behavioral neurologists. Roughly contemporaneous with Luria, the Canadian neurosurgeon Wilder Penfield (1891–1973) presented remarkable observations from awake patients to show convincingly that conscious experiences could be elicited by stimulation of the cerebral cortex (Penfield, 1975).

As neurology gained momentum as a medical specialty in the mid-twentieth century, an unquestioned assumption about the hegemony of the cortex in the organization of cognition steadily became commonplace. One factor supporting this assumption was that laboratory studies using animal models are necessarily limited with respect to the examination of the other major portion of the brain, its white matter. As will be discussed in Chapter 3, nonhuman animals have far less white matter than humans have; in rodents, for example, the laboratory animals studied most often, only about 14% of brain volume is occupied by white matter (Goldberg and Ransom, 2003), whereas in humans this figure is about 50%. Thus the extrapolation of data from rodent studies to humans has led to serious underestimation of the importance of white matter involvement in human disease (Matute and Ransom, 2012). Another development fostering the corticocentric perspective was that, as the technology of clinical neuroscience improved to quantify many aspects of brain structure and function, most methods that came into widespread use – electroencephalography, magnetoencephalography, single photon emission computed tomography, positron emission tomography, and functional magnetic resonance imaging – were not generally applied to the examination of any brain areas except the cerebral cortex (Parvizi, 2009). The oldest of these technologies, electroencephalography, can in fact be employed to study white matter because of the disruption in electrographic coherence caused by white matter lesions (Nunez, Srinivasan, and Fields, 2015), but the primary application of electroencephalography has clearly been in the study of cortical function. Thus the use of available methods for studying the brain further exacerbated the bias toward the cortex and away from other regions. Because the instruments available to study the brain were not developed to probe any region except its outermost layer, it is not surprising that the underlying tissue remained to a large extent understudied. This situation persists to a considerable degree today; despite structural neuroimaging techniques that allow detailed views of subcortical regions, functional imaging studies of the cerebral cortex dominate the field.

A related problem unique to the world of dementia research also deserves comment. As will be discussed in more detail later in this book, the assumption that cortical neuropathology underlies the dementia of AD is so pervasive that it has come to dominate thinking about how dementing disease produces clinical dysfunction. The striking postmortem appearance of cortical neuritic plaques and neurofibrillary tangles in a person who was known to have dementia is indeed compelling, and, drawing from experience with other neuropathological lesions such as atherosclerosis, neoplasia, and viral inclusions that clearly cause clinical illness, neurologists are predisposed to conclude that plaques and tangles cause dementia. Even though this conclusion cannot be indisputably supported, as will be discussed in subsequent chapters, the powerful influence of plaques and tangles further reinforces the view that the cortex is the most essential, or even only, site of cognitive function. Thus a certain circularity of reasoning develops, by which it is claimed that because plaques and tangles in the cortex explain the dementia of AD, the cortex is the only region that matters for cognition (Figure 1.1). Whereas the cortex is undoubtedly important for cognition, to invoke the neuropathology of AD as proof that only the cortex matters runs the risk of oversimplifying the complexity of dementing illness.

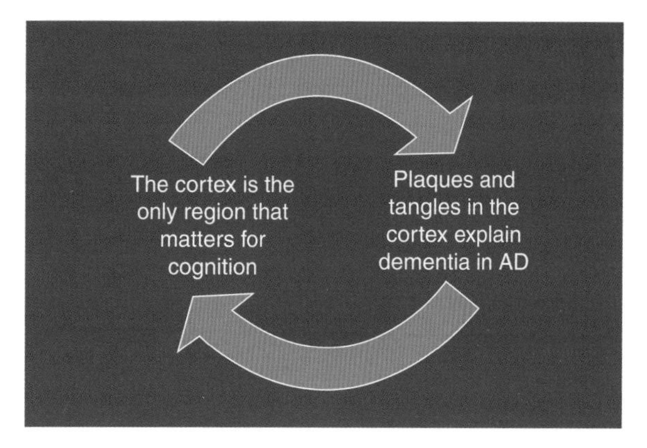

Figure 1.1 Circular reasoning on the structural basis of dementia.

In sum, all of these factors have conspired to concentrate research efforts on the cerebral cortex in the overwhelming majority of current studies in cognitive neuroscience, particularly those devoted to the study of dementia. This situation would seem to be in need of an adjustment that will serve to extend investigation to other regions of the brain that play a key role. It is in this light that the present state of cognitive neuroscience suffers from what has been justifiably termed corticocentric "myopia" (Parvizi, 2009).

If the undue concentration on the cerebral cortex is to be rectified, a comprehensive effort to examine regions subjacent to the cortical mantle is clearly warranted. This directive immediately implicates the impressive array of noncortical structures, which include the deep gray matter of the thalamus, basal ganglia, the cerebellum, and of course the white matter. The subcortical dementias, the most familiar being Huntington's Disease (HD) and Parkinson's Disease (PD), are classically associated mainly with neuropathology in the basal ganglia, and despite some criticism, the concept of subcortical dementia has endured as a useful contrasting clinical syndrome to the cortical dementia of AD (Bonelli and Cummings, 2008). White matter disorders are often included in the subcortical dementias, alternatively known as frontal-subcortical dementias (Bonelli and Cummings, 2008), but uncertainty has lingered about the importance of white matter damage in producing neurobehavioral effects. In part because white matter changes on contemporary neuroimaging are so common, and at times present in normal people of all ages, patients with dementia and white matter lesions are frequently assumed to have coexistent cortical neuropathology to explain their cognitive loss. White matter is not traditionally discussed as a specific foundation of cognitive or emotional operations in curricula or textbooks considering the neural organization of human behavior, and it is not surprising that until recently it has figured only incidentally in research on dementia.

Why white matter matters

White matter merits focused and systematic consideration as a brain component critical not only to the field of dementia but to all of behavioral neurology (Filley et al., 1988; Filley, 2011, 2012). At first glance, it should not be a novel realization that the roughly one half of the human brain occupied by white matter may be important for behavior (Nolte, 2002; Schmahmann and Pandya, 2006). Nature has little use for tissues with no functional significance, and white matter provides the essential macroconnectivity of distributed neural networks coursing within and between the hemispheres to subserve information processing speed and a range of related neurobehavioral functions. Evolution has in fact produced an expansion of white matter volume exceeding that of gray matter in *Homo sapiens*, as will be elaborated in Chapter 3. From a clinical perspective, modern neuroimaging has revealed that white matter lesions with a predilection for the frontal lobes are present in a large proportion of the entire population, and in the vast majority of older adults (Launer, 2004), observations that not only implicate white matter dysfunction in the pathogenesis of cognitive impairment but also underscore the prominence of frontal white matter as a feature of human neuroanatomy (Schoenemann, Sheehan, and Glotzer, 2005). The gray matter, meanwhile, contributes at the level of the synapse via an intricate web of microconnectivity, and is the major locus of much investigation describing the mediation of memory, language, praxis, perception, and other instrumental functions, and, of course, the cognitive impairment related to neuropathology in these regions. White matter functions in parallel with gray matter to expand the operational capacity of neurons by enabling the rapid and efficient transfer of information that complements the information processing of synapses and neuronal cell bodies (Turken et al., 2008; Bartzokis et al., 2010; Kochunov et al., 2010; Kerchner et al., 2012).

These ideas have recently coalesced to foster a new development in neuroscience centered on the concept of the "connectome," generally defined as the totality of neural connections in the human brain (Sporns, 2011). These connections include synaptic contacts in gray matter, often called the microconnectome, and the longer connections made by white matter tracts, which are known as the macroconnectome (Kaiser, 2013), the collection of macroscopic tracts that form the basis of this book. Whereas the history of neuroscience is replete with efforts by many distinguished investigators to map the brain, these attempts most often focus on the cerebral cortex, and the power of advanced neuroimaging now enables the study of what has come to be called connectomics as never before (Catani et al., 2013). Exciting as the prospect may be, however, it is wise to put the topic in perspective: whereas the complete connectome of the nervous system in the nematode *Caenorhabditis elegans* was mapped almost 30 years ago (White et al., 1986), this project involved the analysis of just 302 neurons and 5,000 synapses, and it is a far more daunting task to take on the roughly 100 billion neurons and 100 trillion synapses of the human brain (Catani et al., 2013). Nevertheless, the extraordinary connectivity that subserves the highly integrated phenomena of cognition and emotion calls out for exactly this kind of investigation. To that end, the Human Connectome Project has been launched in the United States, with the assistance of federal funding, with the goal of producing a comprehensive, publicly available map of human brain connectivity (Toga et al., 2012). Impressive progress has already been made in advancing the understanding of connectivity as neuroimaging techniques continue to evolve at a rapid pace.

As will be demonstrated throughout this book, and can be reviewed in a previous monograph (Filley, 2012), the neurobehavioral study of white matter discloses a host of cognitive and emotional deficits that can plausibly be related to tract damage in the subcortex and, to some extent, within the cortex itself. These observations are crucial for clinical neuroscience, including the daily tasks of accurate diagnosis and informed patient care. But it is also worth considering the role of white matter in health, and studies are showing that the functions of white matter as determined by modern neuroimaging correspond well with the loss of functions observed with lesions of those same systems. With the availability of astonishing neuroimaging techniques that can identify regions of white matter and correlate their structure and function with normal cognitive operations, it is becoming clear that cerebral white matter is centrally engaged in cognitive processing speed (Kerchner et al., 2012), mathematical ability (Matejko et al., 2013), measured intelligence (Jung et al., 1999), several traditional neurobehavioral domains such as executive function (Sasson et al., 2013), memory (Fields, 2011), language (Friederici, 2015), and visuospatial skills (Umarova et al., 2010), and in more recently considered areas, including social cognition (Parkinson and Wheatley, 2014) and creativity (Takeuchi et al., 2010). Far from the often expressed view that white matter simply "follows" gray matter as a mere extension of the neuronal cell bodies and synapses in the cerebral cortex that primarily generate the phenomena of higher function, white matter makes its own unique contribution to the multiple distributed neural networks subserving behavior. Moreover, the importance of white matter is apparent across the life span as developmental changes exert selective age-dependent effects (Bartzokis et al., 2001; Bartzokis, 2005). The myelinated tracts of the brain participate in all normal neurobehavioral functions, and their breakdown or dysfunction under abnormal conditions may have profound clinical consequences.

The behavioral neurology of white matter

The many advantages offered by the advent of neuroimaging techniques over the past three decades have allowed clinicians and investigators to examine the white matter using a time-honored approach known as the lesion method. Originating with the work of nineteenth-century neurologists who correlated neurobehavioral deficits seen in life with brain damage seen at autopsy (Benson, 1993), the lesion method has been and remains the major source of information at the core of behavioral neurology (Damasio, 1984; Benson, 1993; Filley, 2011). Yet the data gathered by this method largely focused on gray matter, especially that of the cerebral cortex, and white matter was traditionally not given equal consideration. Conventional magnetic resonance imaging (MRI) directly addresses this deficiency with its remarkable capacity to depict the white matter of the brain in health and disease (Aralasmak et al., 2006). With MRI, white matter findings can be correlated in life with neurobehavioral deficits just as securely as changes within gray matter, and in some cases even more so. Since then, an impressive database has been generated to support the role of white matter in cognition and emotion.

One of the most durable tenets of behavioral neurology, and indeed a principle central to all of neurology, is that the location of a lesion is more clinically revealing than its etiology. That is, the understanding of altered behavior in people with brain damage is fundamentally determined by the site of the damage rather than its cause. Once the correlation of the behavioral change with the area(s) of damage is established, then the critically important tasks of defining the neuropathology as precisely as possible and then treating the problem can proceed. But from a neurobehavioral perspective, localization is paramount. Nonfluent aphasia in a right-handed individual, for example, implies left inferior frontal cortical injury, and similarly, a cerebral disconnection syndrome suggests damage to the corpus callosum; in each case, neuropathological lesions ranging from infarction and trauma to infection and neoplasm may all be responsible.

With the emergence of modern neuroimaging invigorating the study of brain–behavior relationships, interest in white matter steadily mounted. As MRI led to better understanding of old diseases and the discovery of intriguing new ones – many associated with obvious neurobehavioral dysfunction – it became ever more difficult to ignore the impact of white matter lesions on normal cognition and emotion. A good example of this trend was apparent in the understanding of multiple sclerosis (MS); whereas cognitive impairment of any severity was thought to be present in only around 5% of patients in the pre-MRI era (Kurtzke, 1970), careful study of this issue in later years disclosed cognitive impairment in 43% of MS patients (Rao et al., 1991), and figures higher than this are often cited.

MRI, therefore, offered the novel opportunity to examine white matter–behavior relationships. As with cortical diseases, white matter disorders can be investigated by use of the lesion method, and combined with neuropathological methods, MRI and its derivative techniques are steadily establishing the selective role of white matter dysfunction in disturbing normal behavior. Studies of this kind are also helping find a solution to the issue of the potential role of concomitant gray matter neuropathology that may complicate the relationships between white matter and behavior (Stadelmann et al., 2008). Reports have now appeared that demonstrate selective white matter dysfunction – with minimal gray matter involvement, or none at all – that has compelling neurobehavioral relevance. Examples can be found in cases of focal damage detected by MRI (Arnett et al., 1996; Van Zandvoort et al., 1998), volumetric MRI studies demonstrating macrostructural disruption (Juhasz et al., 2007; Northam et al., 2011), advanced neuroimaging with magnetic resonance spectroscopy (MRS; Filley et al., 2009), magnetization transfer imaging (MTI; Iannucci et al., 2001), and diffusion tensor imaging (DTI; Gold et al., 2010) disclosing microstructural disturbances, and neuropathological study of white matter (Filley, Halliday, and Kleinschmidt-DeMasters, 2004; Al-Hajri and Del Bigio, 2010; Del Bigio, 2010). In all of these examples, the relative contributions of white and gray matter have been considered, and the conclusion has been reached that neurobehavioral significance can be attributed to disordered white matter alone. While not likely to come as a surprise to many neurologists and others who examine brain–behavior relationships, the demonstration that white matter by itself disrupts neurobehavioral competence has been uncommon until recently. Studies of this kind are most welcome, as the information generated is crucial for understanding the unique contribution of white matter to behavior.

It has thus become apparent that a behavioral neurology of white matter can be plausibly considered (Filley, 2012). Historically, the development of such a body of knowledge would not be possible without the work of Norman Geschwind (1926–1984; Figure 1.2), recognized as the founder of behavioral neurology, whose most important paper (Geschwind, 1965) emphasized the role of cerebral disconnection in the pathogenesis of neurobehavioral syndromes. The idea of disconnection, which prominently involves cerebral white matter damage or dysfunction, had been introduced by many prominent nineteenth-century European neurologists, and Geschwind vigorously revived and expanded the concept while launching the discipline known as behavioral neurology. Classic syndromes such as conduction aphasia and alexia without agraphia were highlighted as clearly implicating white matter, setting the stage for the detailed analysis of many other syndromes related to white matter lesions that would become possible with neuroimaging. Today the behavioral neurology of white matter includes not only the classic disconnection syndromes of Geschwind and his predecessors, but also a variety of neuropsychiatric conditions, and the syndromes of cognitive impairment that are the subject of this book.

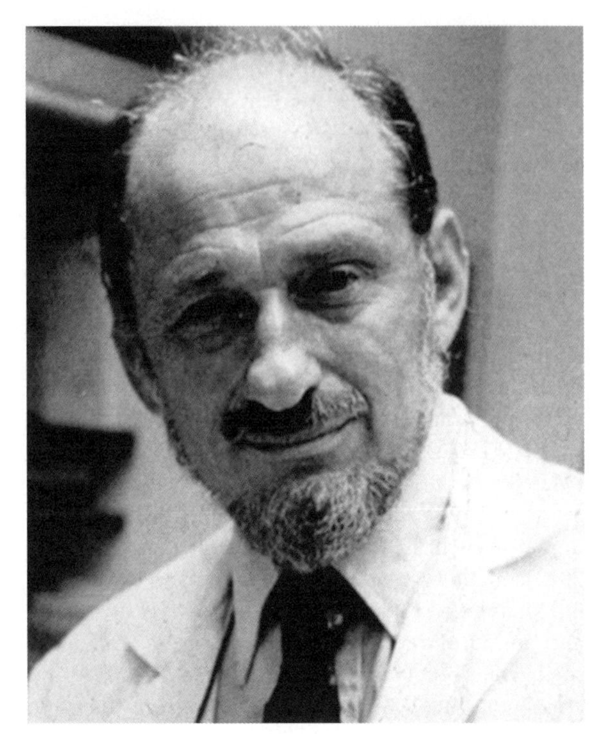

Figure 1.2 Norman Geschwind.

Despite its traditional position as a minor contributor to the mediation of cognition and emotion, white matter can be seen to have a particularly noteworthy position in the study of dementia. Once investigation turns its attention to this part of the brain, a spectrum of intriguing data and implications becomes evident. The neuropathology of white matter disorders is typically diffuse or widespread, thus disrupting many networks simultaneously and producing a multidomain syndrome that merits the term "dementia." Whereas focal neurobehavioral syndromes and various neuropsychiatric syndromes may occur with white matter lesions, dementia is also being recognized as demanding attention, and its importance in behavioral neurology may extend to a broad spectrum of disorders. This book describes the origin and development of the syndrome of white matter dementia, a term introduced nearly three decades ago (Filley et al., 1988) to call attention to the cognitive sequelae of white matter disorders affecting the brain.

References

Al-Hajri Z, Del Bigio MR. Brain damage in a large cohort of solvent abusers. Acta Neuropathol 2010; 119: 435–445.

Alzheimer A. Über eine eigenartige Erkankung der Hirnrinde. Allgemeine Zeitschrift fur Psychiatrie under Psychisch-Gerichtliche Medizin 1907; 64: 146–148. (Trans. Jarvik L, Greenson H. Alzheimer Dis Assoc Disord 1987; 1: 3–8).

Aralasmak A, Ulmer JL, Kocak M, et al. Association, commissural, and projection pathways and their functional deficit reported in literature. J Comput Assist Tomogr 2006; 30: 695–715.

Arnett PA, Rao SM, Hussain M, et al. Conduction aphasia in multiple sclerosis: a case report with MRI findings. Neurology 1996; 47: 576–578.

Bartzokis G. Brain myelination in prevalent neuropsychiatric developmental disorders: primary and comorbid addiction. Adolesc Psychiatry 2005: 29: 55–96.

Bartzokis G, Beckson M, Lu PH, et al. Age-related changes in frontal and temporal lobe volumes in men. Arch Gen Psychiatry 2001; 58: 461–465.

Bartzokis G, Lu PH, Tingus K, et al. Lifespan trajectory of myelin integrity and maximum motor speed. Neurobiol Aging 2010; 31: 1554–1562.

Benson DF. The history of behavioral neurology. Neurol Clin 1993; 11: 1–8.

Bock O. Cajal, Golgi, Nansen, Schäfer and the neuron doctrine. Endeavour 2013; 37: 228–234.

Bonelli RM, Cummings JL. Frontal-subcortical dementias. Neurologist 2008; 14: 100–107.

Catani M, Thiebaut de Schotten M, Slater D, Dell'acqua F. Connectomic approaches before the connectome. Neuroimage 2013; 80: 2–13.

Damasio AR. Behavioral neurology; research and practice. Semin Neurol 1984; 4: 117–119.

Del Bigio MR. Neuropathology and structural changes in hydrocephalus. Dev Disabil Res Rev 2010; 16: 16–22.

Fields RD. Imaging learning: the search for a memory trace. Neuroscientist 2011; 17: 185–196.

Filley CM. *Neurobehavioral anatomy*. 3rd ed. Boulder: University Press of Colorado, 2011.

Filley CM. *The behavioral neurology of white matter*. 2nd ed. New York: Oxford University Press, 2012.

Filley CM, Franklin GM, Heaton RK, Rosenberg NL. White matter dementia: clinical disorders and implications. Neuropsychiatry Neuropsychol Behav Neurol 1988; 1: 239–254.

Filley CM, Halliday W, Kleinschmidt-DeMasters BK. The effects of toluene on the central nervous system. J Neuropathol Exp Neurol 2004: 63: 1–12.

Filley CM, Kozora E, Brown MS, et al. White matter microstructure and cognition in non-neuropsychiatric systemic lupus erythematosus. Cogn Behav Neurol 2009; 22: 38–44.

Friederici AD. White-matter pathways for speech and language processing. Handb Clin Neurol 2015; 129: 177–186.

Gall FJ, Spurzheim JK. *Anatomie et physiologie de systeme nerveux en general et du cerveau en particular*. Paris: Schoell, 1810–1818.

Geschwind N. Disconnexion syndromes in animals and man. Brain 1965; 88: 237–294, 585–644.

Gold BT, Powell DK, Andersen AH, Smith CD. Alterations in multiple measures of white matter integrity in normal women at high risk for Alzheimer's disease. Neuroimage 2010; 52: 1487–1494.

Goldberg MP, Ransom BR. New light on white matter. Stroke 2003; 34: 330–332.

Iannucci G, Dichgans M, Rovaris M, et al. Correlations between clinical findings and magnetization transfer imaging metrics of tissue damage in individuals with cerebral autosomal dominant arteriopathy with subcortical infarcts and leukoencephalopathy. Stroke 2001; 32: 643–648.

Juhasz C, Lai C, Behen ME, et al. White matter volume as a major predictor of cognitive function in Sturge-Weber syndrome. Arch Neurol 2007; 64: 1169–1174.

Jung RE, Brooks WM, Yeo RA, et al. Biochemical markers of intelligence: a proton MR spectroscopy study of normal human brain. Proc Biol Sci 1999; 266: 1375–1379.

Kaiser M. The potential of the human connectome as a biomarker of brain disease. Front Hum Neurosci 2013; 7: 484.

Kandel ER, Schwartz JH, Jessell TM, et al. *Principles of neural science*. 5th ed. New York: McGraw-Hill, 2013.

Kerchner GA, Racine CA, Hale S, et al. Cognitive processing speed in older adults: relationship with white matter integrity. PloS One 2012; 7: e50425.

Kochunov P, Coyle T, Lancaster J, et al. Processing speed is correlated with cerebral health markers in the frontal lobes quantified by neuroimaging. Neuroimage 2010; 49: 1190–1199.

Kurtzke JF. Neurologic impairment in multiple sclerosis and the disability status scale. Acta Neurol Scand 1970; 46: 493–512.

Launer LJ. Epidemiology of white matter lesions. Top Magn Reson Imaging 2004; 15: 365–367.

Luria AR. *Higher cortical functions in man*. New York: Consultants Bureau, 1966.

Matejko AA, Price GR, Mazzocco MM, Ansari D. Individual differences in left parietal white matter predict math scores on the Preliminary Scholastic Aptitude Test. Neuroimage 2013; 66: 604–610.

Matute C, Ransom BR. Roles of white matter in central nervous system pathophysiologies. ASN Neuro 2012; 4. pii: e00079.

Nolte J. *The human brain*. 5th ed. St. Louis: Mosby, 2002.

Northam GB, Liégeois F, Chong WK, et al. Total brain white matter is a major determinant of IQ in adolescents born preterm. Ann Neurol 2011; 69: 702–711.

Nunez PL, Srinivasan R, Fields RD. EEG functional connectivity, axon delays and white matter disease. Clin Neurophysiol 2015; 126: 110–120.

Parkinson C, Wheatley T. Relating anatomical and social connectivity: white matter microstructure predicts emotional empathy. Cereb Cortex 2014; 24: 614–625.

Parvizi J. Corticocentric myopia: old bias in new cognitive sciences. Trends Cogn Sci 2009; 13: 354–359.

Penfield W. *The mystery of the mind*. Princeton: Princeton University Press, 1975.

Querfurth HW, LaFerla FM. Alzheimer's disease. N Engl J Med 2010; 362: 329–344.

Rao SM, Leo GJ, Bernardin L, Unverzagt F. Cognitive dysfunction in multiple sclerosis: I. Frequency, patterns, and prediction. Neurology 1991; 41: 685–691.

Sasson E, Doniger GM, Pasternak O, et al. White matter correlates of cognitive domains in normal aging with diffusion tensor imaging. Front Neurosci 2013; 7: 1–13.

Schmahmann JD, Pandya DN. *Fiber pathways of the brain*. New York: Oxford University Press, 2006.

Schmahmann JD, Smith EE, Eichler FS, Filley CM. Cerebral white matter: neuroanatomy, clinical neurology, and neurobehavioral correlates. Ann N Y Acad Sci 2008; 1142: 266–309.

Schoenemann PT, Sheehan MJ, Glotzer LD. Prefrontal white matter is disproportionately larger in humans than in other primates. Nat Neurosci 2005; 8: 242–252.

Sporns O. The human connectome: a complex network. Ann N Y Acad Sci 2011; 1224: 109–125.

Stadelmann C, Albert M, Wegner C, Brück W. Cortical pathology in multiple sclerosis. Curr Opin Neurol 2008; 21: 239–234.

Takeuchi H, Taki Y, Sassa Y, Hashizume H, et al. White matter structures associated with creativity: evidence from diffusion tensor imaging. Neuroimage 2010; 51: 11–18.

Toga AW, Clark KA, Thompson PM, et al. Mapping the human connectome. Neurosurgery 2012; 71: 1–5.

Turken AU, Whitfield-Gabrieli S, Bammer R, et al. Cognitive speed and the structure of white matter pathways: convergent evidence from normal variation and lesion studies. Neuroimage 2008; 42: 1032–1044.

Umarova RM, Saur D, Schnell S, et al. Structural connectivity for visuospatial attention: significance of ventral pathways. Cereb Cortex. 2010; 20: 121–129.

Van Zandvoort MJ, Kappelle LJ, Algra A, De Haan EH. Decreased capacity for mental effort after single supratentorial lacunar infarct may affect performance in everyday life. J Neurol Neurosurg Psychiatry 1998; 65: 697–702.

White JG, Southgate E, Thomson JN, Brenner S. The structure of the nervous system of the nematode Caenorhabditis elegans. Philos Trans R Soc Lond B Biol Sci. 1986; 314: 1–340.

Chapter 2

The essential contributions of neuroimaging

The increasing interest in white matter within the scope of behavioral neurology has been stimulated by several impressive advances of neuroimaging. The many techniques now available can be divided into those that allow some means by which the structure of white matter itself can be seen, and those that enable the visualization of gray matter regions connected by white matter tracts (Table 2.1). The inaugural event in this sequence of innovations was the introduction of computed tomography (CT) in the late 1970s, which provided the first noninvasive method allowing clinicians to see the brain in a living individual (Oldendorf, 1978). Replacing the painful and often inconclusive procedure of pneumoencephalography that went before, CT of the head offered major advantages in terms of visualizing the brain parenchyma instead of other features of intracranial anatomy (Oldendorf, 1978). An x-ray technique with some degree of radiation risk, CT nevertheless proved to be a tremendous diagnostic advance, and continues today as a routine component of the clinical work of neurologists around the world. Head CT is a standard procedure in the assessment of acute stroke because it can immediately identify hemorrhage and thus avert catastrophic bleeding if thrombolytic therapy is used, and CT is also useful in the evaluation of traumatic brain injury, brain neoplasia, and hydrocephalus. However, whereas CT can readily assess brain tissue in general, its capacity to reveal the details of white matter was, and remains, very limited.

Table 2.1 Neuroimaging methods contributing to the study of white matter

Structural
Computed tomography (CT)
Magnetic resonance imaging (MRI)
Magnetic resonance spectroscopy (MRS)
Magnetization transfer imaging (MTI)
Diffusion tensor imaging (DTI)
Diffusion spectrum imaging (DSI)
Diffusion kurtosis imaging (DKI)
Perfusion-weighted imaging (PWI)
Functional
Positron emission tomography (PET)
Single-photon emission computed tomography (SPECT)
Functional magnetic resonance imaging (fMRI)

Magnetic resonance imaging

As useful as CT became for imaging the brain as a whole, it was the introduction of magnetic resonance imaging (MRI) in the early 1980s that enabled a major step forward in the imaging of white matter (Bradley, 1986). One useful feature of MRI was the absence of radiation risk, an obvious advantage for patient care, but the impressive diagnostic capability of MRI was equally valuable. For the first time, white matter could be visualized and correlated with clinical phenomenology without the need for autopsy. Whereas CT is able to image the brain for many purposes critical for patient care, MRI was a crucial breakthrough, enabling far more detailed views of myelinated systems that could be productively exploited by both clinicians and investigators (Tanridag and Kirshner, 1987; Haller et al., 2009).

MRI proved transformative for clinical neurology, revising the traditional model of detailed history-taking and careful neurologic examination to a scenario in which a review of neuroimaging is a necessary portion of nearly all clinical evaluations involving a patient with known or suspected brain pathology. In the past, neurologic patients were seen with primary attention devoted to the subtleties of the neurologic history and examination because neuroimaging was not available as a component of the evaluation, but now it is expected that review of neuroimaging – most often brain MRI – is a key component of the neurologist's role, often providing the definitive diagnostic information. Neurology is still firmly based on clinical evaluation, and remains justifiably confident that no neuroimaging or other test will ever replace the careful and sensitive approach to the patient together with the many

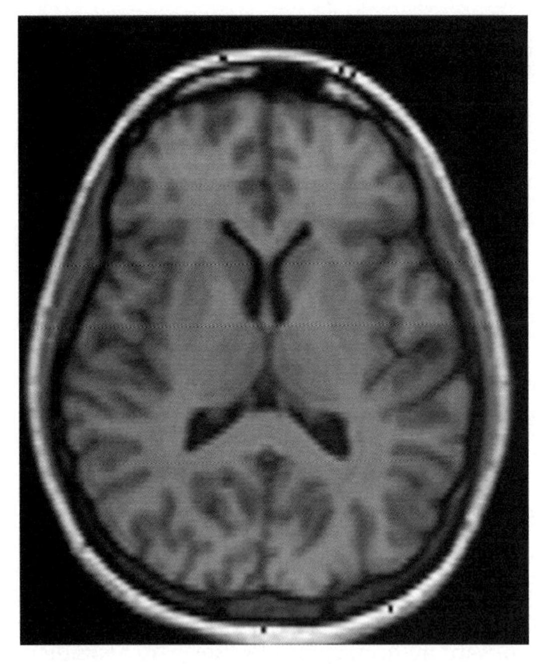

Figure 2.1 Axial T1-weighted MRI scan of a normal adult. The distinction of cortical and subcortical gray matter from cerebral white matter is readily apparent.

complex factors that may influence the clinical picture. But MRI and related techniques are increasingly essential to effective patient care. As will be seen repeatedly in this book, MRI also remains at the center of research on brain–behavior relationships, particularly regarding white matter and its disorders.

By widespread consensus, MRI is the modality of choice in the assessment of brain white matter and the pathology to which it is vulnerable (Haller et al., 2009). The value of MRI in this regard is immediately apparent on seeing a typical axial MRI image, where it is clear that white matter can be distinguished from both cortical and subcortical gray matter (Figure 2.1). The remarkable resolution of brain structures enabled by MRI is nowhere more impressive than in the depiction of white matter. In the most familiar white matter disorder, multiple sclerosis (MS), MRI quickly became an essential tool in the evaluation of affected patients, and remains today the core neuroimaging modality used for the diagnosis and follow-up of this disease (Simon, 2014). A wide range of other white matter disorders have been clarified, and, not surprisingly, improvements in the identification and characterization of white matter pathology quickly followed as MRI was widely implemented.

From its introduction into clinical use, one of the most obvious findings on MRI was the frequent presence of scattered hyperintense changes noted incidentally on the T2-weighted and proton density images of brain MRI from patients with all manner of neurologic presentations. These changes, often known as "unidentified bright objects" (UBOs), were found to be quite common, and their interpretation remains part of the routine work of any practicing neurologist. White matter changes on MRI are highly prevalent in the population, and whereas overall prevalence figures including all ages are unavailable, it is known that the great majority of older adults harbor at least one such lesion. As a general rule, the percentage of people with this finding roughly parallels age, so that 40% of those at age 40, 60% of 60-year-olds, and 90% of those at age 90 have at least one MRI white matter hyperintensity, and often far more (Launer, 2004). UBOs were soon noted to differ from the lesions of recognized white matter diseases such as MS, and with further study it became clear that UBOs usually have an ischemic basis; moreover, important neurobehavioral correlates began to be found, related in large part to the preponderance of UBOs in the frontal lobes (Launer, 2004).

These insights, however, were not readily apparent, at least in the early years of MRI. One of the persistent questions that has proved challenging for the investigation of white matter lesions has been the measurement of their extent in the brain. A more formal descriptor of these lesions was adopted – white matter hyperintensities (WMHs) – but quantification of the burden they impose on the brain has been problematic. As interest in this area grew, a number of visual rating scales appeared that were designed to quantitate WMH location and volume from routine axial MRI images. As well intentioned as these scales were, it soon became apparent after their introduction that considerable inconsistency existed among them, limiting the degree of interrater agreement (Mäntylä et al., 1997). Some of the uncertainty in this area can be ascribed to the continually evolving MRI techniques used in these studies, yielding data that may be difficult to compare across studies. However, the most important problem appears to have been the use of two-dimensional mapping techniques that often fail to characterize the full extent of a given WMH. A major advance in this field was made with the introduction of three-dimensional mapping, which was more capable of determining the precise spatial localization of WMHs (DeCarli et al., 2005). Whereas the everyday clinical assessment of WMH has yet to be affected by this kind of detailed analysis, the formal study of white matter lesions has been considerably improved by this innovation.

In a larger context, the recognition of UBOs and WMHs helped stimulate the investigation of a wide range of both previously known and soon to be discovered white matter disorders with the unmatched descriptive power of MRI. MRI initiated a large body of clinical research, which continues with vigor today, and this book is based largely on the observations of MRI that have radically expanded our knowledge of white matter and its disorders. From the perspective of behavioral neurology and allied disciplines, MRI has been essential to the establishment of a systematic approach to the cognitive and emotional correlates of normal and abnormal white matter structure and function (Filley, 2012).

Advanced structural neuroimaging

As time went on, additional MRI techniques were developed that further refined the detection of white matter damage (Wozniak and Lim, 2006). One of these is magnetic resonance spectroscopy (MRS), based on nuclear magnetic resonance, which identifies and quantifies chemicals in living tissue (Rudkin and Arnold, 1999). MRS findings are displayed in spectra of peaks that represent the chemical structure and concentration of metabolites in the tissue of interest. In the white matter, this technique has been used to detect axonal damage by identifying a decrease in N-acetyl aspartate (NAA), an amino acid regarded as a marker of neuronal integrity (Simmons, Frondoza, and Coyle, 1991), and myelin injury by disclosing an increase in the membrane-associated metabolite choline (Narayana, 2005). MRS has thus been particularly useful in white matter disorders; in MS, for example, reductions in NAA are found not only within plaques, but in white matter areas that appear normal on conventional MRI (Grossman, Kappos, and Wolinsky, 2000); and in systemic lupus erythematosus, elevated choline has been found in frontal lobe white matter that appears otherwise normal (Filley et al., 2009). Thus MRS may enable more sensitive detection of early abnormalities in white matter disorders that can be correlated with clinical variables (Wozniak and Lim, 2006).

Neuroradiologists then began using magnetization transfer imaging (MTI), a technique based on interactions between protons in water and macromolecules in the brain. The combination of a radiofrequency saturation pulse with an imaging sequence enables the derivation of a magnetization transfer ratio (MTR; van Buchem, 1999), the most popular MTI parameter. In white matter, a low MTR reflects damage to myelin and axons, and can be seen in a variety of disorders such as MS (Cercignani et al., 2000) and white matter ischemia (Tanabe et al., 1999); and, as with MRS abnormalities, a low MTR may be seen in the white matter that appears to be normal before conventional MRI discloses any changes (Loevner et al., 1995). The MTR also correlates with the degree of normal myelination, extending the utility of MTI to the study of development and aging (Rademacher et al., 1999). In addition to the use of the MTR in specific regions of interest, which has facilitated study of the evolution of individual white matter lesions, whole brain histograms also allow quantification of total disease burden (van Buchem, 1999). MTI thus has promise for measuring the entire range of white matter neuropathology, macroscopic and microscopic, and for providing a basis for improved correlations with neurobehavioral data (van Buchem, 1999; Wozniak and Lim, 2006).

As further progress was made, MRI soon came to be amplified by the introduction of diffusion weighting, which exploits the diffusion of water in the brain to enable the viewing of normal and damaged structures in greater detail (Horsfield and Jones, 2002). Diffusion weighting, among its other assets, proved most useful for allowing the early identification of ischemia in the brain, especially in the white matter, and thus the evaluation and treatment of cerebrovascular disease was greatly enhanced. From this development arose the possibility that more specific information on white matter tracts could be gathered. A key concept underlying this notion is the property of anisotropy, which refers to the diffusion of water in the direction of the tract being imaged. Anisotropic (directional) diffusion is a normal phenomenon in the white matter, in contrast to the opposite process of isotropic (random) diffusion, which implies that diffusion is more chaotic and less well organized as a result of tract damage.

From these advances, the technique of diffusion tensor imaging (DTI) soon evolved (Wozniak and Lim, 2006; Choudhri et al., 2014), and quickly became

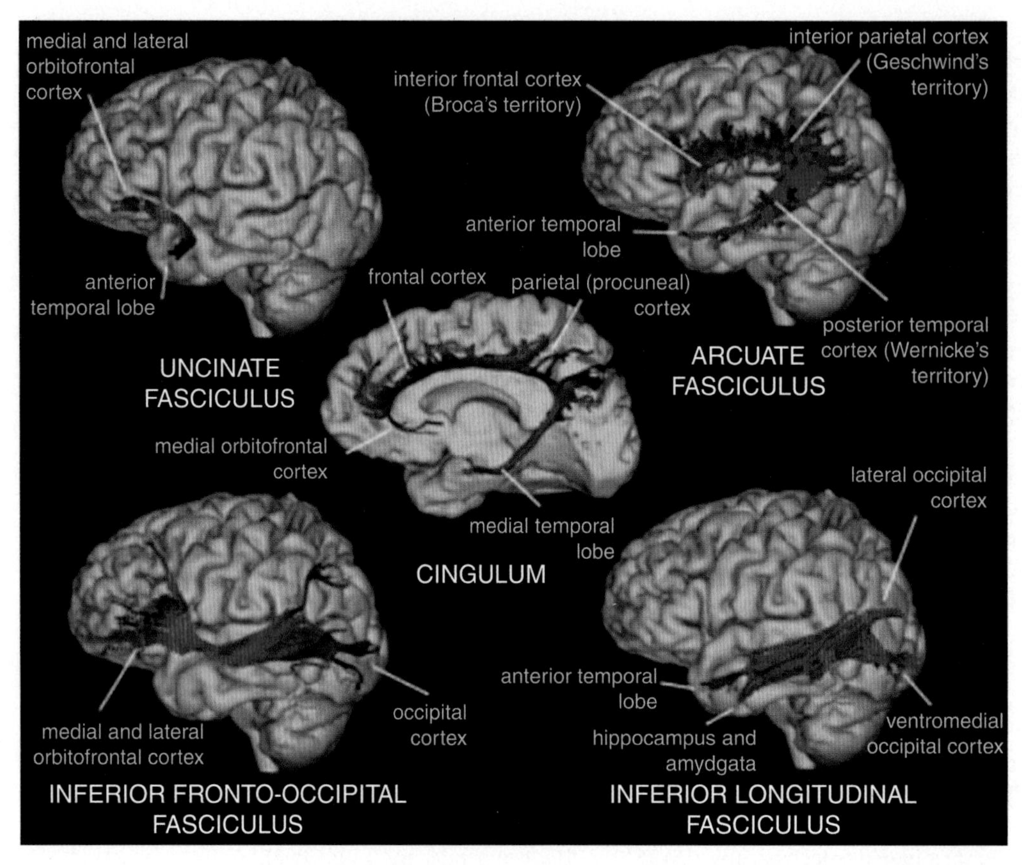

Figure 2.2 DTI tractography reconstruction depicting major association tracts (from Catani and Thiebaut de Schotten, 2012, p. 39).

the most widely used neuroradiological approach to the detailed study of white matter. The identification of specific white matter pathways began to flourish, opening up entirely new ways of identifying the localization of higher functions (Catani et al., 2012). Figures 2.2 and 2.3 demonstrate the remarkable capacity of DTI to reveal the location and course of tracts that cannot be seen by any other method (Catani and Thiebaut de Schotten, 2012). It is clear that the origin, trajectory, and destination of individual tracts can now be seen noninvasively and over longitudinal follow-up, thus offering unique insights into brain circuitry. In addition to the tractography that is enabled by DTI, specific assessment of tract microstructure is possible with measurement of fractional anisotropy (FA) and mean diffusivity (MD), the most commonly used parameters of white matter integrity (Alexander et al., 2007). Initial investigations exploring the measurement of FA and MD were based on a region of interest (ROI) approach, but with further study, an analysis strategy known as tract-based spatial statistics (TBSS) became popular and is now widely used (Smith et al., 2006; Alves et al., 2015).

One of the problems that attends the imaging of white matter tracts with DTI is the phenomenon of crossing fibers. White matter tracts are not typically organized like highways on a map, allowing for clear separation from one another when viewed in vivo. Rather, these tracts are often structurally intermixed, and in some areas intricately intertwined, so that the fibers of one tract will cross over and blend with those of another tract. One approach to this problem has been the technique of diffusion spectrum imaging (DSI), introduced as an experimental technique to deal with this problem (Schmahmann et al., 2007; Wedeen et al., 2008; Granziera et al., 2009). DSI has the capacity to image more complex distributions of fiber orientation, and has been shown to clarify known areas of fiber intersection – such as within the optic chiasm, centrum semiovale, and brain stem – when DTI could not accurately do so (Wedeen et al., 2008). More recently, the technique

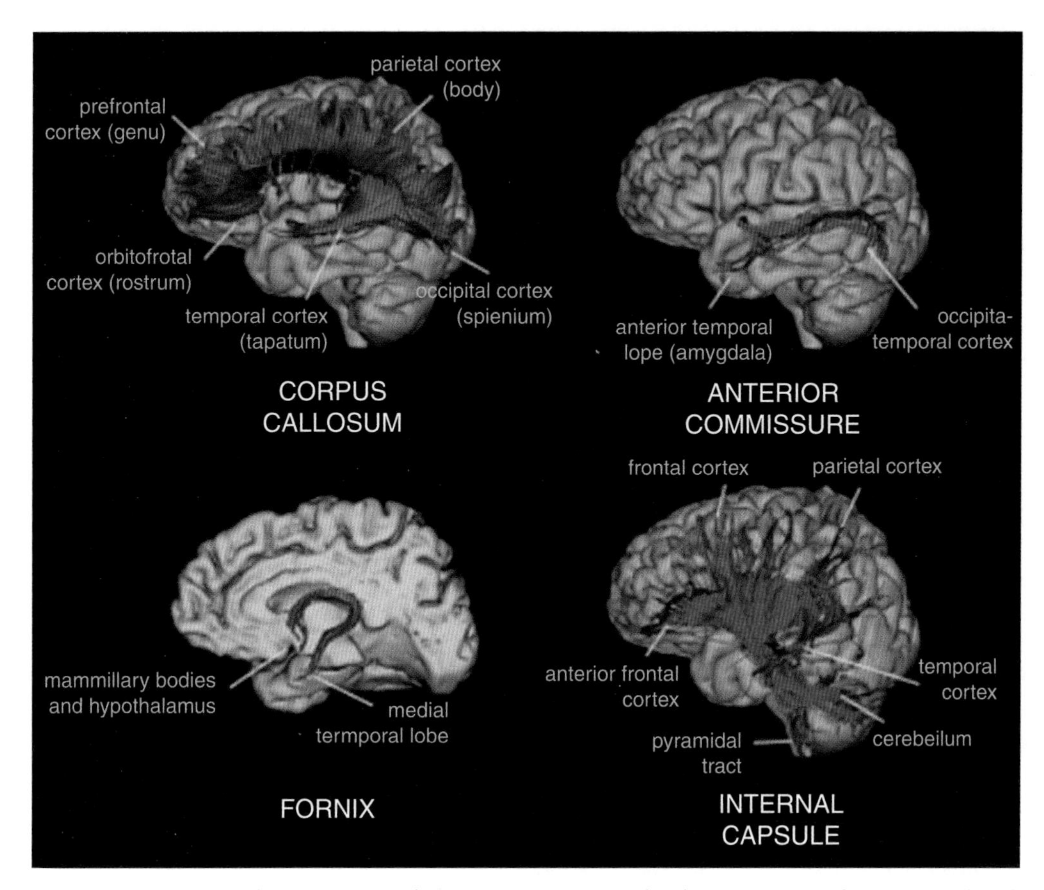

Figure 2.3 DTI tractography reconstruction depicting major commissural and projection tracts (from Catani and Thiebaut de Schotten, 2012, p. 40).

of diffusion kurtosis imaging (DKI) has been investigated as another means of dealing with crossing fibers (Jensen and Helpern, 2010; Fieremans, Jensen, and Helpern, 2011). DKI is an extension of DTI that is capable of extracting more information on the microstructure of white matter. This additional characterization of white matter tracts stems from the capacity of DKI to enable the quantification of non-Gaussian water diffusion, whereas DTI can capture only Gaussian diffusion (Jensen and Helpern, 2010; Fieremans, Jensen, and Helpern, 2011).

All of these newer structural neuroimaging methods led to a remarkable expansion of the ability to visualize white matter that is not overtly affected on conventional MRI. This development quickly focused attention on the microstructure of white matter as well as its macrostructure. What was previously seen as normal tissue began to be suspected of harboring occult lesions that could presumably be detected with more sensitive neuroimaging. The investigation of the normal-appearing white matter (NAWM) thus became relevant, as the areas of white matter that were seemingly unaffected began to attract attention as potentially important. An explosion of research findings quickly appeared to document NAWM abnormalities by MRS, MTI, and DTI in a wide range of disorders. Intriguingly, these disorders included many known white matter diseases, but also what were thought to be gray matter diseases, as well as psychiatric disorders and even normal aging.

Most recently, the technique of perfusion-weighted imaging (PWI) has appeared, allowing for the assessment of white matter perfusion (Haller et al., 2009). Two variants of PWI have been introduced, one (diffusion susceptibility contrast PWI) involving the use of an intravenous contrast agent, and the other (arterial spin labeling PWI) using inflowing blood as an endogenous contrast agent (Haller et al., 2009). In the normal brain, the perfusion of gray matter is about five times greater than that of white matter, and thus

PWI is generally more relevant to the assessment of gray matter and its disorders, but the technique can be helpful in the evaluation of white matter dysfunction or damage related to vascular disease (Haller et al., 2009).

Functional neuroimaging

While white matter structural imaging made remarkable progress over the past 30 years, equally noteworthy has been the advance of functional neuroimaging. The prospect of actually seeing the brain in action is of course compelling to anyone considering the basis of higher functions (Prichard and Cummings, 1997). The first functional imaging method was positron emission tomography (PET) scanning, which employs the injection of radiolabeled glucose molecules to depict cortical activity (Alavi and Hirsch, 1991). A widely used but less precise companion of PET is single-photon emission computed tomography (SPECT; Alavi and Hirsch, 1991). Later, functional MRI (fMRI) was introduced (D'Esposito, 2000), and offered another method for imaging cognitive operations. Today, fMRI has become the preferred functional neuroimaging method (Bandettini, 2009), and hundreds of studies regularly appear using fMRI to map out cortical regions involved in various cognitive tasks. While significant issues still complicate the use of these techniques, including the variability of methodologies across laboratories and the problem of signal-to-noise ratio, functional neuroimaging has had a clear impact on the localization of higher functions.

Functional neuroimaging methods are all designed to provide data on gray matter regions, particularly of the cerebral cortex, because gray matter is more metabolically active than white matter and thus more readily viewed with methods based on the interrogation of cerebral metabolism. Whether the advance of these technologies has been driven by a corticocentric bias is a matter of speculation, and it may be that functional neuroimaging has served to reinforce corticocentrism in neuroscience by offering data on localization that by their very nature preclude the consideration of white matter. But regardless, white matter must be assessed by other means, and techniques such as MRS, MTI, and DTI have provided this opportunity. Many studies are steadily appearing on the localization of specific tracts in health, the alterations seen with tract dysfunction, and the correlation of neuroimaging findings with aspects of higher function.

One of the important results of functional neuroimaging research has been the identification of numerous distributed neural networks in the brain subserving various aspects of cognition. Networks such as these have been identified from clinical studies based on the lesion method, and well-known networks for attention, language, and memory are recognized (Mesulam, 1990). Recently, fMRI studies have provided evidence for other networks, most notably the default mode network (DMN) associated with resting state brain activity (Raichle et al., 2001), and the involvement of the DMN and related networks in neurodegenerative diseases has also been demonstrated (Seeley et al., 2009). From the perspective of white matter disorders, it has been reassuring, although not unexpected, that the functional connectivity shown by regional coactivation of cortical regions in fMRI work generally correlates with what is known of structural connectivity as demonstrated by DTI (Damoiseaux and Greicius, 2009). One of the most critical goals of this work is the understanding of distributed neural networks in all their complexity, which of course includes not only the gray matter hubs of cortical activity but the white matter tracts that connect these areas (Filley, 2012). But there is much more work to be done, as the extraordinary macroconnectivity of the brain has only begun to be appreciated.

A word of caution is that many of these advances are still confined for the most part to the world of neuroscience research. The application of these techniques to the clinical arena must await refinement of methodology to the point where the benefits for patient care justify the costs inherent in sophisticated tasks such as detailed tractography and neural network definition. The effort necessary for identifying an individual tract with DTI, for example, is at present not trivial, even without the presence of neuropathology in the tract that could radically alter its imaging characteristics. Moreover, with respect to the definition of neural networks involved in distributed processing, the relatively long history of fMRI and especially PET scanning has still not seen these modalities introduced into routine clinical practice with the aim of querying the structure and function of large-scale networks with their gray and white matter components. The prospect of introducing white matter neuroimaging into clinical practice entails significant issues of expense, both for the equipment needed for clinical studies and for the time necessary for postacquisition processing. Definitive clinical studies, such as those that have clearly demonstrated the value of conventional MRI in the diagnosis and treatment monitoring of patients with MS (Simon, 2014), will be needed to justify the study of white matter systems in the detail needed to advance understanding of white matter–behavior relationships, especially in view of what appear to be ever-increasing limits on medical spending.

Despite these technical challenges, the role of neuroimaging in the modern investigation of brain–behavior relationships can scarcely be exaggerated. In ways that would have astonished the early investigators whose only avenue toward expanded neurobehavioral knowledge was correlation of behavior in life with pathoanatomical alterations seen post-mortem, modern structural and functional neuroimaging has forever changed the landscape of human neuroscience. This development is as relevant for white matter as for gray. Whereas it is doubtless true that clinicians remain essential in any medical encounter – and indeed, neuroimaging often raises more questions than it answers – the arrival of advanced neuroimaging has revolutionized behavioral neurology as it has neurology and medicine in general.

References

Alavi A, Hirsch LJ. Studies of central nervous system disorders with single photon emission computed tomography and positron emission tomography. Semin Nucl Med 1991; 21: 58–81.

Alexander AL, Lee JE, Lazar M, Field AS. Diffusion tensor imaging of the brain. Neurotherapeutics 2007; 4: 316–329.

Alves GS, Oertel Knöchel V, Knöchel C, et al. Integrating retrogenesis theory to Alzheimer's disease pathology: insight from DTI-TBSS investigation of the white matter microstructural integrity. Biomed Res Int 2015; 2015: 291658.

Bandettini PA. What's new in neuroimaging methods? Ann NY Acad Sci 2009; 1156: 260–293.

Bradley WG Jr. Magnetic resonance imaging in the central nervous system: comparison with computed tomography. Magn Res Ann 1986; 81–122.

Catani M, Dell'acqua F, Bizzi A, et al. Beyond cortical localization in clinico-anatomical correlation. Cortex 2012; 48: 1262–1287.

Catani M, Thiebaut de Schotten M. *Atlas of human brain connections*. Oxford: Oxford University Press, 2012.

Cercignani M, Iannucci G, Rocca MA, et al. Pathologic damage in MS assessed by diffusion-weighted and magnetization transfer MRI. Neurology 2000; 54: 1139–1144.

Choudhri AF, Chin EM, Blitz AM, Gandhi D. Diffusion tensor imaging of cerebral white matter: technique, anatomy, and pathologic patterns. Radiol Clin North Am 2014; 52: 413–425.

Damoiseaux JS, Greicius MD. Greater than the sum of its parts: a review of studies combining structural connectivity and resting-state functional connectivity. Brain Struct Funct 2009; 213: 525–533.

DeCarli C, Fletcher E, Ramey V, et al. Anatomical mapping of white matter hyperintensities (WMH): exploring the relationships between periventricular WMH, deep WMH, and total WMH burden. Stroke 2005; 36: 50–55.

D'Esposito M. Functional neuroimaging of cognition. Semn Neurol 2000; 20: 487–498.

Fieremans E, Jensen JH, Helpern JA. White matter characterization with diffusional kurtosis imaging. Neuroimage 2011; 58: 177–188.

Filley CM. *The behavioral neurology of white matter*. 2nd ed. New York: Oxford University Press, 2012.

Filley CM, Kozora E, Brown MS, et al. White matter microstructure and cognition in non-neuropsychiatric systemic lupus erythematosus. Cogn Behav Neurol 2009; 22: 38–44.

Granziera C, Schmahmann JD, Hadjikhani N, et al. Diffusion spectrum imaging shows the structural basis of functional cerebellar circuits in the human cerebellum in vivo. PloS One 2009; 4: e5101.

Grossman RI, Kappos L, Wolinsky JS. The contribution of magnetic resonance imaging in the differential diagnosis of the damage of the cerebral hemispheres. J Neurol Sci 2000; 172: S57–S62.

Haller S, Pereira VM, Lazeyras F, et al. Magnetic resonance imaging techniques in white matter disease: potentials and limitations. Top Magn Reson Imaging 2009; 20: 301–312.

Horsfield MA, Jones DK. Applications of diffusion-weighted and diffusion tensor MRI to white matter diseases – a review. NMR Biomed 2002; 15: 570–577.

Jensen JH, Helpern JA. MRI quantification of non-Gaussian water diffusion by kurtosis analysis. NMR Biomed 2010; 23: 698–710.

Launer LJ. Epidemiology of white matter lesions. Top Magn Reson Imaging 2004; 15: 365–367.

Loevner LA, Grossman RI, Cohen JA, et al. Microscopic disease in normal-appearing white matter on conventional MR imaging in patients with multiple sclerosis: assessment with magnetization-transfer measurements. Radiology 1995; 196: 511–515.

Mäntylä R, Erkinjuntti T, Salonen O, et al. Variable agreement between visual rating scales for white matter hyperintensities on MRI: comparison of 13 rating scales in a poststroke cohort. Stroke 1997; 28: 1614–1623.

Mesulam M-M. Large-scale neurocognitive networks and distributed processing for attention, language, and memory. Ann Neurol 1990; 28: 597–613.

Narayana PA. Magnetic resonance spectroscopy in the monitoring of multiple sclerosis. J Neuroimaging 2005; 15 (4 Suppl): 46S–57S.

Oldendorf WH. The quest for an image of brain: a brief historical and technical review of brain imaging techniques. Neurology 1978; 28: 517–533.

Prichard JW, Cummings JL. The insistent call from functional MRI. Neurology 1997; 48: 797–800.

Rademacher J, Engelbrecht V, Burgel U, et al. Measuring in vivo myelination of human white matter fiber tracts with magnetization transfer MR. Neuroimage 1999; 9: 393–406.

Raichle ME, MacLeod AM, Snyder AZ, et al. A default mode of brain function. Proc Natl Acad Sci 2001; 98: 676–882.

Rudkin TM, Arnold DL. Proton magnetic resonance spectroscopy for the diagnosis and management of cerebral disorders. Arch Neurol 1999; 56: 919–926.

Schmahmann JD, Pandya DN, Wang R, et al. Association fibre pathways of the brain: parallel observations from diffusion spectrum imaging and autoradiography. Brain 2007; 130: 630–653.

Seeley WW, Crawford RK, Zhou J, et al. Neurodegenerative diseases target large-scale human brain networks. Neuron 2009; 62: 42–52.

Simmons M, Frondoza C, Coyle J. Immunocytochemical localization of N-acetyl-aspartate with monoclonal antibodies. Neuroscience 1991; 45: 37–45.

Simon JH. MRI outcomes in the diagnosis and disease course of multiple sclerosis. Handb Clin Neurol 2014; 122: 405–425.

Smith SM, Jenkinson M, Johansen-Berg H, et al. Tract-based spatial statistics: voxelwise analysis of multi-subject diffusion data. Neuroimage 2006; 31: 1487–1505.

Tanabe JL, Ezekiel F, Jagust WJ, et al. Magnetization transfer ratio of white matter hyperintensities in subcortical ischemic vascular dementia. AJNR 1999; 20: 839–844.

Tanridag O, Kirshner HS. Magnetic resonance imaging and CT scanning in neurobehavioral syndromes: comparative neuroradiologic findings. Psychosomatics 1987; 28: 517–528.

Van Buchem MA. Magnetization transfer: applications in neuroradiology. J Comp Assist Tomogr 1999; 23 (Suppl 1): S9–S18.

Wedeen VJ, Wang RP, Schmahmann JD, et al. Diffusion spectrum magnetic resonance imaging (DSI) tractography of crossing fibers. Neuroimage 2008; 41: 1267–1277.

Wozniak JR, Lim KO. Advances in white matter imaging: a review of in vivo magnetic resonance methodologies and their applicability to the study of development and aging. Neurosci Biobehav Rev 2006; 30: 762–774.

Chapter 3

White matter neurobiology

To consider how a given component of the brain might be involved in the vast array of human behavior, both normal and otherwise, a focused review of relevant neurobiology is in order as an introduction. Standard textbooks of neuroscience offer elegant and detailed accounts of gray matter structure and function, highlighting the role of the cerebral cortex in neurobehavioral operations, and white matter receives less attention (Kandel et al., 2013). However, much information about the white matter of the brain is available, much of it relevant to the higher functions, and this chapter will endeavor to distill key concepts that are required to understand the role of myelinated systems in normal cognition and emotion. From this background, the disorders considered in subsequent chapters will be more readily recognized as disturbing the many functions arising from the normal organization of brain white matter.

Anatomy

White matter makes up about 50% of the human brain (Miller, Alston, and Corsellis, 1980; Filley, 2012). Coursing within the white matter of the forebrain are vast numbers of myelinated fibers, with an estimated combined length of 135,000 km (Saver, 2006) to 176,000 km (Marner et al., 2003), meaning that the myelinated fibers in one human brain could encircle the earth more than three times (Walhovd, Johansen-Berg, and Káradóttir, 2014). These observations alone argue strongly for the notion that myelinated tracts are important for higher functions, and evidence supporting this view steadily mounts. Yet the relationships of white matter structure and function to cognition and emotion are not easily understood. Students of neuroanatomy are dutifully informed of various white matter tracts and their connections, but beyond the general impression that these tracts link together gray matter structures through the brain, little detail is typically imparted. Similarly, to clinicians accustomed to seeing standard brain imaging studies, the white matter appears to be an undifferentiated mass of tissue lying between the cerebral cortex and the lateral ventricles, and the complexity and significance of its connectivity are not readily apparent. Less metabolically active than gray matter, white matter cannot be meaningfully studied with functional neuroimaging. Maps of the brain white matter that could be compared to the long-familiar Brodmann areas of the cerebral cortex have not yet been widely disseminated, and indeed many details of white matter anatomy remain to be fully described. However, largely propelled by advances in structural neuroimaging, including diffusion tensor imaging (DTI), a more complete understanding of white matter is now emerging. This work is a major contributor to the idea of the "connectome" (Sporns, 2011), now being intensively mapped with DTI and other neuroimaging techniques.

White matter is found throughout the central nervous system (CNS), and that within the brain is pertinent to higher function. The descriptor "cerebral" is often used to refer to the white matter of the brain, although tracts in the brain stem and cerebellum should also be included in a complete account, and indeed evidence supports the importance of all white matter rostral to the spinal cord in the organization of cognition and emotion (Schmahmann and Pandya, 2008). White matter tracts vary greatly in their size, some large enough to be grossly visible and others only identifiable with microscopic examination. The larger tracts have attracted the most attention by investigators, but the smaller ones are currently being studied in more detail with the use of newer neuroimaging methods. Table 3.1 lists the tracts most clearly implicated in brain–behavior relationships.

The traditional account of brain white matter designates three categories of tracts – association, commissural, and projection – and for most purposes these distinctions are still useful (Nolte, 2002; Catani and Thiebaut de Schotten, 2012). Figure 3.1 shows DTI reconstruction of these general categories. However, white matter anatomy is being steadily revised with improvements in modern neuroimaging and neuroanatomic investigation (Aralasmak et al., 2006; Schmahmann and Pandya, 2006). Association and commissural tracts are most crucial for cognition and emotion, as projection fiber systems are devoted mainly to elemental sensory and motor functions. Association tracts are either long (serving to connect distant regions) or short (linking adjacent gyri), and interconnect intrahemispheric gray matter structures. The major, but not only, commissural tract is the corpus callosum, which links the entire cerebrum via a large mass of fibers traversing the midline of the hemispheres. Together, the association and commissural tracts make up the foundation of brain connectivity that integrates cerebral gray matter regions into functional neuronal ensembles (Geschwind, 1965; Filley, 2012).

Table 3.1 White matter tracts most relevant to behavioral neurology

Cerebral hemispheres	Association
	Arcuate fasciculus
	Superior occipitofrontal fasciculus
	Inferior occipitofrontal fasciculus
	Uncinate fasciculus
	Cingulum
	Short association (U) fibers
	Commissural
	Corpus callous
	Anterior commissure
	Hippocampal commissure
	Projection
	Optic radiations
	Thalamocortical radiations
	Internal capsule
Limbic system	Fornix
	Fimbria
	Alveus
Cerebral cortex	Outer band of Baillarger
	Inner band of Baillarger
Basal ganglia and thalamus	Ansa lenticularis
	Lenticular fasciculus
	Thalamic fasciculus
	Subthalamic fasciculus
Cerebellum	Superior cerebellar peduncle
	Middle cerebellar peduncle
	Inferior cerebellar peduncle

Another major tract with important neurobehavioral implications is the fornix, which, together with its companions the fimbria and the alveus, serves as the major efferent pathway for the hippocampus (Nolte, 2002). The fornix occupies a central neuroanatomic position in both the limbic system and the Papez circuit (Mega et al., 1997), and its role in memory and emotion is increasingly appreciated. In recent years, the fornix has attracted additional attention because of its relevance to Alzheimer's Disease (AD), as will be discussed later in this book.

A less often appreciated feature of white matter is that it is also found within the gray matter of both the cerebral cortex and many subcortical gray matter structures (Nolte, 2002). In the cortex, classic neuroanatomy has long recognized that horizontal white matter fascicles – the outer and inner bands of Baillarger – travel in layers IV and V, respectively (Nolte, 2002). In the occipital cortex, a particularly

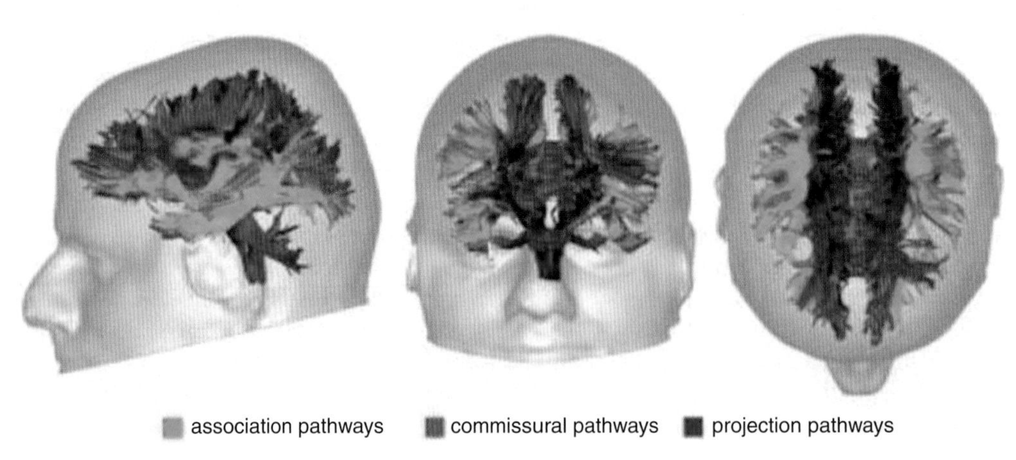

Figure 3.1 DTI reconstruction of the association, commissural, and projection pathways in the brain (from Catani and Thiebaut de Schotten, 2012, p. 38).

large segment of the outer band of Baillarger can be seen on gross inspection as the line of Gennari (Nolte, 2002). White matter also courses through the thalamus and basal ganglia, and recognized tracts in these areas include the ansa leticularis and the lenticular, thalamic, and subthalamic fasciculi (Nolte, 2002).

Finally, white matter tracts connect the cerebellum with the rest of the brain via three peduncles (Nolte, 2002). The largest of these, the middle cerebellar peduncle (also known as the brachium pontis), receives input from the contralateral cerebral hemisphere, while the inferior cerebellar peduncle (the restiform body) contains afferents from the spinal cord and brain stem, and the superior cerebellar peduncle (the brachium conjunctivum) conveys cerebellar output to more rostral structures.

The smaller fiber systems have received relatively little investigation in the neuroanatomic literature on white matter, and their neurobehavioral significance has not been studied in any detail. Neurologists and many neuroscientists have long been accustomed to thinking only of large tracts below the cortical mantle when the topic of white matter is raised. Currently, however, the less obvious fiber tracts are beginning to attract attention as powerful magnetic resonance imaging (MRI) techniques permit the visualization of fascicles far smaller than those within the major white matter regions of the brain (Grydeland et al., 2013; Van Essen and Glasser, 2014; Kleinnijenhuis et al., 2013), and the cerebral cortex has been a major focus of these studies.

More than a century ago, the neuroanatomists Oskar and Cecile Vogt undertook the task of parcellating the cerebral cortex in terms of its patterns of myelination (Nieuwenhuys, 2013). Their study of *myeloarchitectonics* paralleled the study of *cytoarchitectonics* that was pursued by the Vogts' noted contemporary Korbinian Brodmann, whose areas of the neocortex are well known (Nieuwenhuys, 2013). Figure 3.2 depicts the remarkable symmetry of investigation carried out by these investigators as they sought to develop detailed maps of the cerebral cortex (Catani and Thiebaut de Schotten, 2012). Whereas the mapping of cortical white matter did not stimulate nearly the interest of Brodmann's areas, the Vogts conducted impressive studies to show that white matter fascicles can be found in all six neocortical layers, and that the various

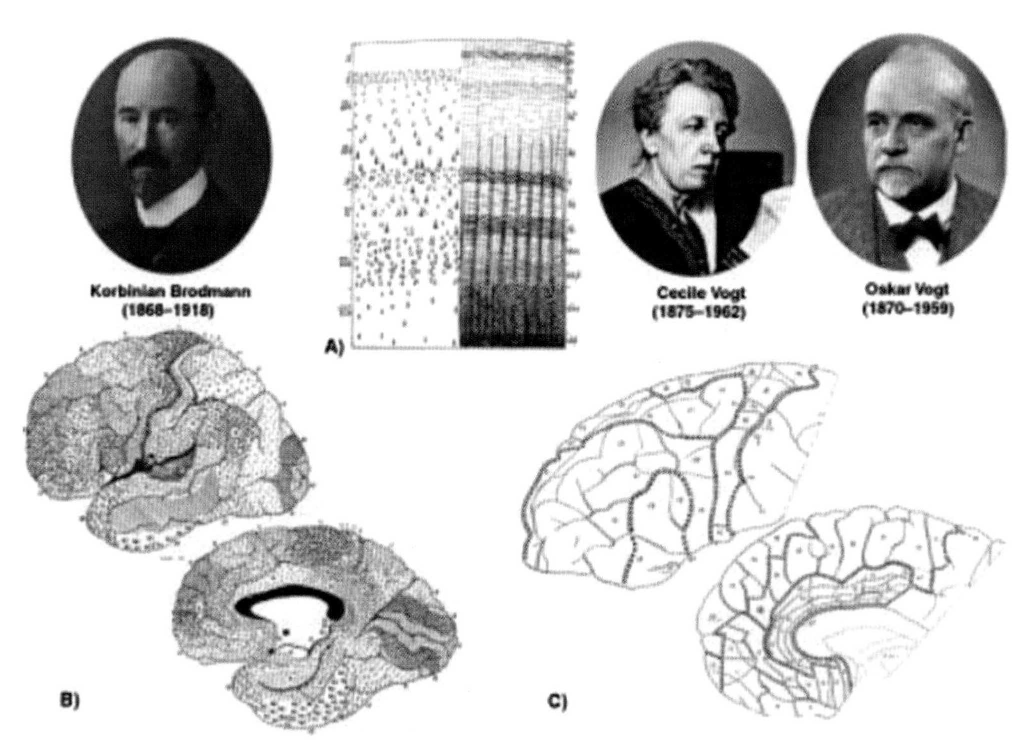

Figure 3.2 Comparison of the work of Korbinian Brodmann and that of Oskar and Cecile Vogt in mapping the cytoarchitectonics and myeloarchitectonics of the cerebral cortex (from Catani and Thiebaut de Schotten, 2012, p. 31).

patterns of cortical myelination delineate roughly 200 myeloarchitectonic areas (Nieuwenhuys, 2013).

Modern neuroimaging is now building on these observations. Studies of the postmortem human neocortex with 11.7 T MRI, for example, have demonstrated laminar patterns of white matter microstructure (Kleinnijenhuis et al., 2013), consistent with the Vogts' finding that cortical myelination exists in all neocortical layers. Intracortical myelin has attracted some interest and attention among neurologists, as it is known that cortical plaques occur in multiple sclerosis (MS) (Brownell and Hughes, 1962), and that intracortical myelin appears to be a target of the inflammatory attack (Kutzelnigg et al., 2005). The idea has since been suggested that cognitive dysfunction in MS is related to cortical demyelination (Stadelmann et al., 2008). Whereas the potential neurobehavioral consequences of cortical demyelination merit continued investigation, it is premature to assume that this phenomenon adequately accounts for cognitive disability. Much more work is necessary before the relative contributions of cortical and large tract demyelination – in MS or any similar disorder – can be determined. Indeed, while the cortical and deep gray matter fascicles of white matter may eventually blur the clinical distinctions between white and gray matter as commonly understood, the role of these fascicles in cognition and emotion is not possible to infer from present data. For the purposes of this book, the term *white matter*, unless otherwise specified, will be used to refer to major tracts within and between the cerebral hemispheres.

The signature neuroanatomic feature of any white matter tract is myelin, the fatty insulation that coats most axons in the brain and dramatically increases neuronal conduction velocity (Baumann and Pham-Dinh, 2001). Myelin, a complex mixture of about 70% lipid and 30% protein, encircles axons after being laid down by oligodendrocytes (Bennaroch, 2009); the white hue of the cut brain at autopsy in fact derives from myelin. At the neuronal level, myelin forms a concentric sheath along the length of the axon, leaving small unmyelinated nodes of Ranvier that permit the phenomenon of saltatory conduction (Baumann and Pham-Dinh, 2001). The nodes of Ranvier thus allow the action potential to jump from one node to the next as it rapidly traverses the length of the axon to the terminal dendrites and synapses (Baumann and Pham-Dinh, 2001). The result of this arrangement is that white matter dramatically accelerates the transfer of information in the brain.

Physiology

Axons are essential for signaling between neurons, and the axonal cytoskeleton contains microtubules and other structures responsible for, among other tasks, the transport of neurotransmitters synthesized in the cell body to the synapse (Kandel et al., 2013). These neurotransmitters serve as chemical messengers between neurons, and the electrical activity of the axon stimulates synaptic transmission (Kandel et al., 2013). Two mechanisms have evolved that enhance the speed of electrical conduction along axons: an increase in the size of axons and the phenomenon of myelination (Hartline and Colman, 2007). Small axons devoid of myelin are capable of comparatively slow electrical transmission, a situation not conducive to adaptation in a demanding environment. Thus the crucial physiologic aspect of white matter is its greatly enhanced speed of electrical conduction, as action potentials or "spikes" are conducted as much as 100 times faster in large myelinated axons than in their small unmyelinated counterparts (Kandel et al., 2013). Whereas the large white matter tracts of the human brain contain some unmyelinated axons, most are myelinated (Hildebrand et al., 1993), and these account for the increase in conduction velocity within association and commissural tracts critical for higher functions. The brain contains some 100 billion neurons, many of which are distant from each other, and the capacity of the brain to "talk to itself" is essential for the seamless and efficient operations of evolved complex behavior (Filley, 2012). Whereas it may seem overly simplistic to assert that slower electrical conduction of brain axons means slowed mentation, much evidence now demonstrates exactly this; the more myelin is engaged in a given function, the faster the speed with which the processes supporting that function are performed (Turken et al., 2008; Bartzokis et al., 2010; Kochunov et al., 2010; Venkatraman et al., 2011).

The enhanced electrical conduction enabled by white matter appears to have evolutionary importance. Myelin is a relatively recent development in phylogeny, and is almost exclusively confined to the nervous systems of vertebrate species (Baumann and Pham-Dinh, 2001). This feature of more highly evolved brains has central importance for human behavior, as will be considered further later. Intriguing comparative neuroanatomic data also indicate a selective increase in prefrontal white matter volume in humans compared to nonhuman primates, whereas gray matter volume is not significantly different (Schoenemann, Sheehan, and Glotzer 2005; Smaers et al., 2010). This finding has recently been disputed (Barton and Venditti, 2013), but the measurement of gray and white matter volumes is notably imprecise, and despite this uncertainty, wide agreement exists that frontal lobe connectivity is fundamental to the unique cognitive repertoire of *Homo sapiens* (Sherwood and Smaers, 2013). These observations suggest that the myelin within white matter has a special role in enhancing neuronal conduction velocity not only generally within the brain, but specifically within frontal networks devoted to the most highly evolved human behaviors.

New data on synaptic function and neurotransmitter signaling within white matter also exist that are radically changing the traditional view of white matter function (Wake, Lee, and Fields, 2011; Alix and Domingues, 2011; Matute and Ransom, 2012). Neurons are now known to communicate with glial cells in white matter via axo-oligodendroglial synapses (Wake, Lee, and Fields, 2011). Glutamatergic transmission is prominent at these synapses, and other neurotransmitters also appear to be involved (Matute and Ransom, 2012). These observations have many implications for white matter physiology under normal and abnormal conditions, as white matter signaling may be crucial in the pathophysiology of many white matter disorders (Matute and Ransom, 2012) and in the plasticity of myelination that is increasingly thought to occur in health and after injury (Wake, Lee, and Fields, 2011). Thus, whereas conventional synapses are still a key feature of gray matter, the traditional view that synapses appear *only* within gray matter needs revision. A wide range of new ideas on the etiopathogenesis and treatment of neurologic disorders can be imagined in light of the concept of synaptic activity within white matter, and these will be taken up later in these pages.

A discussion of brain white matter physiology would not be complete without considering the role of myelinated systems in the connectome. This concept refers to the totality of neuronal connections in the brain (Sporns, 2011), and thus includes both the macroconnectivity of visible white matter tracts and the microconnectivity enabled by the trillions of synapses in the brain. All of these connections combine to effect the continuously proceeding operations of cognition and emotion, during wakefulness and sleep, and even at the lowest functional levels of severe dementia, the minimally conscious state, and the vegetative state. Determining the functional state of the organism as it derives from the structural connectivity of the brain is a most worthy goal, and the contributions of both white and gray matter are critical. However, it is humbling to reflect on this topic and realize that the brain is a dynamic organ, changing every moment under countless environmental stimuli that produce structural alterations in both white and gray matter. The connectome with which one goes to sleep is not the same as the one that is present on awakening, and even a single conversation, perception, or experience causes structural change in the brain. The breathtaking complexity of unraveling the operations of cognition and emotion becomes still more accentuated in this light, but the quest to pursue the details of brain connectivity is no less enticing as a result.

Development and aging

The processes of brain development and aging show markedly different trajectories for white and gray matter. The entire brain complement of neurons, the cell bodies of which are the central constituent of gray matter, is formed during the first half of gestation, whereas white matter is only beginning to develop at birth, and myelination occurs mainly in postnatal life (Baumann and Pham-Dinh, 2001). Myelin is in fact laid down steadily for many years, particularly in childhood and adolescence but even into the sixth decade, and reaches its maximal volume in midlife (Yakovlev and Lecours, 1967; Benes et al., 1994; Miller et al., 2012). Recent evidence has confirmed a "quadratic" or inverted *U* pattern of brain white matter development whereby myelination proceeds to expand white matter until about the age of 45, after which this volume slowly declines (Bartzokis et al., 2001).

In early life, the cerebral commissures and association tracts are among the latest to develop, and myelination as a delayed maturational event in ontogeny corresponds with the emergence of the mature adult brain and its associated behaviors (Bartzokis, 2005; Filley, 2012). Also contributing to the development of maturity is the appearance of intracortical myelin, which also occurs well into adulthood (Miller et al., 2012). Given that the addition of brain volume associated with myelination continues well past the time in childhood when the skull becomes rigid and further brain expansion is precluded, some reduction of other brain regions must occur to permit myelination. Importantly, myelin expansion is temporally associated with the recently recognized "pruning" of cortical synapses during development (Petanjek et al., 2011). Hence cortical synaptic density is reduced by roughly 50% between childhood and age 30 (Petanjek et al., 2011), while at the same time brain myelination is steadily increasing to its adult maximum (Bartzokis and Lu, 2014). In this way, the brain can accommodate the need for more myelin by sacrificing cortical gray matter volume (Bartzokis and Lu, 2014). Still more intriguingly, the loss of synapses in adolescence and young adulthood does not compromise cognition, as might be expected from a corticocentric perspective. On the contrary, the maturing individual actually acquires cognitive and emotional competence while synapses are being lost and myelin is being acquired (Bartzokis and Lu, 2014). These observations provide yet more support for the critical importance of white matter in cognition and emotion (Bartzokis and Lu, 2014).

In late life, loss of white matter, most notably in the frontal lobes, has been associated with age-related changes in cognition (Sullivan and Pfefferbaum, 2006; Bennett and Madden, 2014). At the same time, the much-feared loss of cortical neurons that occurs with normal aging, formerly well accepted, may have been overestimated (Filley, 2012). This temporal profile of myelination over the life span suggests that, perhaps even more than gray matter, the cerebral white matter may influence the most highly evolved human behaviors (Bartzokis, 2005; Bartzokis and Lu, 2014). Moreover, a wide range of neurobehavioral disorders of early and late life – from autism to Alzheimer's Disease – may relate in some manner to the altered formation of myelin before maturity, or changes in white matter with aging (Bartzokis, 2005; 2011; Filley, 2012). While parallel developments in gray matter, such as synaptic pruning in development and neuronal cell body loss in aging, cannot be overlooked, the white matter exerts its own unique effects on normal mentation throughout life.

The evolution of white matter

With this brief review of white matter neurobiology as a summary, it is useful to step back and consider how the white matter came to be what it is. If white matter has an important role in the operations of cognition and emotion, the course of its phylogenetic development over time should naturally reflect its steadily growing contribution. As a means of taking on this task, the evolutionary background of brain development offers an instructive perspective.

Any discussion of evolution must immediately involve the work of the great biologist Charles Darwin. Using his legendary skills as both an observer and a synthesizer, Darwin was interested in the development of all manner of traits displayed by living organisms, and human intelligence was no exception. In his 1871 book *The Descent of Man*, he offered an opinion that has served to reflect and organize neuroscientific thinking about the brain and intelligence for more than a century:

> No one, I presume, doubts that the large size of the brain in man, relatively to his body, in comparison with that of the gorilla or orang, is closely connected with his higher mental powers.

In this statement, Darwin expressed what is widely regarded as the primary reason for the presumed superiority of the human intellect over that of all other creatures. Whereas no reliable metric exists with which to compare the intelligence of humans with that possessed by other animals such as great apes, whales, and elephants – and respect for the often impressive cognitive capabilities of such animals should be maintained – the singular capacity of *Homo sapiens* for both creative ability and, regrettably, destructive power cannot be denied. While human intelligence may produce a panoply of negative consequences as well as many positive sequelae, its superiority among the animals seems undeniable.

Evidence for the use of the human intellect for malevolent purposes is abundantly available, but a striking example is directly relevant to this discussion. Subsequent to Darwin's manifestly apolitical assertion, the notion that brain size predicts intelligence was subsequently employed to motivate an egregious scientific racism based on faulty craniometric comparisons purporting to demonstrate racial differences based on head size and shape (Gould, 1981). This appalling attitude was most notoriously promoted in the Germany of Adolf Hitler, where extreme racial prejudice was promulgated by the assertion that differences in head morphology could be used to establish differences among races in terms of desirable traits. Revulsion against the idea of considering brain size in relation to intelligence quickly led to a virtual standstill of work in this field.

With the arrival of modern structural neuroimaging some decades later, however, a more accurate and objective approach to this difficult issue was made possible. Beginning in the early 1990s, many studies of normal subjects using computed tomography (CT) and MRI were conducted that enabled the actual measurement of the brain itself. Consistent with Darwin's original idea, a review of 28 CT and MRI scans found that among 1,389 normal subjects, brain size was modestly but significantly correlated with "general mental ability" (GMA), meaning performance on standard measures of intelligence such as the Wechsler tests and their relatives (Rushton and Ankney, 2009). Of note, both brain size and GMA are also significantly correlated with age, socioeconomic position, gender, and population group differences, suggesting that many factors contribute to the relationship between brain size and intelligence (Rushton and Ankney, 2009).

If a bigger brain is in general more intelligent, what is the basis for this relationship? Rushton and Ankney (2009) offer a reasonable, although very cautious, explanation: "The number of neurons available to process information may mediate the correlation of brain size and GMA." At first glance, this statement seems uncontroversial. Indeed, few would take issue, for example, with the idea that a muscle or a bone is stronger if it has more of its basic functional units – its cells. As for the brain, the corticocentric bias of contemporary neuroscience (Parvizi, 2009) would of course prompt an unquestioned leap to the idea that more neurons means more intelligence – and these neurons would naturally reside within the cerebral cortex (Chapter 1).

But there may be much more to this story. As so often happens, the brain turns out to be more complex than organs elsewhere in the body. In mammalian evolution, comparative neuroanatomic studies have disclosed a selective enlargement of cerebral white matter that follows a universal scaling law by which white matter expansion exceeds that of cortical gray matter by a ratio of 4:3 (Zhang and Sejnowski, 2000). Figure 3.3 depicts the increase in white matter relative to cortical volume in a smaller brain compared to a larger one. As brains became larger over an evolutionary course that can be traced back at least

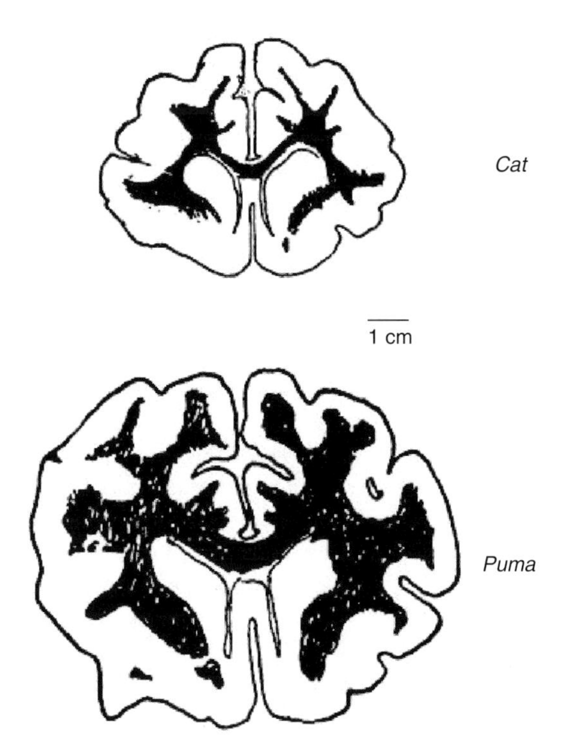

Figure 3.3 Comparison diagram showing the disproportionate enlargement of white matter in a larger brain (from Zhang and Sejnowski, 2000).

570 million years (Rushton and Ankney, 2009), the neocortex expanded its area by folding into many gyri in which cell bodies became densely aggregated. These adaptations led to an impressive increase in the number of cortical neurons. However, the scaling ratio of 4:3 means that the white matter volume expanded more than gray matter volume as larger distances were created between the cell bodies of cortical neurons, and thicker, more heavily myelinated axons were required to support faster conduction velocity and integrated network activity (Zhang and Sejnowski, 2000). Myelination of cerebral axons was accompanied by the heightened capacity for saltatory conduction, which allows for decreased conduction time between cortical regions as well as decreased metabolic demand (Wang et al., 2008). These advantages require a greater percentage of intracranial volume being devoted to white matter, since the wider diameter of myelinated axons occupies more space than that needed for the more compact expansion of the neocortex. Thus white matter is hyperscaled compared to cortical gray matter across the entire cerebrum (Zhang and

Sejnowski, 2000), and the main reason for the increased cranial size of humans over other primates is white matter expansion. In view of accumulating evidence that brain size is correlated with intelligence (Rushton and Ankney, 2009), the selective expansion of white matter over millions of years is another strong argument supporting the importance of myelinated systems in the brain with regard to cognition.

The evolution of myelination in the brain may have initially enhanced the function of motor and sensory systems before cognitive function was a primary selective advantage. It has been suggested that faster central axonal conduction velocity served to facilitate escape reflexes and hunting behaviors, allowing early primates the adaptive advantages of more efficiently avoiding predators and acquiring sustenance to survive and reproduce (Harris and Attwell, 2012). As brain size and neuronal numbers further increased, myelination increased disproportionately, most prominently in the frontal lobes, and cognitive function became more important as an adaptive advantage in higher primates, reaching its highest expression in *Homo sapiens.*

If bigger brains are correlated with higher intelligence, and white matter expansion is the primary reason for the enlargement of the human brain, it might be speculated that neurons are not as crucial as commonly believed in the phylogeny of human intelligence. The cortex and its neurons, however, must not be neglected in this discussion. If brain enlargement were enough by itself to assure the superiority of intelligence, then whales and elephants would surpass humans because their brains are much larger than those of humans – the whale can have a brain as large as 9,000 grams, more than six times the weight of an average adult human brain (Roth and Dicke, 2005).

The resolution of these issues seems to be that both the number of neurons and the degree of myelination play critical roles in the mediation of human intelligence. Humans do indeed possess the most cortical neurons of any animal, and they also have the most extensive myelination (Roth and Dicke, 2005). While whales and elephants have much larger brains and nearly as many cortical neurons, the myelin of these animals is much thinner (Roth and Dicke, 2005). A reduction of conduction velocity between gray matter regions results from this relative paucity of myelin, and is further exacerbated by the much longer intracranial distances that must be traversed by action potentials (Roth and Dicke, 2005).

The accumulated evidence documenting white matter expansion in evolution, and the highest degree of myelination in humans, strongly supports the premise of this book that white matter in the brain is as important for cognition as is gray matter. Simply put, the best brains have the most neurons and the most myelin. It now becomes our task to consider how loss or dysfunction of white matter can be as determinative in the syndrome of dementia as the much better appreciated syndromes of gray matter involvement.

References

Alix JJ, Domingues AM. White matter synapses: form, function, and dysfunction. Neurology 2011; 76: 397–404.

Aralasmak A, Ulmer JL, Kocak M, et al. Association, commissural, and projection pathways and their functional deficit reported in literature. J Comput Assist Tomogr 2006; 30: 695–715.

Barton RA, Venditti C. Human frontal lobes are not relatively large. Proc Natl Acad Sci 2013; 110: 9001–9006.

Bartzokis G. Brain myelination in prevalent neuropsychiatric developmental disorders: primary and comorbid addiction. Adolesc Psychiatry 2005; 29: 55–96.

Bartzokis G. Alzheimer's disease as homeostatic responses to age-related myelin breakdown. Neurobiol Aging 2011; 32: 1341–1371.

Bartzokis G, Beckson M, Lu PH, et al. Age-related changes in frontal and temporal lobe volumes in men. Arch Gen Psychiatry 2001; 58: 461–465.

Bartzokis G, Lu PH, Tingus K, et al. Lifespan trajectory of myelin integrity and maximum motor speed. Neurobiol Aging 2010; 31: 1554–1562.

Bartzokis G, Lu PH. Degenerative brain diseases and white matter injury. In: Baltan S, Carmichael ST, Matute C, Xi G, Zhang JH, eds. *White matter injury in stroke and CNS disease.* New York: Springer, 2014: 281–319.

Baumann N, Pham-Dinh D. Biology of oligodendrocyte and myelin in the mammalian nervous system. Physiol Rev 2001; 81: 871–927.

Benes FM, Turtle M, Khan Y, Farol P. Myelination of a key relay zone in the hippocampal formation occurs in the human brain during childhood, adolescence, and adulthood. Arch Gen Psychiatry 1994; 51: 477–484.

Bennaroch EF. Oligodendrocytes: susceptibility to injury and involvement in neurologic disease. Neurology 2009; 72: 1779–1785.

Bennett IJ, Madden DJ. Disconnected aging: cerebral white matter integrity and age-related differences in cognition. Neuroscience 2014; 276: 187–205.

Brownell B, Hughes JT. The distribution of plaques in the cerebrum in multiple sclerosis. J Neurol Neurosurg Psychiatry 1962; 25: 315–320.

Catani M, Thiebaut dc Schotten M. *Atlas of human brain connections.* New York: Oxford University Press, 2012.

Filley CM. *The behavioral neurology of white matter.* 2nd ed. New York: Oxford University Press, 2012.

Geschwind N. Disconnexion syndromes in animals and man. Brain 1965; 88: 237–294, 585–644.

Gould SJ. *The mismeasure of man.* New York: W.W. Norton, 1981.

Grydeland H, Walhovd KB, Tamnes CK, et al. Intracortical myelin links with performance variability across the human lifespan: results from T1- and T2-weighted MRI myelin mapping and diffusion tensor imaging. J Neurosci 2013; 33: 18618–18630.

Harris JJ, Attwell D. The energetics of CNS white matter. J Neurosci 2012; 32: 356–371.

Hartline DK, Colman DR. Rapid conduction and the evolution of giant axons and myelinated fibers. Curr Biol 2007; 17: R29–R35.

Hildebrand C, Remahl S, Persson H, Bjartmar C. Myelinated nerve fibres in the CNS. Prog Neurobiol 1993; 40: 319–384.

Kandel ER, Schwartz JH, Jessell TM, et al. *Principles of neural science.* 5th ed. New York: McGraw-Hill, 2013.

Kleinnijenhuis M, Zerbi V, Küsters B, et al. Layer-specific diffusion weighted imaging in human primary visual cortex in vitro. Cortex 2013; 49: 2569–2582.

Kochunov P, Coyle T, Lancaster J, et al. Processing speed is correlated with cerebral health markers in the frontal lobes quantified by neuroimaging. Neuroimage 2010; 49: 1190–1199.

Kutzelnigg A, Lucchinetti CF, Stadelmann C, et al. Cortical demyelination and diffuse white matter injury in multiple sclerosis. Brain 2005; 128: 2705–2712.

Marner L, Nyengaard JR, Tang Y, Pakkenberg B. Marked loss of myelinated nerve fibers in the human brain with age. J Comp Neurol 2003; 462: 144–152.

Matute C, Ransom BR. Roles of white matter in central nervous system pathophysiologies. ASN Neuro 2012; 4. doi: pii: e00079.

Mega MS, Cummings JL, Salloway S, Malloy P. The limbic system: an anatomic, phylogenetic, and clinical perspective. J Neuropsychiatry Clin Neurosci 1997; 9: 315–330.

Miller AKH, Alston RL, Corsellis JAN. Variation with age in the volumes of grey and white matter in the cerebral hemispheres of man: measurements with an image analyser. Neuropathol Appl Neurobiol 1980; 6: 119–132.

Miller DJ, Duka T, Stimpson CD, et al. Prolonged myelination in human neocortical evolution. Proc Natl Acad Sci 2012; 109: 16480–16485.

Nieuwenhuys R. The myeloarchitectonic studies on the human cerebral cortex of the Vogt-Vogt school, and their significance for the interpretation of functional neuroimaging data. Brain Struct Funct 2013; 218: 303–352.

Nolte J. *The human brain.* 5th ed. St. Louis: Mosby, 2002.

Parvizi J. Corticocentric myopia: old bias in new cognitive sciences. Trends Cogn Sci 2009; 13: 354–359.

Petanjek Z, Judaš M, Šimic G, et al. Extraordinary neoteny of synaptic spines in the human prefrontal cortex. Proc Natl Acad Sci 2011; 108: 13281–13286.

Roth G, Dicke U. Evolution of the brain and intelligence. Trends Cogn Sci 2005; 9: 250–257.

Rushton JP, Ankney CD. Whole brain size and general mental ability: a review. Int J Neurosci 2009; 119: 691–731.

Saver JL. Time is brain – quantified. Stroke 2006; 37: 263–266.

Schmahmann JD, Pandya DN. *Fiber pathways of the brain.* New York: Oxford University Press, 2006.

Schmahmann JD, Pandya DN. Disconnection syndromes of basal ganglia, thalamus, and cerebrocerebellar systems. Cortex 2008; 44: 1037–1066.

Schoenemann PT, Sheehan MJ, Glotzer LD. Prefrontal white matter is disproportionately larger in humans than in other primates. Nat Neurosci 2005; 8: 242–252.

Sherwood CC, Smaers JB. What's the fuss over human frontal lobe evolution? Trends Cogn Sci 2013; 17: 432–433.

Smaers JB, Schleicher A, Zilles K, Vinicius L. Frontal white matter volume is associated with brain enlargement and higher structural connectivity in anthropoid primates. PloS One 2010; 5: e9123.

Sporns O. The human connectome: a complex network. Ann N Y Acad Sci 2011; 1224: 109–125.

Stadelmann C, Albert M, Wegner C, Brück W. Cortical pathology in multiple sclerosis. Curr Opin Neurol 2008; 21: 239–234.

Sullivan EV, Pfefferbaum A. Diffusion tensor imaging and aging. Neurosci Biobehav Rev 2006; 30: 749–761.

Turken AU, Whitfield-Gabrieli S, Bammer R, et al. Cognitive speed and the structure of white matter pathways: convergent evidence from normal variation and lesion studies. Neuroimage 2008; 42: 1032–1044.

Van Essen DC, Glasser MF. In vivo architectonics: a cortico-centric perspective. Neuroimage 2014; 93: 157–164.

Venkatraman VK, Aizenstein HJ, Newman AB, et al. Lower digit symbol substitution score in the oldest old is related to magnetization transfer and diffusion tensor imaging of the white matter. Front Aging Neurosci 2011; 3: 11.

Wake H, Lee PR, Fields RD. Control of local protein synthesis and initial events in myelination by action potentials. Science 2011; 333: 1647–1651.

Walhovd KB, Johansen-Berg H, Káradóttir RT. Unraveling the secrets of white matter – bridging the gap between cellular, animal and human imaging studies. Neuroscience 2014; 276: 2–13.

Wang SS-H, Schultz JR, Burish MJ, et al. Shaping of white matter composition by biophysical scaling constraints. J Neurosci 2008; 28: 4047–4056.

Yakovlev PI, Lecours AR. The myelogenetic cycles of regional maturation of the brain. In: Minkowski A, ed. *Regional development of the brain in early life*. Oxford: Blackwell Scientific Publications, 1967: 3–79.

Zhang K, Sejnowski TJ. A universal scaling law between gray matter and white matter of cerebral cortex. Proc Natl Acad Sci 2000; 97: 5621–5626.

Chapter 4

A neuroanatomic overview of dementia

The word *dementia* literally means "down from the mind" (from the Latin *de* and *mens*), and this broad concept implicates a long and continually expanding list of disorders that diminish intellect to a level lower than expected. The syndrome of dementia can result from many diseases within the brain, or from many others originating elsewhere in the body that exert secondary effects on the brain. The acquired loss of cognitive competence meant by the term *dementia* implies that brain function is compromised to the extent that multiple cognitive domains are affected and neither normal cognition nor customary social and occupational function can be maintained (McKhann et al., 1984; Mendez and Cummings, 2003). The recently updated *Diagnostic and Statistical Manual of Mental Disorders* (*DSM-V*) proposes the entity of "major neurocognitive disorder" to designate what is essentially the same syndrome (American Psychiatric Association, 2013). The term *dementia* is widely used and has served well as a descriptor of clinically significant cognitive dysfunction, and both clinicians and researchers have derived benefit from the organizing framework this notion implies. In the clinic, establishing the presence of dementia impels a critical search for reversible causes of the syndrome, correction of which can lead to a cure. The regrettably far more common scenario of finding an irreversible cause can still prove helpful with respect to the provision of information on prognosis, avoidance or mitigation of medical problems that can worsen the dementia, use of carefully selected medications for behavioral problems that may arise, and counseling as the disease progresses to its end. For researchers, the concept of dementia means the persistent if not permanent failure of brain systems devoted to normal cognition, and detailed investigation of the basis for this failure can proceed.

One approach to the understanding of the neurologic basis of dementia, therefore, can begin with the brain regions in which cognitive dysfunction is thought to occur (Filley, 2011). This method is well established in neurology and has proven effective for identifying and classifying the steadily increasing numbers of dementing disorders (Mendez and Cummings, 2003; Miller and Boeve, 2009). Neuropathological identification of specific disorders, particularly at postmortem examination, has traditionally stood as the gold standard of neurologic diagnosis, allowing clinicians to know the extent to which the clinical impression in life was accurate. In addition, the recognition of characteristic findings associated with various dementias keenly focuses the investigator on visible abnormalities that may provide clues to etiopathogenesis and ultimately treatment. The classic works of Alois Alzheimer, Arnold Pick, Otto Binswanger, and others more than a century ago have clearly stimulated a great deal of work on neuropathological findings in the dementias as potential avenues to understanding.

A related aspect of the neuropathological method is that this approach has greatly advanced the study of brain–behavior relationships pertinent to dementia. Although the well-known lesion method of behavioral neurology (Damasio, 1984) has been seen by many as best applied to focal cerebral lesions such as those produced by stroke, pursuing alterations in behavior can also be understood by attention to the structural lesions underlying the dementia syndromes. Application of the lesion method has in fact disclosed that a single lesion can produce dementia, as dementia has been noted to follow isolated vascular lesions of the thalamus, left angular gyrus, medial frontal lobe, and basal forebrain (Szirmai et al., 2002; Auchus et al., 2002). Yet such cases of "strategic infarct dementia" are rare, and the usual dementia syndrome involves a more complex picture of brain damage featuring more widespread neuropathology disturbing multiple distributed neural networks. Still, the principle of the lesion method remains valid, and the distribution of

Table 4.1 Traditional dementia categories and examples of specific diseases

Cortical
Alzheimer's Disease
Frontotemporal lobar degeneration
Subcortical
Huntington's Disease
Parkinson's Disease
Progressive supranuclear palsy
Wilson's Disease
Toxic and metabolic disorders
Mixed
Multi-infarct dementia
Creutzfeldt-Jakob disease
Lewy body dementia
Corticobasal degeneration
Neurosyphilis
Subdural hematoma
Hypoxic-ischemic encephalopathy
Autoimmune dementia

neuropathological involvement in dementia cases can be usefully conceptualized in view of the behavioral alterations produced. It is in this light that the information to follow is presented (see Table 4.1).

A complete description of the many disorders to be discussed is beyond the scope of this chapter, and recent textbooks provide complete and authoritative accounts (Mendez and Cummings, 2003; Miller and Boeve, 2009). Rather, the objective here is to offer an overview of how the dementias can be classified by their localization in the brain. As a reliance on the differences between cortical and subcortical dementia will be readily apparent, a point worth emphasizing is that this dichotomy provides an essential foundation for a specific focus on the white matter and its disorders. The cortical-subcortical dementia distinction has both advocates and critics, and controversy surrounding the idea will be considered. The intent of this chapter is not to claim that all the dementias can be neatly classified within this framework, but that the broad categories discussed can serve to organize a rational approach with respect to the primary targets of neuropathology that can lead to dementia.

Cortical dementia

The cerebral cortex – measuring just a few millimeters in thickness – enjoys a time-honored position in neuroscience whereby it is seen as the most important region of the brain for the operations of cognition. Indeed, a wealth of clinical and experimental support can be invoked to support the prominence of this thin ribbon of gray matter comprising the outermost surface of the brain (Kandel et al., 2013). The locus of billions of neuronal cell bodies, each making thousands of connections to other neurons, is indeed impressive for its biological complexity and computational capacity, and naturally leads to the assumption that cognitive operations are firmly, if not exclusively, rooted in the cerebral cortex.

The cortical dementias were for many years listed as Alzheimer's Disease (AD) and its far less common relative Pick's Disease (Koranyi, 1988). These two diseases were the best examples of dementing illness in which microscopic and histologic neuropathology were most apparent in the cortex, specifically the neocortex and the hippocampus. Without question, AD remains today the classic cortical dementia, and is widely recognized as a looming threat to the medical system and society in general because of its high prevalence, incurability, and enormous burden of emotional distress and financial costs (Cummings, 2004; Querfurth and LaFerla, 2010).

The recognition of AD as a major problem occurred, however, only with increasing life expectancy in the developed world. For many decades after its introduction to medical readers by the German neurologist and neuropathologist Alois Alzheimer (1907), the disease that came to bear his name was a relatively obscure neurologic disorder thought to afflict only a small number of adults who were diagnosed at autopsy, but this situation dramatically changed with the aging of the population over the course of the twentieth century. Alzheimer described the now classic neuropathogy of neuritic (senile) plaques and neurofibrillary tangles, both of which were mainly situated in the cerebral cortices (Alzheimer, 1907), and to this day these collections of proteins fascinate researchers who find it difficult to avoid the presumption that damage to the cortex is entirely responsible for the clinical features and etiopathogenesis of AD. As Alzheimer's 1907 report attracted more attention, many older adults gradually came to be identified as suffering from a dementing illness that featured the same neuropathology as that of the first case, a 55-year-old woman named Auguste Deter (Alzheimer, 1907). Thus the distinction between "presenile dementia" – Alzheimer's 1907 term – and "senile dementia" was abandoned, and all cases were called simply AD.

Memory loss became well known as the usual presenting symptom of the disease, and with increasing knowledge of the importance of the hippocampus and adjacent cortical regions in learning and memory, the location of neuropathology in these areas was plausible as an important explanation for the clinical presentation. Then, in 1984, standard diagnostic criteria for AD were established that led to many more people being accurately diagnosed in life (McKhann et al., 1984). A recent revision of the 1984 criteria incorporated biomarker evidence to assist with research, but retained the core features of the original publication because of their well-established utility (McKhann et al., 2011). Today there are thought to be more than 5 million Americans living with AD, most of whom are over 65 years of age, and many millions more around the world (Thies et al., 2013).

Pick's Disease, first described as lobar atrophy in the nineteenth century (Pick, 1892), has been recast as frontotemporal lobar degeneration (FTLD), itself a collection of several complex disorders that all involve more restricted areas of cortical degeneration than is seen in AD. Pick actually described the disease as "lobar atrophy," an apt designation that is echoed in the current terminology. In contrast to its former status as a very rare disease, recent studies indicate that FTLD accounts for at least 5% of all neuropathological diagnoses of dementia (Rabinovici and Miller, 2010). Although clinical recognition of FTLD was long felt to be dauntingly difficult, many neurologists believing that only autopsy could distinguish this entity from AD, the various behavioral and language presentations of the disease are becoming better appreciated (Rabinovici and Miller, 2010). Unlike AD, FTLD leaves memory unaffected early in the course, and instead poses unique challenges to patients, families, and clinicians coping with often disruptive behaviors and severe language disturbances. Both diseases pose vexing challenges to investigators attempting to understand the basis of disease, and the still unmet need for more effective treatments.

AD and FTLD both manifest most prominent neuropathology in the cerebral cortex, but it is worth keeping in mind that they also feature less obvious neuropathology in subcortical regions such as the basal forebrain, basal ganglia, and thalamus (Mendez and Cummings, 2003). Nevertheless, the key distinctions between these diseases can be seen as beginning with their characteristic abnormalities in the cerebral cortex. As is true in all of behavioral neurology, the clinical manifestations of disease are explained by the location of the neuropathology. Thus cortical degeneration in AD, which primarily targets the hippocampus and parietotemporal cortices, has been associated with amnesia, aphasia, apraxia, and agnosia, whereas in FTLD the frontal and temporal cortices are damaged while the hippocampus is spared until later, producing the early behavioral dysfunction or aphasia of this disease in the absence of amnesia (Filley, 2011).

Support for the role of cortical damage in causing the clinical features of dementia has been adduced in both diseases. In AD (Terry et al., 1991) as well as FTLD (Lippa, 2004), the most likely problem underlying neurobehavioral decline is synaptic and neuronal loss in relevant neocortical and allocortical regions. But the loss of synapses and cortical neurons is a later event in cortical degeneration, and likely a marker of some earlier neuropathological process, so that what happens in the brain to produce the loss of synapses and neurons is fundamental. At the microscopic level, intense effort is being directed to understanding the origin and significance of cortical histopathological changes that may hold the key to understanding. Neuritic plaques and neurofibrillary tangles are the cortical hallmarks of AD (Cummings, 2004; Querfurth and LaFerla, 2010), whereas tau-positive (FTLD-TAU) or TAR DNA-binding protein 43 (TDP-43)-positive (FTLD-TDP) inclusion bodies are primarily found in FTLD (Rabinovici and Miller, 2010). Investigations focused on these proteins are in turn closing in on many genetic and environmental factors that underlie the cortical alterations. Most investigators would agree that genetic predisposition is modified by environmental influences to determine the appearance of clinical illness. It is likely that both nature and nurture contribute to the expression of the cortical dementias, and AD in particular demands attention as an increasingly threatening medical and societal challenge. Yet major gaps in our knowledge remain, as will be considered later in this book.

Subcortical dementia

Brain regions that lie subjacent to the cerebral cortex are generally known as subcortical. This large expanse of neural tissue actually occupies the great majority of the brain volume, as it consists of the many deep gray matter nuclei within the basal ganglia, diencephalon, and brain stem, as well as the cerebellum and all the larger white matter tracts coursing within the brain. Considering all of these structures as sharing a set of common functions may seem misguided, as these diverse regions must surely have a multitude of different contributions to behavior. However, a significant tradition in behavioral neurology and neuropsychology has supported and kept alive the maintenance of a distinction between dementia related to cortical disease and dementia that can be ascribed to subcortical dysfunction. Clinical and theoretical reasons can both be implicated for the establishment of this dichotomy. For the purposes of diagnosis, a general categorization of cognitive deficits related to cortical versus noncortical disease is often helpful in directing the evaluation toward specific neuropathologies. In terms of research, the cortical-subcortical distinction helps refine investigation of how distributed neural networks operate and what role is played by brain connectivity.

The concept of subcortical dementia was first developed in the early twentieth century, when investigators began to examine the possibility that disorders involving selective lesions of subcortical structures such as the basal ganglia and thalamus could disrupt normal cognition and emotion. In 1922, "bradyphrenia" was described in patients with postencephalitic parkinsonism, who presumably had primary damage to the substantia nigra and related subcortical regions (Naville, 1922). This observation would prove prescient for later work on Parkinson's Disease (PD), a common movement disorder in which dementia came to be increasingly recognized as a major cause of disability. The term subcortical dementia was introduced 10 years after Naville's observation to characterize postencephalitic patients with a similar mental slowness who also had personality and affective disturbances (Von Stockert, 1932). These developments were largely ignored, however, as were concepts of cerebral localization in general during the first half of this century. The ascendancy of Freudian interpretations of behavior in those years, as well as an emphasis on holistic or Gestalt thinking about brain–behavior relationships, were powerful factors diverting attention away from efforts to identify the specific details of the neural basis of behavior, whether cortical or subcortical (Benson, 1993).

Many decades later, however, after behavioral neurology had become established as a distinct discipline, the concept of subcortical dementia was revived. The work of two groups in the 1970s was critical in this process, as each published remarkably similar clinical observations independent of the other. Martin Albert and colleagues (1974), studying five patients with progressive supranuclear palsy (PSP), described a pattern of cognitive impairment consistent with subcortical dementia, while Paul McHugh and Marshall Folstein (1975) presented a nearly identical syndrome in eight patients with Huntington's Disease (HD). These investigators extended the old idea of bradyphrenia and emphasized cognitive slowing, forgetfulness, and personality and emotional changes as typical of subcortical dementias, in contrast to the amnesia, aphasia, apraxia, and agnosia traditionally associated with cortical dementias. Subcortical dementia was theorized to disrupt the "fundamental" functions of arousal, attention, motivation, and mood that underlie the timing and activation of cortical processes, whereas cortical dementia was conceptualized as interfering with the "instrumental" functions of memory, language, praxis, and perception primarily associated with the neocortex (Albert, 1978). An analogous distinction was drawn between the idea of "channel" functions, meaning the specific domains of cognition, and "state" functions, those that maintain the state of information processing in the brain (Mesulam, 2000). Based on these formulations, descriptive clinical work in the dementias flourished, and subcortical dementia became a widely used, if not universally accepted, term for the dementia that manifests in patients with a variety of subcortical diseases (Cummings and Benson, 1984). As further data appeared, the clinical resemblance of subcortical disease with frontal lobe disease was recognized, and the alternate terms "fronto-subcortical dementia" and "frontal systems dementia" were suggested (Freedman and Albert, 1985), although subcortical dementia remains the most commonly used descriptor for this syndrome.

The subcortical dementias include a wide range of neuropathological entities (Table 4.1). The category is perhaps best exemplified by two neurodegenerative diseases: HD and PD, in which major neuropathology is found in deep gray matter nuclei. Among many such regions involved, the caudate nucleus is prominently affected in HD, and in PD the substantia nigra is severely damaged. Whereas dementia is seen by some as an undifferentiated syndrome of brain failure, the neurobiology of diseases such as HD and PD differs markedly from others such as AD and FTLD, and group comparisons can be pursued with these diseases that can inform the understanding of how dementia develops. Central to this approach is the eminently reasonable proposition that different sites of cerebral pathology will lead to different clinical presentations.

The notion of subcortical dementia, however, has encountered considerable opposition (Mayeux et al., 1983; Whitehouse, 1986; Tierney et al., 1987; Brown and Marsden, 1988). One problem with the idea as first proposed was that the descriptions of mental status changes were generally impressionistic, and few data were introduced to permit quantification of the various deficits and strengths, and the degree to which a given impairment was present. Clinical features in the initial reports of the 1970s such as the "impaired ability to manipulate acquired knowledge" (Albert et al., 1974) and "apathy and inertia" (McHugh and Folstein, 1975) were subjective and difficult to quantitate, leading to uncertainty about how these problems were unique to diseases such as PSP and HD. As clinicians' time to examine patients with attention to these subtleties steadily shrank with changes in the health care system, the usefulness of gathering detailed but relatively nonquantifiable clinical information became increasingly questioned. This issue was confounded by the recognition of overlap in the neuropathological features of cortical and subcortical dementias. Clinically, it is indeed the case that any patient with dementia may have bradyphrenia, and distinguishing forgetfulness from amnesia can be challenging. Similarly, it is true that cortical dementia can feature coexistent neuropathology in subcortical regions while the converse can also be seen in many cases.

However, considerable evidence indicates that subcortical dementias can often be clinically distinguished from those involving cortical damage, and the subcortical dementias tend to resemble each other more than they do the cortical dementias (Huber et al., 1986; Pillon et al., 1991; Drebing et al., 1994; Darvesh and Freedman, 1996; Savage, 1997; Salmon and Filoteo, 2007; Bonelli and Cummings, 2008). The neocortex and the subcortical regions appear to make distinctly different contributions to cognition and emotion (Albert, 1978; Mesulam, 2000). Despite considerable overlap with other dementias that should be acknowledged, the cortical-subcortical distinction has continued to be frequently invoked by many neurologists and in neuropsychological testing and its interpretation, helping to organize thinking about the clinical classification and neuropathological basis of dementing illness.

In defense of the concept, subcortical dementia represents an early phase that is required in any field of study involving natural systems: the description of phenomenology. The defining feature of individuals afflicted with dementia is disturbed mentation, and careful elucidation of that disturbance is fundamental in investigating the underlying cause. Clinical phenomena are essential in understanding the basis of clinical syndromes, and the gathering of phenomenological detail, in addition to facilitating optimal patient care, is crucial before any more focused effort to probe more deeply into the neurobiological basis of the problem is possible. The proposal of subcortical dementia was an earnest and systematic attempt to make sense of one of the most vexing problems in medicine: the progressive decline in intellect that has no obvious medical or psychiatric cause. Criticisms of the idea were easy to mount from the perspective of "hard" science, with its reliance on measurement and reductionism, and the concept proved to be a ready target for those who demand irrefutable data. Such data are of course most desirable. But without careful clinical description as a first step, the syndrome of dementia remains frustratingly opaque.

Today, the idea of subcortical dementia is still alive, continuing to organize thinking about the dementias and their neurobiological basis. The concept is recognized to be most appropriately used in a general sense, and many advances since the 1970s have led to a more nuanced understanding of all the dementias. But broad categorizations such as this one often remain foundational in the challenging task of diagnosis. Neuropsychologists in clinical practice regularly invoke the cortical-subcortical distinction, classifying patients according to whether their cognitive deficits point to involvement of the cerebral cortex and hippocampus or to deeper structures of the brain (Rizzo and Eslinger, 2004; Morgan and Ricker, 2008). Many neurologists also find the dichotomy helpful, and the most recent edition of a widely read and highly respected neurology textbook comments that "the clinical distinction between cortical and subcortical dementia based on a relative sparing of core cortical functions is very useful" (Ropper, Samuels, and Klein, 2014).

In retrospect, the lasting contribution of the idea of subcortical dementia is likely to be that a group of diseases exists that alter intellect by disrupting the timing and activation of cognition (Albert, 2005). The cortex subserves the specific operations of cognition known as instrumental functions – memory, language, praxis, perception – but the subcortical regions provide fundamental neural input that enables these operations to proceed in an efficient and integrated fashion (Albert, 1978). This insight has proven crucial in further work on the dementias, and indeed all neurobehavioral syndromes, as the role of cognitive speed has assumed recent prominence in neurobiology. As this book aims to show, subcortical dementia was a necessary precursor of the idea of white matter dementia, which can be seen as a refinement of the idea using the many advances in clinical neuroscience that have occurred in recent decades.

Mixed dementia

Before proceeding to the white matter disorders, another group of dementias should be considered. To supplement the traditional cortical-subcortical distinction discussed previously, a third category must necessarily be invoked to do justice to a neuropathological classification of the dementias. This category can be named mixed dementia, as it includes many disorders featuring pathology that does not fall predominantly in either the cerebral cortex or the subcortical regions (Filley, 2011). Stated another way, many patients are rendered demented by disorders that exert their ill effects on *both* cortical and subcortical structures. Mixed dementia as a category lacks specificity, and unavoidably involves a group of conditions that do not naturally fit within other, better-specified categories, but it does serve the purpose of including the wide range of dementia neuropathologies within the scheme presented in this book. Examples include multi-infarct dementia, Creutzfeldt-Jakob disease, Lewy body dementia, corticobasal degeneration, neurosyphilis, subdural hematoma, neoplasms with increased intracranial pressure, hypoxic-ischemic encephalopathy, and, most recently recognized, autoimmune dementia that may be paraneoplastic or non-paraneoplastic.

Mixed dementia as defined here thus highlights the presence of overlapping regions of neuropathology rather than specific types of neuropathology. Although clinically useful for interpreting many clues to etiology – stepwise strokes, myoclonus, parkinsonism, visual hallucinations, fluctuating confusion, abnormal cerebrospinal fluid, trauma history, headache, fever, meningismus, papilledema, rapid progession, and so on – the neurologic and neurobehavioral aspects of these disorders are so diverse as to preclude a general categorization. When neuropathology can involve any combination of cortical, subcortical gray matter, or white matter damage in protean fashion, no unifying theme of brain–behavior correlation can be expected to emerge. Patients may have a highly variable combination of cortical signs, such as amnesia, aphasia, and seizures, along with subcortical features, including cognitive slowing, inattention, and extrapyramidal dysfunction. In such cases the neurobehavioral profile typically precludes a convenient classification on a neuroanatomic basis.

In addition to the imprecision of neurobehavioral classification inherent in the mixed dementias, this label may also seem unsatisfying because it includes disease entities that blur neuropathological distinctions. Recent autopsy findings, however, have cast new light on this problem. It is becoming clear with more comprehensive investigation that dementia, at least in older people, is in fact usually related to more than a single cause. For example, the commingling of AD changes with other neuropathological findings, including Lewy bodies and Pick bodies, is increasingly evident as a general phenomenon, and especially important is the coexistence of AD and vascular disease (Langa, Foster, and Larson, 2004; Schneider and Bennett, 2010). In a recent autopsy study of community-dwelling older people, the majority of dementia was found to be attributable to mixed neuropathology and not to a single etiology (Schneider et al., 2007). The most common cause of dementia was in fact AD in combination with vascular dementia, and, remarkably, AD changes in isolation were often found to be compatible with normal cognition (Schneider et al., 2007). Intuitively, it is not surprising that, as people age, they are more likely to display evidence of more than one neuropathology. A long life, however well lived, renders an individual susceptible to a host of illnesses, injuries, and intoxications from which a younger person might be spared. As experienced clinicians are well aware, it is often impossible to attribute dementia to a single cause, and the phenomenon of multiple dementia etiologies in the same patient should not be unexpected.

Mixed dementia, therefore, may have a far more profound impact than as a mere catchall category for dementias that do not fit tidily into one category. If dementia has more than one cause, new avenues for research and treatment are immediately apparent. In contrast to the assumption of recent decades that AD alone accounts for the majority of dementia in the elderly, for example, it may be crucial to consider other comorbidities, most obviously vascular, in the etiopathogenesis of the disease. It may thus now be prudent to expand thinking about AD as a genetic amyloidopathy to include consideration of vascular compromise as a key environmental risk factor. As often happens in the history of medicine and science, the pendulum of thought is swinging back again to a previous paradigm: in this case, that AD is in fact based to a significant extent on vascular disease. The genetic basis of AD remains an important area of study (Querfurth and LaFerla, 2010), but may be most relevant in the context of early-onset familial AD, in which a gene mutation is associated with cortical pathology in the absence of other brain disease. Indeed, the new and intriguing observations of a decline in dementia incidence and prevalence suggest that the treatment of vascular disease may be leading to fewer older people developing dementia, be it what neurologists label AD or otherwise (Larson, Yaffe, and Langa, 2013).

These ideas are all relevant to white matter and cognition. Conventional thinking regards pure AD as the major contributor to the dementia epidemic. However, if neuritic plaques and neurofibrillary tangles are often accompanied by white matter changes, and dementia is declining in older people because of medical attention to cerebrovascular disease, then perhaps avoidance of cerebrovascular white matter disease may be a potential solution to the problem of dementia in the elderly. Evidence for this possibility is indeed available. A large population-based study from the Netherlands found that as dementia risk declined in elders, so too did the burden of cerebral small vessel vascular disease (Schrijvers et al., 2012). These issues will be more fully addressed later in this book, but it is clear that the time has come to adopt a more nuanced view of dementia that considers the interactions of more than a single etiology. In this light, the white matter disorders can be seen to be of central importance.

References

Albert ML. Subcortical dementia. In: Katzman R, Terry RD, Bick KL, eds. *Alzheimer's disease: senile dementia and related disorders*. New York: Raven Press, 1978: 173–180.

Albert ML. Subcortical dementia: historical review and personal view. Neurocase 2005; 11: 243–245.

Albert ML, Feldman RG, Willis AL. The "subcortical dementia" of progressive supranuclear palsy. J Neurol Neurosurg Psychiatry 1974; 37: 121–130.

Alzheimer A. Über eine eigenartige Erkankung der Hirnrinde. Allgemeine Zeitschrift fur Psychiatrie under Psychisch-Gerichtliche Medizin 1907; 64: 146–148. (Trans. Jarvik L, Greenson H. Alzheimer Dis Assoc Disord 1987; 1: 3–8).

American Psychiatric Association. *Diagnostic and statistical manual of mental disorders*. 5th ed. *DSM-V*. Arlington, VA: American Psychiatric Association, 2013.

Auchus AP, Chen CP, Sodagar SN, et al. Single stroke dementia: insights from 12 cases in Singapore. J Neurol Sci 2002; 203–204: 85–89.

Benson DF. The history of behavioral neurology. Neurol Clin 1993; 11: 1–8.

Bonelli RM, Cummings JL. Frontal-subcortical dementias. Neurologist 2008 Mar; 14(2): 100–107.

Brown RG, Marsden CD. "Subcortical dementia": the neuropsychological evidence. Neuroscience 1988; 25: 363–387.

Cummings JL. Alzheimer's disease. N Engl J Med 2004; 351: 56–67.

Cummings JL, Benson DF. Subcortical dementia: review of an emerging concept. Arch Neurol 1984; 41: 874–879.

Damasio AR. Behavioral neurology: theory and practice. Semin Neurol 1984; 4: 117–119.

Darvesh S, Freedman M. Subcortical dementia: a neurobehavioral approach. Brain Cogn 1996; 31: 230–249.

Drebing CE, Moore LH, Cummings JL, et al. Patterns of neuropsychological performance among forms of subcortical dementia. Neuropsychiatry Neuropsychol Behav Neurol 1994; 7: 57–66.

Filley CM. *Neurobehavioral anatomy*. 3rd ed. Boulder: University Press of Colorado, 2011.

Freedman M, Albert ML. Subcortical dementia. In: Vinken PJ, Bruyn VW, Klawans H, Frederiks JAM, eds. *Handbook of clinical neurology*. Vol. 46. *Neurobehavioral disorders*. Amsterdam: Elsevier Science Publishers, 1985: 311–316.

Huber SJ, Shuttleworth EC, Paulson GW, et al. Cortical vs subcortical dementia: neuropsychological differences. Arch Neurol 1986; 43: 392–394.

Kandel ER, Schwartz JH, Jessell TM, et al. *Principles of neural science*. 5th ed. New York: McGraw-Hill, 2013.

Koranyi EK. The cortical dementias. Can J Psychiatry 1988; 33: 838–845.

Langa KM, Foster NL, Larson EB. Mixed dementia: emerging concepts and therapeutic implications. JAMA 2004; 292: 2901–2908.

Larson EB, Yaffe K, Langa KM. New insights into the dementia epidemic. N Engl J Med 2013; 369: 2275–2277.

Lippa CF. Synaptophysin immunoreactivity in Pick's disease: comparison with Alzheimer's disease and dementia with Lewy bodies. Am J Alzheimers Dis Other Demen 2004; 19: 341–344.

Mayeux R, Stern Y, Rosen J, Benson F. Is "subcortical dementia" a recognizable clinical entity? Ann Neurol 1983; 14: 278–283.

McHugh PR, Folstein MF. Psychiatric symptoms of Huntington's chorea: a clinical and phenomenologic study. In: Benson DF, Blumer D, eds. *Psychiatric aspects of neurologic disease.* Vol. 1. New York: Grune and Stratton, 1975: 267–285.

McKhann G, Drachman D, Folstein M, et al. Clinical diagnosis of Alzheimer's disease: report of the NINCDS-ADRDA Work Group under the auspices of Department of Health and Human Services Task Force on Alzheimer's Disease. Neurology 1984; 34: 939–944.

McKhann GM, Knopman DS, Chertkow H, et al. The diagnosis of dementia due to Alzheimer's disease: recommendations from the National Institute on Aging–Alzheimer's Association workgroups on diagnostic guidelines for Alzheimer's disease. Alzheimers Dement 2011; 7: 263–269.

Mendez MF, Cummings JL. *Dementia, a clinical approach.* 3rd ed. Philadelphia: Butterworth Heinemann, 2003.

Mesulam M-M. Behavioral neuroanatomy: large-scale neural networks, association cortex, frontal systems, the limbic system, and hemispheric specializations. In: Mesulam M-M. *Principles of behavioral and cognitive neurology.* 2nd ed. New York: Oxford University Press, 2000: 1–120.

Miller BL, Boeve BF, eds. *The behavioral neurology of dementia.* Cambridge: Cambridge University Press, 2009.

Morgan JE, Ricker JH, eds. *Textbook of clinical neuropsychology.* New York: Taylor and Francis, 2008.

Naville F. Etudes sur les complications et les séquelles mentales de l'encéphalite épidémique: la bradyphrénie. L'Encéphale 1922; 17: 369–375, 423–436.

Pick A. Über die beziehungen der senilin hirnatrophie zur aphasie. Prager Med Wochenschr 1892; 17: 165–167.

Pillon B, Dubois B, Ploska A, Agid Y. Severity and specificity of cognitive impairment in Alzheimer's, Huntington's, and Parkinson's diseases and progressive supranuclear palsy. Neurology 1991; 41: 634–643.

Querfurth HW, LaFerla FM. Alzheimer's disease. N Engl J Med 2010; 362: 329–344.

Rabinovici GD, Miller BL. Frontotemporal lobar degeneration: epidemiology, pathophysiology, diagnosis and management. CNS Drugs 2010; 24: 375–398.

Rizzo M, Eslinger PJ, eds. *Principles and practice of behavioral neurology and neuropsychology.* Philadelphia: W.B. Saunders, 2004.

Ropper AH, Samuels MA, Klein JP. *Adams and Victor's principles of neurology.* 10th ed. New York: McGraw-Hill, 2014.

Salmon DP, Filoteo JV. Neuropsychology of cortical versus subcortical dementia syndromes. Semin Neurol 2007; 27: 7–21.

Savage CR. Neuropsychology of subcortical dementias. Psychiatr Clin North Am 1997; 20: 911–931.

Schneider JA, Arvanitakis Z, Bang W, Bennett DA. Mixed brain pathologies account for most dementia cases in community-dwelling older persons. Neurology 2007; 69: 2197–2204.

Schneider JA, Bennett DA. Where vascular meets neurodegenerative disease. Stroke 2010; 41 (10 Suppl): S144–S146.

Schrijvers EM, Verhaaren BF, Koudstaal PJ, et al. Is dementia incidence declining? Trends in dementia incidence since 1990 in the Rotterdam Study. Neurology 2012; 78: 1456–1463.

Szirmai I, Vastagh I, Szombathelyi E, Kamondi A. Strategic infarcts of the thalamus in vascular dementia. J Neurol Sci 2002; 203–204: 91–97.

Terry RD, Masliah E, Salmon DP, et al. Physical basis of cognitive alterations in Alzheimer's disease: synapse loss is the major correlate of cognitive impairment. Ann Neurol 1991; 30: 572–580.

Thies W, Bleiler L. Alzheimer's Association. 2013 Alzheimer's disease facts and figures. Alzheimers Dement 2013; 9: 208–245.

Tierney MC, Snow WG, Reid DW, et al. Psychometric differentiation of dementia: replication and extension of the findings of Storandt and coworkers. Arch Neurol 1987; 44: 720–722.

Von Stockert PG. Subcorticale demenz. Arch Psychiatry 1932; 97: 77–100.

Whitehouse PJ. The concept of subcortical and cortical dementia: another look. Ann Neurol 1986; 19: 1–6.

Chapter 5

Expanding the concept of dementia

From the three categories of dementia discussed in the previous chapter, a fourth naturally suggests itself, although it is surely the least familiar. This is the form characterized by significant pathology in the brain's white matter, and the topic of this book: the category of white matter dementia (WMD). As discussed in Chapter 3, most of the white matter in the brain is found in large tracts within and between the cerebral hemispheres, and in prior accounts, white matter disorders would logically be considered to fit within the category of subcortical dementia. Indeed, the initial formulations of the varieties of subcortical dementia included disorders of white matter as entries on this list (Cummings and Benson, 1983, 1984). For a time, this approach seemed acceptable, as there was a certain clinical commonality among all the dementias that could be traced to primary neuropathology in regions subjacent to the cerebral cortex. But the sizable portion of the brain occupied by white matter could not be ignored, particularly as modern neuroimaging increasingly expanded its visualization, and attention gradually turned toward the study of myelinated fibers in relation to cognition. As this research began to gain momentum, new data disclosed the need for more specificity and precision in the study of dementia, and a finer tuning of the idea of subcortical dementia was necessary. Thus the white matter disorders came to be seen as deserving their own category within the broad range of afflictions causing dementia.

What lies between

The most obvious fact thrusting white matter squarely in the midst of the study of dementia is its sheer volume – about half of the brain. To illustrate the neuroanatomic relevance of white matter in the pathogenesis of dementia, Figure 5.1 schematically depicts the position of white matter as a brain region interposed between the gray matter of the cerebral cortex and the nuclei of the subcortex. While this

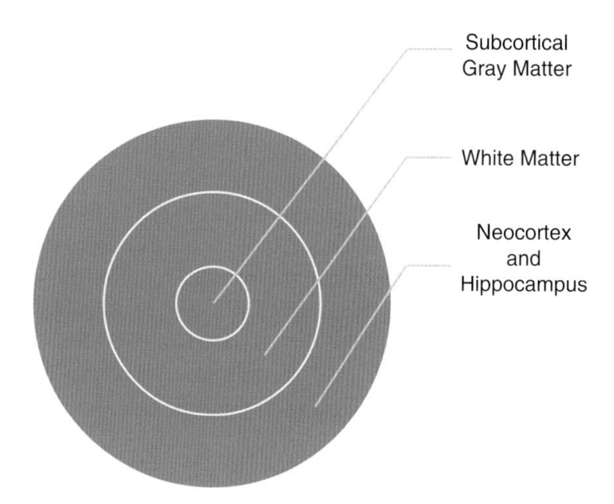

Figure 5.1 Schematic view of major brain regions in which dementia can originate.

depiction is obvious to any student of neuroscience, the prominence of white matter deserves special notice in view of how often it is overlooked. White matter is not simply the passive conduit between neuronal cell bodies (Fields, 2008), and myelin is not just the insulation of axons (Fields, 2014). Nowhere is the problem of corticocentric myopia (Parvizi, 2009) more striking and restrictive than in the neglect of myelinated systems by which the cerebral cortex communicates with the rest of the brain. That this neglect is a serious oversight seems fundamental and inescapable, as it is unimaginable that a brain could function normally with all its gray matter intact but devoid of white matter. In the context of white matter and its disorders, the study of the impact of brain connectivity on cognition can be seen as an important expansion of the idea of subcortical dementia, which encouraged neuroscientists to refine their thinking about the subtleties of dementing illness (Albert, 1978, 2005).

Beyond this self-evident observation, many seasoned clinicians are aware that neurobehavioral impairment can arise from damage or dysfunction of white matter tracts alone. Neurologists have recognized this phenomenon for well over a century (Charcot, 1877), and the advent of magnetic resonance imaging (MRI) facilitated this awareness by disclosing detailed in vivo structural data on the location and nature of all manner of white matter lesions. Moreover, even the white matter that appears normal on MRI has been found to harbor microstructural changes of neurobehavioral significance. By inadvertently reverting to corticocentrism, the clinician who omits the investigation of possible cognitive dysfunction in a patient with white matter disease risks a perilous omission. Inclusion of white matter and its disorders in the study of dementia seems not just reasonable but necessary.

As this discussion proceeds in the pages to follow, the presence of white matter damage should be seen as a general observation that naturally calls out for more detailed description. The clinician who sees an impaired person's brain MRI, and is impressed by the number of white matter lesions, cannot usually know with certainty what neuropathology explains these findings, or even what components of white matter are affected. Damage to white matter tracts that disturbs cognition can always be assumed to impact neuronal function, but not by involving the neuronal cell body or conventional synapses. Rather, the neuropathology that will mainly be considered here implicates the myelinated axons of inter- and intrahemispheric tracts, and, variably, neighborhood pathology involving unmyelinated axons, blood vessels, and glial cells. In many disorders, the precise details of white matter damage are not well understood, but it will become apparent that efforts to tease out the microstructural aspects of damage are well underway. The additional problem of myelinated tracts within gray matter – both of the cerebral cortex and of the deep gray matter of the brain – can only be approached in a preliminary manner, although this neuoranatomic feature beckons as an interesting aspect of white matter that may prove to complicate distinctions between cortical and other forms of dementia.

While all the neuropathological categories of dementia are considered, however, it is wise to bear in mind that all dementias ultimately result from damage to or dysfunction of neurons in the brain. As the neuron doctrine dictates, neurons are the essential signaling units of the nervous system (Chapter 1), and, in the brain, they are the basic elements of the distributed neural networks subserving cognition and emotion. Whereas glial cells and blood vessels perform crucial supportive functions, brain neurons are the sine qua non of human behavior. Thus the distinctions between cortical, subcortical, mixed, and white matter dementia are all to a degree arbitrary, as each one implies neuronal involvement of some kind. Indeed, neurologists working in the dementia clinic soon realize that all the progressive dementias increasingly resemble each other as they evolve to greater severity, reflecting the fact that intellectual competence ultimately depends on the number of brain neurons that are effectively operating. Wherever a dementing disorder begins, therefore, its advance to more severe stages implies a greater degree of neuronal damage. The progression of neuropathology from an initial site to more widespread brain areas is well illustrated by the observation that the advance of ischemic white matter lesions – the most common neuropathology to affect this region of the brain – is associated in most studies with global brain atrophy (Appelman et al., 2009), which can mean either ventricular enlargement (Inatomi et al., 2008) or cortical atrophy (Tuladhar et al., 2015).

The justification for dividing the dementias into the categories presented in this book is that clinical sequelae of neuronal failure – particularly early in the illness – differ markedly depending on which neurons are targeted, and what specific components are affected (Lafosse et al. 2007; Kozora and Filley, 2011; Filley, 2012). Thus the cortical dementias of Alzheimer's Disease (AD) and frontotemporal lobar degeneration (FTLD) reflect damage to specific cortical networks and implicate synapses and neuronal cell bodies, while WMD results from variable damage to association and commissural tracts and involves myelin, axons, or both. All dementia, therefore, reflects compromise of brain neurons, but the manner in which this functional decline occurs is crucial for assessing the etiopathogenesis of cognitive loss, improving the care of individuals with dementia syndromes, and understanding how the normal brain is organized.

Broad implications

While the notion that white matter is relevant to cognition is central to the idea of WMD, other implications are also apparent. In light of recent information, white matter neurobiology is becoming increasingly relevant for the problem of dementia developing early in life, and in the realm of psychiatric dysfunction.

To begin, expanding the concept of dementia to white matter disorders finds utility with regard to the problem of early-onset dementia. As will be seen later in this book, many white matter disorders arising well before the adult and geriatric age ranges can be sufficiently severe to result in dementia. While relatively rare, these disorders can be challenging diagnostically, and highly disruptive to patients and their families because of onset at a time when intellect is ordinarily expanding rather than declining. However, as dementia is widely regarded as a syndrome affecting older people, primarily if not exclusively, less attention is paid to dementia occurring in younger adults.

The term *dementia* can even be considered in the years of childhood and adolescence. While at times the term *regression* may be used by pediatric neurologists and psychologists for whom the word "dementia" conjures up the notion of older adults with degenerative disease (Thomas, Knowland, and Karmiloff-Smith, 2011), dementia is nevertheless an apt descriptor for disabling cognitive loss in a previously normal child or adolescent. These considerations bring up an interesting question: at what point in development can dementia be regarded as a meaningful construct? The idea of dementia in infancy is of course not tenable. Moreover, whereas childhood and adolescence each feature a level of age-appropriate intellectual ability from which disease can produce a decline that could be termed dementia, it can be difficult to establish dementia in children and adolescents undergoing rapid and sometimes turbulent developmental changes. Still, dementia does occur in children and adolescents, even if the term is rarely used in the lexicon of child neurology.

The published literature typically avoids the term *dementia* until considering the late teenage years or later, when the confounding issues posed by the variable developmental changes of children and adolescents have mostly subsided. As adulthood is approached, the determination of a normal cognitive profile becomes more secure, and departures from this state become more reliably determined. As only scant information on dementia in childhood is available, this book will consider dementia beginning as early as in adolescence, and many of the etiologies in these age ranges do in fact implicate damage to or dysfunction of white matter. Furthermore, most of these white matter disorders can present later in life, necessitating an understanding of these problems in the practice of adult neurology as well.

The category known as young-onset dementia has been recently invoked as an organizing principle for this area of research (Mendez, 2006; Kelley, Boeve, and Josephs, 2008; Rossor et al., 2010; Kuruppu and Matthews, 2013). Definitions vary, with some authorities defining this syndrome as beginning before age 65 (Mendez, 2006; Rossor et al., 2010; Kuruppu and Matthews, 2013), and others using a cutoff of less than 45 years of age at onset (Kelley, Boeve, and Josephs, 2008). Dementia beginning between 40 and 65 is most often due to cerebrovascular disease, AD, traumatic brain injury, or FTLD (Mendez, 2006), but this is not the case in younger adults, many of whom have reversible etiologies (Rossor et el., 2010). The early onset of AD was made famous by Alzheimer's report of Auguste Deter, who presented in her early 50s, and genetic AD can develop as young as age 24 (Filley et al., 2007), but below age 40 the neurodegenerative diseases make up a minority of dementia cases (Kelley, Boeve, and Josephs, 2008).

Neurologists often identify white matter disorders when evaluating dementia with onset in adolescence or young adulthood, and indeed leukodystrophies, for example, can present well beyond infancy and childhood (Gray et al., 2000). Other white matter disorders can also be encountered. In a study of 235 cases of dementia with onset between age 17 and 45, neurodegenerative disease accounted for 31%, while 26% of cases were due to a variety of white matter disorders; multiple sclerosis accounted for 11%, and the remainder resulted from leukodystrophies, human immunodeficiency virus infection, progressive multifocal leukoencephalopathy, alcohol, radiation, cerebral autosomal-dominant arteriopathy with subcortical infarcts and leukoencephalopathy (CADASIL), normal pressure hydrocephalus, and unspecified leukoencephalopathy (Kelley, Boeve, and Josephs, 2008). MRI is helpful in detecting these disorders, and is a critical component of the diagnostic evaluation (Rossor et al., 2010).

Inclusion of white matter in considering the organization of cognition is also important with reference to psychiatric disease. It has long been known that the disabling mental illnesses of depression, bipolar disorder, and schizophrenia may feature cognitive impairment or dementia at some point in the course, and this aspect of the disease, as well as others, may find its explanation in dysfunction of the white matter (Bartzokis, 2005; Walterfang et al., 2005; Filley, 2005, 2011; Haroutunian et al., 2014; Mighdoll et al., 2015). Common neuropsychiatric problems in younger people with major cognitive dimensions include autism, attention-deficit/hyperactivity disorder, developmental dyslexia, and addiction, all of which may also find an explanation in white matter derangement (Bartzokis, 2005). Notable in this context, for example, are recent data from dyslexia research documenting left hemisphere white matter abnormalities (Peterson and Pennington, 2012). As the etiopathogenesis of these often disabling diseases has thus far proven elusive, a query of white matter may be revealing in view of the as yet unfulfilled promise of examining gray matter dysfunction as fundamental. Instead of focusing on cortical function as the assumed locus of cognitive disturbance, investigating the involvement of connectivity within distributed neural networks may be more useful.

With these considerations in mind, a detailed account of WMD can be plausibly assembled. While variable degrees of overlap undoubtedly exist between cortical dementia, subcortical dementia, mixed dementia, and WMD, to some extent blurring distinctions, this structurally based classification assists in understanding the diagnosis, etiopathogenesis, and treatment of dementia in all its forms. WMD will first be considered in the next chapter by reviewing many disorders in a variety of neuropathological categories that can generate sufficient white matter damage to produce dementia. Perusal of current neurologic literature quickly discloses the breadth and depth of the investigations now being conducted. A particularly vigorous research area is cerebrovascular disease, and the phenomenon of leukoaraiosis has stimulated much study as a cause of cognitive dysfunction (Inzitari et al., 2009; Debette and Markus, 2010), but all the areas to be reviewed support the notion of WMD.

Then, in the chapters that follow, the syndrome and its many implications will be discussed in detail based on the common features that emerge from study of these disorders. The proposed precursor syndrome of mild cognitive dysfunction will be introduced as a means of conceptualizing the early stages of white matter disease (Kozora and Filley, 2011), and its utility as a clinical and research construct will be considered. Particularly intriguing aspects of the participation of white matter in dementia will also be considered in the context of AD (Bartzokis, 2011) and the problem of chronic traumatic encephalopathy (McKee et al., 2013).

The process of integrative review

At this point, a discussion is in order regarding what is involved in the actual conduct of the scholarly work to be presented herein. Analogous to the Methods section of a research article, a description of the process by which the content of this book was developed will foster a deeper understanding of the main points to be made. To organize this discussion, the concept of integrative review is central.

As a first point, it is crucial to emphasize that this book is essentially a large-scale descriptive study (Grimes and Schulz, 2002). Descriptive studies occupy a valuable and secure position in science, and they are central not only to medicine but also to esteemed disciplines such as astronomy, archaeology, and paleontology (Casadevall and Fang, 2008). Indeed, the work of Charles Darwin, universally acclaimed in biology, was founded on careful description of natural phenomena. Descriptive studies play a crucial role in the progress of science, particularly in the first explorations of observations enabled by new technologies (Casadevall and Fang, 2008), which in the case of white matter neurobiology was clearly the advent of MRI. Whereas the mechanisms by which white matter dysfunction and damage disrupt cognition vary according to which particular disorder is involved, the main objective of this book is the gathering together of descriptive information that will enable the consideration of white matter–behavior relationships with particular attention to dementia. Major opportunities afforded by descriptive studies of this kind include trend analysis, health care planning, and hypothesis generation (Grimes and Schulz, 2002); these objectives are familiar from epidemiology but also apply to the subject matter of this book. As the data supporting the information that follows are derived from descriptive studies, this book offers a large-scale review of a wide variety of primary investigations in many subspecialties of neurology and related fields. A previous work of this kind used the same approach to consider the behavioral neurology of white matter as a broader topic (Filley, 2012). However, as dementia associated with white matter involvement is a novel area of neurology and cognitive neuroscience with its own unique implications, the descriptive review presented here can be seen as a monograph representing the "first scientific toe in the water" (Grimes and Schulz, 2002) addressing this topic.

Like any medical or scientific review, this one is based entirely on prior published information, and offers no new empirical data. It is, therefore, a work of what has recently been termed "knowledge synthesis" (Whittemore et al., 2014). This broad category of scholarship implies that a summary of pertinent studies is provided to synthesize knowledge in a manner that cannot be gleaned from a single study or a limited number of studies. For medical and scientific accounts, two general categories of knowledge synthesis are recognized: quantitative and qualitative. A quantitative review is so named because it includes the statistical combination of the results of primary studies (Cook, Mulrow, and Haynes, 1997), and the best-known method of quantitative review is the popular meta-analysis (Bangert-Drowns, 1995; Whittemore et al., 2014). In contrast, a qualitative review, also known as a narrative review, considers relevant information without statistical analysis, relying instead on careful comparison of data across fields where statistical comparison is not feasible (Bangert-Drowns, 1995). One type of qualitative review is the meta-synthesis, in which results from different but related empirical studies are combined qualitatively to generate a new and presumably higher conceptual understanding of a given phenomenon (Whittemore et al., 2014). A closely related form of knowledge synthesis is the integrative review (Whittemore et al., 2014), in which both empirical and theoretical literature are used to contribute to the synthesis. This book, with its consideration of empirical data within a larger conceptual framework of white matter neurobiology, can be envisioned as a large-scale integrative review.

As is true for any form of knowledge synthesis based on descriptive studies, integrative review has both advantages and drawbacks. A clear advantage is that the information to be reviewed is already available and readily accessible (Grimes and Schulz, 2002). Another is that access to prior published information typically involves no ethical restrictions. Integrative review also offers the only mechanism whereby heterogeneous literatures can be unified (Whittemore et al., 2014), counteracting the understandable tendency for specialty information to be isolated from broader consideration. A drawback is the possibility of bias in the selection of articles to be reviewed, which is particularly an issue without the rigor of meta-analysis (Cook et al., 1997). Another potential problem is "overstepping the data," meaning the unwarranted attribution of cause and effect, an issue captured by the phrase *post hoc, ergo propter hoc* ("after which, therefore because of which"), a common logical fallacy by which an observation is prematurely linked to a subsequent event (Grimes and Schulz, 2002).

As a method intended for the study of white matter and dementia, however, integrative review offers the most productive approach to establishing an initial overview and suggestions for further study. As a complement to the reductionism of many scientific disciplines such as molecular biology, this approach is also allied with holism, a concept recently recast in terms of systems biology (Fang and Casadevall, 2011). Indeed, much of contemporary neuroscience is preoccupied with the organization of neural systems subserving cognition, including the vast collection of brain connections recently dubbed the connectome. Given the widely diverse primary literature devoted to white matter disorders across many areas of neurology and medicine, and the necessity to integrate both empirical and theoretical accounts in reaching a new synthesis, integrative review in fact seems to be the *only* suitable method for the task ahead. This process is closely allied with the exploitation of what has been termed "big data" in the study of dementia – meaning the use of epidemiology and biostatistics to understand key risk factors – and the inclusion of much empirical information is critical (DeKosky, 2014).

Behavioral neurology, like all of medicine, is practiced and studied as an art as much as a science, and a careful iterative review based on a broad knowledge of many fields need not stand behind seemingly more rigorous methods such as meta-analysis (Bangert-Drowns, 1995). Statistical analysis and quantitative rigor surely have their place, but for some endeavors – particularly those making a first comprehensive foray into an area as little explored as white matter–cognition relationships – a broadly synthetic perspective is most useful. In this process, as in clinical medicine with all its inherent uncertainty and nuance, the objective and subjective, the quantitative and qualitative, will be integrated into a synthetic account aimed to discover a first approximation of the truth and inspire further study. As Albert Einstein is reputed to have commented: "Not everything that can be counted counts, and not everything that counts can be counted."

References

Albert ML. Subcortical dementia. In: Katzman R, Terry RD, Bick KL, eds. *Alzheimer's disease: senile dementia and related disorders*. New York: Raven Press, 1978: 173–180.

Albert ML. Subcortical dementia: historical review and personal view. Neurocase 2005; 11: 243–245.

Appelman AP, Exalto LG, van der Graaf Y, et al. White matter lesions and brain atrophy: more than shared risk factors? A systematic review. Cerebrovasc Dis. 2009; 28: 227–242.

Bangert-Drowns RL. Misunderstanding meta-analysis. Eval Health Prof 1995; 18: 304–314.

Bartzokis G. Brain myelination in prevalent neuropsychiatric developmental disorders: primary and comorbid addiction. Adolesc Psychiatry 2005; 29: 55–96.

Bartzokis G. Alzheimer's disease as homeostatic responses to age-related myelin breakdown. Neurobiol Aging 2011; 32: 1341–1371.

Bonelli RM, Cummings JL. Frontal-subcortical dementias. Neurologist 2008; 14: 100–107.

Casadevall A, Fang FC. Descriptive science. Infect Immun 2008; 76: 3835–3836.

Charcot JM. *Lectures on diseases of the nervous system delivered at La Salpêtrière*. London: New Sydenham Society, 1877.

Cook DJ, Mulrow CD, Haynes RB. Systematic reviews: synthesis of best evidence for clinical decisions. Ann Intern Med 1997; 126: 376–380.

Cummings JL, Benson DF. *Dementia: a clinical approach*. Boston: Butterworths, 1983.

Cummings JL, Benson DF. Subcortical dementia: review of an emerging concept. Arch Neurol 1984; 41: 874–879.

Debette S, Markus HS. The clinical importance of white matter hyperintensities on brain magnetic resonance imaging: systematic review and meta-analysis. BMJ 2010; 341: c3666.

DeKosky ST. The role of big data in understanding late-life cognitive decline. JAMA Neurology 2014; 71: 1476–1478.

Fang FC, Casadevall A. Reductionistic and holistic science. Infect Immun 2011; 79: 1401–1404.

Fields RD. White matter in learning, cognition and psychiatric disorders. Trends Neurosci 2008; 31: 361–370.

Fields RD. Neuroscience. Myelin – more than insulation. Science 2014; 344: 264–266.

Filley CM. Neurobehavioral aspects of cerebral white matter disorders. Psychiatr Clin North Am 2005; 28: 685–700.

Filley CM. White matter: beyond focal disconnection. Neurol Clin 2011; 29: 81–97.

Filley CM. *The behavioral neurology of white matter*. 2nd ed. New York: Oxford University Press, 2012.

Filley CM, Rollins YD, Anderson CA, et al. The genetics of very early onset Alzheimer's Disease. Cogn Behav Neurol 2007; 20: 149–156.

Gray RG, Preece MA, Green SH, et al. Inborn errors of metabolism as a cause of neurological disease in adults: an approach to investigation. J Neurol Neurosurg Psychiatry 2000; 69: 5–12.

Grimes DA, Schulz KF. Descriptive studies: what they can and cannot do. Lancet 2002; 359: 145–149.

Haroutunian V, Katsel P, Roussos P, et al. Myelination, oligodendrocytes, and serious mental illness. Glia 2014; 62: 1856–1877.

Inatomi Y, Yonehara T, Hashimoto Y, et al. Correlation between ventricular enlargement and white matter changes. J Neurol Sci 2008; 269: 12–17.

Inzitari D, Pracucci G, Poggesi A, et al. Changes in white matter as determinant of global functional decline in older independent outpatients: three year follow-up of LADIS (leukoaraiosis and disability) study cohort. BMJ 2009; 339: b2477.

Kelley BJ, Boeve BF, Josephs KA. Young-onset dementia: demographic and etiologic characteristics of 235 patients. Arch Neurol 2008; 65: 1502–1508.

Kozora E, Filley CM. Cognitive dysfunction and white matter abnormalities in systemic lupus erythematosus. J Int Neuropsychol Soc 2011; 22: 1–8.

Kuruppu DK, Matthews BR. Young-onset dementia. Semin Neurol 2013; 33: 365–385.

Lafosse JM, Corboy JR, Leehey MA, et al. MS vs. HD: Can white matter and subcortical gray matter pathology be distinguished neuropsychologically? J Clin Exp Neuropsychol 2007; 29: 142–154.

McKee AC, Stein TD, Nowinski CJ, et al. The spectrum of disease in chronic traumatic encephalopathy. Brain 2013; 136: 43–64.

Mendez MF. The accurate diagnosis of early-onset dementia. Int J Psychiatry Med 2006; 36: 401–412.

Mighdoll MI, Tao R, Kleinman JE, Hyde TM. Myelin, myelin-related disorders, and psychosis. Schizophr Res 2015; 161: 85–93.

Parvizi J. Corticocentric myopia: old bias in new cognitive sciences. Trends Cogn Sci 2009; 13: 354–359.

Peterson RL, Pennington BF. Developmental dyslexia. Lancet 2012; 379: 1997–2007.

Rossor MN, Fox NC, Mummery CJ, et al. The diagnosis of young-onset dementia. Lancet Neurol 2010; 9: 793–806.

Thomas MS, Knowland VC, Karmiloff-Smith A. Mechanisms of developmental regression in autism and the broader phenotype: a neural network modeling approach. Psychol Rev 2011; 118: 637–654.

Tuladhar AM, Reid AT, Shumskaya E, et al. Relationship between white matter hyperintensities, cortical thickness, and cognition. Stroke 2015; 46: 425–432.

Walterfang M, Wood SJ, Velakoulis D, et al. Diseases of white matter and schizophrenia-like psychosis. Aust N Z J Psychiatry 2005; 39: 746–756.

Whittemore R, Chao A, Jang M, et al. Methods for knowledge synthesis: an overview. Heart Lung 2014; 43: 453–461.

Chapter 6

White matter disorders

The prominence of white matter as a structural component of the brain suggests that it is a frequent target of neuropathology, and indeed this is the case. A wide range of disorders can involve the white matter, producing a plethora of elemental neurologic deficits and neurobehavioral manifestations. White matter dementia (WMD) can be caused by disorders within ten broad categories of neuropathology, including a broad array of conditions that feature highly differing neuropathological characteristics. The notable exception to this list is neurodegenerative disease, a category generally referring to the progressive loss of neurons in gray matter, but, as will be considered later in this book, intriguing data are beginning to implicate white matter in this category as well. Well over 100 diseases, intoxications, and injuries can lead to WMD, a list that is constantly expanding as magnetic resonance imaging (MRI) discloses new entities and improves the understanding of older ones (Filley, 2012). These disorders may occur at any age and in a wide variety of medical settings, highlighting the broad relevance of the WMD concept. A detailed discussion of all these entities can be found elsewhere (Filley, 2012), and it is not our purpose here to offer an exhaustive compendium. Rather, this chapter will be confined to the major causes of dementia within each of the ten categories that most securely make the case for WMD. This account will highlight the remarkable similarity of the dementia syndrome despite the wide diversity of neuropathology that is responsible.

Vascular diseases

Vascular disease of the brain is one of the most important areas of clinical medicine, and stroke remains a major concern of neurologists, both as a common source of disability from physical and neurobehavioral dysfunction, and as a leading cause of death in the United States. One of the most feared consequences of stroke is vascular dementia, a syndrome perhaps best known for its imprecise definition. Some clarification of the idea of vascular dementia can be offered, however, in light of recent findings on the origin and significance of white matter changes often seen on the neuroimaging scans of older individuals. Among the many forms of cerebrovascular disease that prominently involve the white matter, reflecting a wide range of neuropathology (Box 6.1), the entities Binswanger's Disease (BD) and its close relative leukoaraiosis (LA) merit special attention with respect to dementia.

Focal cerebral infarctions are well understood to produce a wide range of neurologic deficits that can affect both sensorimotor and neurobehavioral function. As greater sophistication has come to be applied to the neurobehavioral sequelae of stroke and related pathology, considerable confusion has been generated about the classification of patients with cerebrovascular disease and cognitive impairment or dementia. Yet despite much effort, no widely accepted agreement has been reached on either clinical or neuropathological diagnostic criteria for vascular dementia. This lack of consensus invites a novel approach based on the location of neuropathology, and white matter is an appropriate site for the investigation of how vascular disease interferes with normal cognition.

The scattered, focal white matter changes often noted on computed tomography (CT) and MRI scans of older people, for which the term leukoaraiosis (LA) was introduced (Hachinski, Potter, and Merskey, 1987), have focused much interest on the dementia first described in the nineteenth century known as BD (Babikian and Ropper, 1987; Caplan, 1995). BD is a dementia syndrome putatively attributed to widespread white matter infarction and ischemia, but the disease has been controversial because uncertainties in the original case reports have led to concerns about whether BD merits recognition as a distinct disease (Hachinski, 1991). Still, BD has persisted as a neuropathological,

BOX 6.1 Vascular diseases of white matter

- Binswanger's Disease
- Leukoaraiosis
- Cerebral amyloid angiopathy
- White matter disease of prematurity
- Migraine

and sometimes clinical, diagnosis that can arguably be considered one of the most frequent causes of vascular dementia.

With the application of modern neuroimaging, the relationship of LA to BD has become highly relevant. Although it has become clear that the two phenomena are not synonymous, LA has come to be appreciated as a vascular disorder (Pantoni and Garcia, 1997), and a continuum of severity likely exists from the mild changes of LA to the more pervasive pathology of BD (Román, 1996; Libon et al., 2004; Debette and Markus, 2010). In part because of continuing uneasiness associated with the use of BD, the more inclusive term subcortical ischemic vascular dementia (SIVD) has been introduced as a way to include both BD and a close clinical-pathological relative called the lacunar state (Román et al., 2002). Whatever terminology is used, however, considerable evidence favors the existence of a variety of vascular dementias characterized primarily by white matter infarction and ischemic demyelination (Román et al., 1993; Román et al., 2002). This entity will now be considered in some detail, with a discussion of LA serving as an appropriate point of departure.

Leukoaraiosis

The advent of modern neuroimaging has had an enormous impact on the study of vascular white matter disease (Román, 1996; Jones et al., 1999). The era began with clinicians often encountering unexpected white matter changes on neuroimaging scans of older persons, which were somewhat tentatively ascribed to ischemia. Figure 6.1 is an axial MRI scan from an older person depicting a typical example of LA. As these changes were found to be common in older people with apparently intact cognitive and emotional function, they were often regarded as no more than a feature of normal aging. Even when the neuroimaging findings were extensive, reluctance to diagnose a specific disorder persisted. In contrast, however, some began

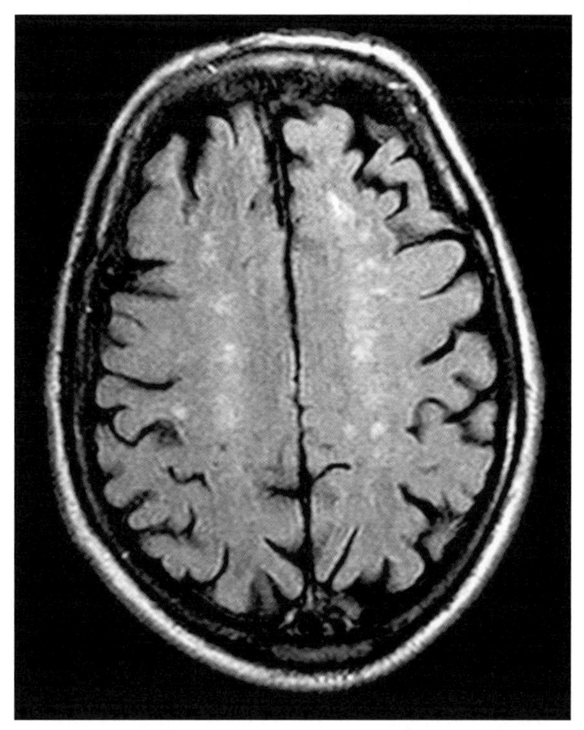

Figure 6.1 Axial fluid-attenuated inversion recovery (FLAIR) MRI scan of an older person with leukoaraiosis. Patchy white matter hyperintensties are scattered throughout the white matter.

to interpret these changes as a problem of epidemic proportions in the elderly mandating a vigorous effort by the medical community (van Gijn, 1998). It was clear that more sophisticated understanding was needed.

The concept of LA was introduced by Hachinski and colleagues to designate the white matter "rarefaction" frequently seen on CT and especially MRI scans of older individuals with or without symptoms and signs of cerebral impairment (Hachinski, Potter, and Merskey, 1987). These changes appear as low-density white matter areas on CT and white matter hyperintensities on MRI, and the term "unidentified bright objects" was popular for several years in reference to the MRI changes (Román, 1996). The intent of the term LA was to provide a purely descriptive word for brain white matter abnormalities (Hachinski, Potter, and Merskey, 1987), which at that time were not well understood in terms of pathogenesis and clinical correlates. The caution embodied by the use of the term was indeed appropriate, as some quickly made the premature assumption that the changes of LA represented BD (Kinkel et al., 1985). With further work, however, both the origin and the significance of LA began to be understood, and the emerging information directly indicated a relationship to vascular compromise and BD.

As for pathogenesis, support for the ischemic origin of LA steadily accumulated (Pantoni and Garcia, 1997; Pantoni, Poggesi, and Inzitari, 2007; O'Sullivan, 2008). Neuropathological studies consistently found arteriosclerotic changes within areas of LA (Leifer, Buonanno, and Richardson, 1990; Fazekas et al., 1993). The small penetrating arterioles supplying the white matter were noted to manifest narrowing of the lumen secondary to the accumulation of hyaline material, and the sparing of subcortical U fibers further argued for selective small vessel involvement (Pantoni and Garcia, 1997). Gradually a consensus grew that LA reflects recurrent transient hypotension leading to incomplete infarction that damages the oligodendrocytes, myelin, and axons of cerebral white matter (Pantoni and Garcia, 1997; Román et al., 2002; O'Sullivan, 2008). Cerebral blood flow studies have supported this proposed pathogenesis by showing reduced white matter perfusion in areas of LA while gray matter is normally perfused (Markus et al., 2000). Studies of clinical populations found strong correlations between LA and cerebrovascular risk factors such as hypertension, diabetes mellitus, cardiovascular disease, and past history of stroke (Gerard and Weisberg, 1986; Inzitari et al., 1987) and, more recently, smoking (Fukuda and Kitani, 1996), obesity (Jagust et al., 2005), and the metabolic syndrome (Park et al., 2007). As helpful as these advances have proven, however, it must be remembered that LA remains a neuroradiological finding that may reflect physiologic changes such as dilation of perivascular Virchow-Robin spaces (*état criblé*) or periventricular caps and bands – all of which are benign – or other neuropathology such as the demyelinative plaques of multiple sclerosis (MS) (Merino and Hachinski, 2000; Barkhof and Scheltens, 2002).

As the ischemic origin of LA has been amply documented, and it has become clear that environmental factors play an important role in pathogenesis, a genetic contribution to LA has also been observed. A recent large European genome-wide association study (GWAS) involving more than 9,000 subjects identified a novel locus on chromosome 17 as associated with LA (Fornage et al., 2011). This discovery helps explain the considerable heritability of LA, reported as ranging from 55% to 80% (Fornage et al., 2011). As the first substantial evidence of a genetic influence on LA, these findings invite further investigation of what is becoming a complex pathogenesis. In this light, it is noteworthy that some evidence also supports an association of the apolipoprotein E ε4 allele with a higher burden of LA (Godin et al., 2009). Data now appearing therefore suggest that nature and nurture both contribute to the origin of LA.

The specific cerebral location of LA has attracted some attention, and evidence exists that the pathogenesis and sequelae of LA may differ depending on where it is found. From neuropathological studies of older people with incidental white matter hyperintensities, Fazekas and colleagues (1993) proposed that while subcortical lesions were ischemic, periventricular lesions were related to altered fluid dynamics producing white matter edema and subsequent demyelination. The functional consequences of lesions in these locations may differ as well, with subcortical lesions associated with cognitive dysfunction (Soumaré et al., 2009), and periventricular lesions associated with gait disorder (Blahak et al., 2009). Others have pointed out, however, that subcortical and periventricular lesions are highly correlated with each other, and thus a categorical distinction between them may be arbitrary; in this light, the clinical implications of subcortical versus periventricular lesions remain tentative (DeCarli et al., 2005).

The neurobehavioral significance of LA has come to be understood from many studies that have steadily yielded an ever more coherent account. Early investigations using low-field-strength MRI magnets and standard neuropsychological measures found no correlation of LA with cognitive dysfunction, suggesting that improved imaging and more specific cognitive measures might prove more useful (Rao et al., 1989c; Filley et al., 1989a). Subsequent research found that such correlations could indeed be detected, and the primary cognitive domains affected in LA were attention and cognitive speed (Junqué et al., 1990; van Swieten et al., 1991; Schmidt et al., 1993; Ylikoski et al., 1993). Large-scale MRI studies of older individuals began to appear, and correlations continued to be found between the severity of LA and cognitive dysfunction (Longstreth et al., 1996; de Groot et al., 2000; Au et al., 2006; Inzitari et al., 2007; Murray et al., 2010). More recently, longitudional study has documented that the advance of LA produces more severe cognitive dysfunction (Smith et al., 2015). With these impressive data sets, a consistent pattern has emerged of slowed processing speed and executive dysfunction, deficits found regardless of white matter lesion location, an observation that may be explained by the substantial convergence of numerous association tracts on the frontal lobes (Tullberg et al., 2004). To sum up a large body of work, comprehensive reviews have concluded that LA has been convincingly shown to have effects on cognition, with major effects on processing speed and executive function (O'Sullivan, 2008; Debette and Markus, 2010).

Most recently, newer neuroimaging techniques now in use have disclosed abnormalities in the normal-appearing white matter (NAWM) of people with LA. Perhaps not surprisingly, much of the brain in LA is affected beyond the extent of the obvious lesions seen on conventional MRI. Magnetic resonance spectroscopy (MRS) was found to reveal neurometabolite changes in the NAWM of individuals with LA consistent with myelin damage (Firbank, Minett, and O'Brien, 2003; Charlton et al., 2006). Diffusion tensor imaging (DTI) has been still more informative, with studies showing microstructural white matter abnormalities to correlate with impaired global cognition, processing speed, attention, working memory, and executive function (Jones et al., 1999; Charlton et al., 2006; Vernooij et al., 2009; van Norden et al., 2012). DTI changes have also been suggested to be more sensitive to longitudinal cognitive decline than the advance of LA on MRI (Charlton et al., 2010).

These studies on the NAWM in LA inform previous work on the idea of a threshold effect for cognitive decline. Boone and colleagues (1992) reported that a threshold of 10 cm^2 of affected white matter on MRI was required before cognitive dysfunction could be detected. A 1993 consensus statement suggested that cognitive impairment occurred when LA involved 25% of the cerebral white matter (Román et al., 1993). Libon and colleagues (2008) extended this work by showing that only severe LA was associated with executive dysfunction. These studies recall similar observations in other white matter disorders that a certain threshold of disease burden is required before cognitive impairment occurs (Filley, 2012). The notion of a threshold effect is indeed plausible, but it is clear that LA seen on conventional MRI does not represent the entirety of ischemic neuropathology within the cerebral white matter. The NAWM data introduce considerably more complexity into this issue since the true extent of disease may be unclear. Moreover, as will be discussed, the impact of LA can also be mitigated by cognitive reserve, further confounding the interpretation of this finding.

It has also become clear that additional neurologic morbidity and mortality are associated with LA. Briley and colleagues (2000) found that LA predicts morbidity and mortality independent of previous neurologic deficits. An early MRI study found a significant association of LA with gait disorder (Longstreth et al., 1996), and longitudinal MRI has clearly documented progressive slowing of gait with the advance of LA (Smith et al., 2015). Smith (2010) summarized evidence that LA is important for determining stroke outcome as well as stroke incidence. Recent findings have also suggested that LA may increase the risk of anticoagulant-related hemorrhage in patients with atrial fibrillation or other conditions requiring anticoagulation (O'Sullivan, 2008). In view of the wide distribution of cerebral white matter, and the probability of multifocal white matter involvement interfering with the operations of multiple distributed neural networks, it should not be surprising that LA of sufficient magnitude can disrupt elemental as well as higher neurologic functions and compromise other important determinants of brain health.

Another intriguing aspect of the work on LA is that education appears to protect against the cognitive dysfunction produced by white matter lesions. A population-based study showed that an association between LA and cognitive dysfunction was present in individuals with lower education but not in more educated people (Dufouil, Alpérovitch, and Tzourio, 2003). These findings are similar to recent observations in other white matter disorders (Filley, 2012), and support the hypothesis that cognitive reserve conferred by education, which is plausibly mediated by increased cortical synaptic density, can mitigate the detrimental cognitive consequences of LA (Dufouil, Alpérovitch, and Tzouri, 2003).

The accumulated evidence now justifies the statement that LA is a largely ischemic phenomenon that predicts an increased risk of cognitive dysfunction, dementia, gait disorder, stroke, and mortality (Debette and Markus, 2010; Smith et al., 2015). The pattern of cognitive dysfunction in LA most typically implicates processing speed and executive function (O'Sullivan, 2008; Debette and Markus, 2010). These conclusions, combined with neuroradiological and neuropathological commonalities, lend support to the contention that LA lies on the same clinical-pathological spectrum as BD (Filley et al., 1988; van Swieten et al., 1991; Román, 1996; Libon et al., 2004; Debette and Markus, 2010). One important implication of this connection is that vigorous treatment of LA by modification of many well-recognized cerebrovascular risk factors may significantly impact the onset and manifestations of age-related cognitive decline. This and other implications of the relationship of LA to BD will now be taken up.

Binswanger's Disease

In 1894, the Swiss neuropathologist Otto Binswanger sparked what became more than a century of controversy on white matter disease and dementia. In a three-part article on the differential diagnosis of general paresis of the insane, a common dementing disease of that time, Binswanger presented gross neuropathology from eight patients who had progressive dementia associated with marked white matter atrophy. The cortex was spared, but there was prominent atherosclerosis; he called this disease "encephalitis subcorticalis chronica progressiva" and related it to insufficient blood supply of the cerebral white matter (Blass, Hoyer, and Nitsch, 1991). Binswanger thus offered the seminal proposal that ischemic damage to white matter alone could lead to progressive cognitive decline.

Eight years later, Alois Alzheimer presented additional cases similar to those of Binswanger but with histologic observations supporting the idea that arteriosclerotic white matter disease could produce dementia (Alzheimer, 1902). It was in fact Alzheimer who linked the name Binswanger with this disorder (Román, 1987), thus establishing BD in the medical literature. Other names appeared, however, as time progressed. In 1962, Olszewski translated the articles of Binswanger and Alzheimer and presented two new cases emphasizing the importance of lacunar infarction, offering the alternative name "subcortical arteriosclerotic encephalopathy" (Olszewski, 1962). Today, many avoid the use of BD and prefer the more generic subcortical ischemic vascular dementia (SIVD) as a category of vascular dementia that includes both BD and the lacunar state (*état lacunaire*) of Pierre Marie (Román et al., 2002).

BD has been questioned as a clinical-pathological entity because Binswanger may not have been the first to describe the disorder, and because he provided no microscopic data in his reports to complement the gross neuropathologic findings (Hachinski, 1991). Olszewski (1962) even speculated that Binswanger's cases could have had neurosyphilis. However, several authoritative reviews have endorsed the eponymic terminology (Babikian and Ropper, 1987; Fisher, 1989; Bennett et al., 1990; Caplan, 1995; Hurley et al., 2000; Román et al., 2002; Caplan and Gomes, 2010; Huisa and Rosenberg, 2014), and BD persists as a clinical entity in major neurology textbooks (Ropper, Samuels, and Klein, 2014). In this book, while the controversy about this disease will be acknowledged, the term BD will be used because Binswanger deserves credit for associating diffuse ischemic white matter disease with progressive dementia (O'Sullivan, 2008), and because the specific impact of BD on white matter renders the term most appropriate for our purposes.

BD can be considered a form of vascular dementia characterized by prominent involvement of the cerebral white matter. Its prevalence is not known because no definitive diagnostic test is available during life; although white matter lesions on neuroimaging scans of older people are suggestive, such lesions alone are insufficient for the diagnosis because they can be seen in many other diseases and in normal aging. Moreover, many neurologists are influenced by their corticocentric bias to make the diagnosis of coexisting Alzheimer's Disease (AD) in patients with white matter lesions suggestive of BD. Despite these issues, BD may nevertheless be common. Nearly all older people have one or more ischemic white matter lesions on MRI (Román et al., 2002), and whereas most do not have BD, some autopsy studies have found that up to 35% of older dementia patients may have BD lesions at postmortem examination (Santamaria Ortiz and Knight, 1994). Evidence for BD existing as a dementia distinct from AD comes from study of patients with SIVD and severe white matter disease who also had Pittsburgh compound B (PiB) imaging with positron emission tomography to assess the burden of amyloid: More than two-thirds of these patients did not have cortical PiB retention (Lee et al., 2011), suggesting that BD may be more common than often thought. More satisfactory answers to the question of BD prevalence must await further study.

Clinically, BD is strongly associated with hypertension and other cerebrovascular risk factors, and

Table 6.1 Three sets of clinical and imaging criteria for the ante-mortem diagnosis of Binswanger's Disease

	Bennett et al. (1990)	Caplan (1995)	Huisa and Rosenberg (2014)
Clinical	Dementia on clinical examination and by neuropsychology Any two of the following: A vascular risk factor or evidence of systemic vascular disease Focal cerebrovascular disease Subcortical cerebral dysfunction (parkinsonian, magnetic, or senile gait; rigidity; *gegenhalten*; incontinence related to a spastic bladder)	Usual onset 55–75 years of age Men = women Acute strokes, often lacunar infarcts Subacute onset of focal signs Seizures during subacute progression Stepwise progression of motor, cognitive, and behavioral deficits Periods of stabilization, plateaus, and even improvement Pyramidal signs Extrapyramidal signs Abnormal gait Pseudobulbar signs Apathy, inertia, disinterest, abulia Poor judgment, lack of insight, altered affective responses Variable deficits in memory, language, and visuospatial function	Cognitive impairment Pyramidal signs Extrapyramidal signs Hypertension Ataxia, balance disturbance, falls Progressive symptoms
Imaging	Bilateral LA on CT, or Bilateral, multiple, or diffuse subcortical T2 lesions on MRI	Patchy, irregular PV WM attenuation Irregular focal PV and subcortical WM lesions Lesions in corona radiata and centrum semiovale, often large and confluent Multiple lacunar infarcts Hydrocephalus	WM hyperintensities Brain atrophy, mild to moderate Lacunar infarcts Microbleeds Enlarged perivascular spaces Intracranial atherosclerosis High pulsatility index by transcranial Doppler

LA – leukoaraiosis, CT- computed tomography, PV– periventricular, WM – white matter, MRI – magnetic resonance imaging

presents in middle to late life as progressive neurologic and neurobehavioral dysfunction, sometimes, but not always, following a stepwise course (Babikian and Ropper, 1987; Fisher, 1989; Bennett et al., 1990; Caplan, 1995; Caplan and Gomes, 2010; Huisa and Rosenberg, 2014). Table 6.1 displays three approaches to the clinical diagnosis of BD. Neurologic features include focal corticospinal dysfunction, extrapyramidal signs, acute lacunar syndromes, gait disorder, and pseudobulbar affect. A useful sign of BD is diffuse hyperreflexia, a finding not typically present in AD patients with a comparable degree of dementia. Neurobehavioral manifestations include apathy, inertia, abulia, memory impairment, visuospatial dysfunction, depression, poor judgment, loss of insight, and relatively preserved language. The diagnosis may be difficult in early stages, when all of these features may be less apparent. Psychiatric dysfunction may develop before cognitive deterioration and neurologic signs (Lawrence and Hillam, 1995), a sequence typical of many other white matter disorders (Filley, 2012). Apathy and inertia can be mistaken for the cognitive slowing that is commonly seen in normal aging. Together with CT or MRI evidence of white matter vascular disease (Figure 6.2), however, BD can usually be diagnosed in life with considerable confidence (Bennett et al., 1990; Caplan, 1995; Huisa and Rosenberg, 2014). Whereas some clinicians hesitate to make this diagnosis because of the absence of accepted diagnostic criteria, and select instead SIVD or vascular dementia, inspection of Table 6.1 discloses that various sets of clinical and imaging criteria for BD actually have much in common.

Neuropathological observations constitute the basis for understanding the origin of dementia in BD. Hypertension is the most powerful risk factor,

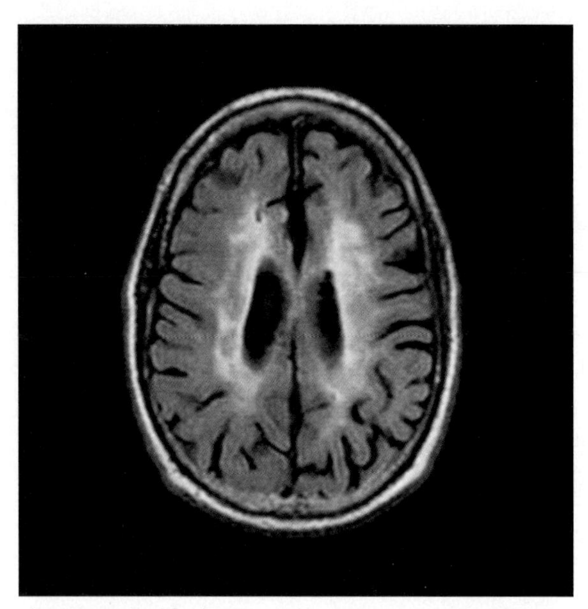

Figure 6.2 Axial fluid-attenuated inversion recovery (FLAIR) MRI scan of a patient with Binswanger's Disease. Extensive periventricular hyperintensity is present.

and the long penetrating arterioles of the deep cerebral white matter are invariably damaged by thickening and hyalinization of the vessel walls (Román et al., 2002). This arteriosclerosis in turn leads either to BD, in which hypoperfusion produces incomplete infarction of the white matter, or to the lacunar state, with occlusion of small vessels and completed infarcts leaving encephalomalacia (Román et al., 2002). The brain stem may be affected in BD (Pullicino et al., 1995), but the cortex is spared from the neuropathological process, and the subcortical gray matter is less affected than the white matter (Caplan, 1995; Caplan and Gomes, 2010). It has been shown in both human studies (Brown and Thore, 2011) and nonhuman animal studies (Pantoni, Garcia, and Gutierrez, 1996) that a high vulnerability of cerebral white matter to ischemia exists because of compromised perfusion from long penetrating arterioles superiorly and lenticulostriate arteries inferiorly. Microscopic findings early in the course of BD may be limited to myelin pallor, but in advanced cases there is loss of oligodendrocytes, myelin, and axons along with astrocytic gliosis; the subcortical U fibers are typically spared in BD, as they are in LA (Román et al., 2002). To summarize, BD can be seen to develop as complete and incomplete white matter infarctions accumulate (Román et al., 2002), sufficient to cause dementia from selective white matter injury and not because of comorbid neuropathology from AD (Lee et al., 2011).

Not surprisingly, the neuroradiology of BD is controversial because of unresolved questions about the nosologic status and diagnosis of the disease. CT initially provided some idea of lesion burden, and the use of MRI improved the identification of white matter changes to such an extent that many were led to conclude that these lesions establish the presence of BD (Kinkel et al., 1985). However, this view was soon abandoned as it was realized that white matter changes are not always associated with dementia. Currently, BD is a diagnosis suggested, but not confirmed, by the MRI white matter findings, and clinical correlation is essential. The ultimate decision about whether an older demented patient has BD can be made only at autopsy, and MRI is most useful in showing the type, location, and extent of white matter disease in vivo.

Recent advances in neuroimaging have led to more detailed studies designed to evaluate microvascular alterations within the white matter. As in LA, investigation has led to the recognition that the NAWM may not be normal in BD. MRS has documented microstructural changes in the NAWM of patients with vascular dementia (Jones and Waldman, 2004). Similarly, magnetization transfer imaging (MTI) of vascular dementia patients has shown reduced magnetization transfer ratio (MTR) most prominent within periventicular white matter lesions (Tanabe et al., 1999), and other investigators correlated decreased MTR with cognitive dysfunction in BD (Hanyu et al., 1999). DTI has also shown its value, disclosing that NAWM abnormalities in SIVD are more sensitive to early cognitive impairment than conventional MRI findings (Xu et al., 2010).

The characterization of cognitive dysfunction in BD has been clarified to some extent. Babikian and Ropper (1987) called attention to memory loss, confusion, apathy, and changes in mood and behavior that were typically not accompanied by aphasia, apraxia, and movement disorder. Román (1987) classified BD as a subcortical dementia because of the frequency of personality change, forgetfulness, and confusion, and the relative rarity of aphasia, apraxia, and agnosia. Stuss and Cummings (1990) endorsed this opinion, adding that the neurobehavioral profile of BD reflects frontal-subcortical dysfunction. Several clinical studies have also supported this characterization, with detailed mental status or neuropsychological examinations in BD patients documenting impaired executive function, attention, memory, visuospatial ability, and abstract thinking in the presence of relatively spared language, praxis, and gnosis (Kinkel et al., 1985; Sacquena et al., 1989; Lee et al., 1989; Caplan, 1995; Libon et al., 2004; Huisa and Rosenberg, 2014). Evidence thus exists to show that cognitive and emotional dysfunction in BD can be attributed to subcortical or frontal-subcortical pathology.

The specific contribution of the white matter disease to the dementia of BD is more difficult to establish, reflecting the generalization that white matter is more challenging to examine. But evidence has steadily accumulated. In early studies, lowered IQ scores were correlated with white matter lesions on CT scans (Loizou, Kendall, and Marshall, 1981), and correlations of cognitive decline with ischemic white matter changes were shown using MRI (Révész et al., 1989). Later, neuropsychological evaluation of BD patients found poor concentration, apathy, and cognitive slowing consistent with frontal lobe disturbance and white matter dysfunction (Bogucki et al., 1991). An important contribution came from study of stroke patients who were found to have limiting neurobehavioral dysfunction even after a single white matter lacunar infarct (Van Zandvoort et al., 1998). The gradual accumulation of incomplete infarctions within white matter in BD was found to have similar effects on cognition, as shown in a quantitative MRI study of vascular dementia patients that found a strong correlation between white matter lesion area and dementia (Liu et al., 1992). Further study of MRI white matter lesions led to the view that these lesions exert prominent effects on frontal-subcortical circuits and produce executive dysfunction (Desmond, 2002). More recent evidence supports a deficit profile in BD patients characterized by cognitive slowing, executive dysfunction, and impaired memory retrieval with sparing of language (Román et al., 2002; Libon et al., 2004; Huisa and Rosenberg, 2014).

Despite these advances, BD remains a controversial entity that serves to underscore several unresolved questions in the relationship between vascular white matter disease and dementia. Whereas neurologists have long understood the potential for cortical and subcortical gray matter infarcts to impact cognitive function, acceptance of the view that ischemic white matter lesions alone can produce dementia has at times been grudging. Clinicians can rightly point out that solitary white matter lacunes and even numerous MRI white matter hyperintensities may have no apparent cognitive correlates. In addition, the possibility that gray matter disease – cerebrovascular, degenerative, or both – exists in patients with numerous white matter hyperintensities produces continued reluctance to ascribe cognitive dysfunction to white matter lesions. However, more detailed study of cerebrovascular disease has disclosed important white matter–behavior relationships, and BD can be seen as a useful, albeit imperfect, example of how white matter disease can produce dementia (Filley et al., 1988; Filley, 1998, 2012).

Toxic Leukoencephalopathy

Neurotoxicology, the study of the effects of toxic agents on the nervous system, encompasses a wide and diverse range of toxins. Some exert their effects on the peripheral nervous system (PNS), and others damage the central nervous system (CNS), including the brain white matter. Many physical and chemical toxins have a predilection for producing white matter damage, and this selective toxic effect led to the recognition of a division of neurotoxicology called toxic leukoencephalopathy (Filley and Kleinschmidt-DeMasters, 2001). MRI has been central to the discovery and characterization of many of these intoxications, often enabling detection of subtle white matter involvement that was previously unappreciated. Four categories of toxic leukoencephalopathy can be distinguished: drugs of abuse, cranial irradiation, therapeutic drugs, and environmental toxins (Filley and Kleinschmidt-DeMasters, 2001). Table 6.2 lists the best-known white matter toxins within these categories. In this section, toluene abuse, radiation, and cancer chemotherapy will be discussed as particularly illustrative examples of how toxic injury illuminates the function of normal and abnormal white matter.

Toluene leukoencephalopathy

Drugs of abuse are well known to cause injury to the nervous system, but the characterization of these intoxications has been been difficult because drug abusers are often exposed to more than one agent, and there exists a relative paucity of neuropathological studies of individuals with single exposures. As a general rule, brain injury from drugs of abuse features

Table 6.2 White matter toxins

Drugs of abuse
Toluene
Alcohol
Cocaine
Heroin
Cocaine
MDMA (3,4-methylenedioxy-methamphetamine)
Psilocybin
Radiation
Therapeutic drugs
Cancer chemotherapeutic agents
Cyclosporine
Tacrolimus
Amphotericin B
Hexachlorophene
Environmental toxins
Carbon monoxide
Arsenic
Carbon tetrachloride

a wide spectrum of neuropathology, including ischemia, cerebrovascular disease, and a range of neuronal changes implicating additional inflammatory and degenerative mechanisms (Büttner, 2011). Specific white matter changes can be seen that suggest a direct leukotoxic effect, although much remains to be clarified (Büttner, 2011). The discussion to follow will consider a commonly abused drug for which substantial neuroimaging evidence, and in some cases neuropathological evidence, exists to document selective effects on white matter with neurobehavioral sequelae.

One of the more intriguing discoveries made possible by the application of MRI is toluene leukoencephalopathy, which convincingly illustrates the capacity for pure white matter damage to produce dementia (Hormes, Filley, and Rosenberg, 1986; Rosenberg et al., 1988a; Rosenberg et al., 1988b; Filley, Heaton, and Rosenberg, 1990). Toluene (methylbenzene) is a common household and industrial solvent that is also popular as a drug of abuse among millions of people in the United States and in many countries around the world. Inhalant abuse is a highly prevalent but underappreciated form of drug abuse; it is estimated that 9% of the United States population has experimented with inhalants, and that as many as 50% of these individuals are at risk of abuse (Filley, 2013). The abuse of toluene is practiced by the inhalation of solvent vapors derived mainly from spray paint, which leads to rapid inebriation and euphoria without a notable withdrawal state (Filley, Halliday, and Kleinschmidt-DeMasters, 2004). The solvent may be inhaled to achieve this effect on a daily basis for years without respite. If exposure is heavy and prolonged, a dramatic neurologic syndrome appears in which dementia is the most prominent component of a clinical proflile that also includes ataxia, corticospinal dysfunction, and various brain stem and cranial nerve abnormalities (Hormes, Filley, and Rosenberg, 1986). These effects may be persistent in many abusers even after abstinence is achieved, and the pattern of dementia in these individuals resembles that described in subcortical dementia (Hormes, Filley, and Rosenberg, 1986) and, more specifically, the profile of WMD (Filley, Rosenberg, and Heaton, 1990; Filley, Halliday, and Kleinschnidt-DeMasters, 2004). MRI scans of toluene abusers display diffuse T2 hyperintensity in the cerebral and cerebellar white matter, and the degree of cerebral involvement strongly correlates with the severity of dementia, the most prominent clinical manifestation (Filley, Heaton, and Rosenberg, 1990). Autopsy studies confirm the MRI findings by revealing selective myelin loss with sparing of the cerebral cortex, neuronal cell bodies, and even axons in all but the most severe cases (Rosenberg et al., 1988b; Kornfeld et al., 1994; Fornazzari et al., 2003; Filley, Halliday, and Kleinschmidt-DeMasters, 2004). A recent review of 30 studies of toluene misuse concluded that white matter is indeed the likely target of toluene, and that observed cognitive deficits are consistent with white matter damage (Yücel et al., 2008). Toluene leukoencephalopathy thus serves as a model of the toxic white matter disorders, and as a convincing example of how white matter disease can lead to dementia.

Early MRI studies of toluene abuse investigating the pathogenesis of dementia proved invaluable in documenting diffuse leukoencephalopathy in the cerebrum and cerebellum. Several findings were revealed, including diffusely increased periventricular white matter signal on T2-weighted images, loss of differentiation between the gray and white matter, and diffuse cerebral atrophy (Rosenberg et al., 1988b), and these observations were amply confirmed (Caldemeyer et al., 1993; Xiong et al., 1993; Yamanouchi et al., 1997). Some cases have shown T2 hypointensities in the thalamus and basal ganglia, which were initially attributed to iron deposition but later attributed to the partitioning of toluene in lipids within these areas (Unger et al., 1994). The leukotoxic predilection of toluene is also consistent with documented neuropsychological defcitis in processing speed, sustained attention, memory retrieval, and executive function (Yücel et al., 2008). Preliminary DTI studies have found that microstructural white matter abnormalities can also be detected in inhalant abusers (Yücel et al., 2010).

Neuropathological investigation of toluene leukoencephalopathy has established the selectivity of white matter involvement. Initial autopsy studies consistently disclosed widespread white matter changes in the brain that spared cortical and subcortical gray matter as well as axons (Rosenberg et al., 1988b; Kornfeld et al., 1994). Whereas true demyelination was not observed, an increase in very long-chain fatty acids in the cerebral white matter suggested a neuropathological commonality with adrenoleukodystrophy (Kornfeld et al., 1994). More recently, further evidence was presented from a large neuropathological study that discovered selective white matter damage in 22 of 75 solvent abusers, with sparing of gray matter and axons within the injured white matter; the 22 affected brains were from people who had undergone longer periods of abuse (Al-Hajri and Del Bigio, 2010).

The neurobehavioral sequelae of extended toluene abuse are clear, but the impact of low-level occupational exposure to toluene and other solvents remains uncertain (Filley, Halliday, and Kleinschmidt-DeMasters, 2004; Filley, 2013). Exposure to toluene and similar solvents is common in the household, and there is little reason for concerns about leukotoxicity in this setting, Workers exposed to solvents in industrial settings, however, often have a variety of neurobehavioral complaints that could be a result of exposure, but their symptoms, which typically include fatigue, poor concentration, memory loss, depression, and sleep disturbance, are nonspecific and frequently unaccompanied by neurologic findings or evidence of neuropsychological dysfunction. Moreover, determining a cause-and-effect relationship in this situation is difficult because many individuals are exposed to multiple solvents, suffer depression or anxiety, struggle with concurrent alcohol or other drug issues, or are involved in often protracted litigation. The issue has been controversial since the 1970s, when reports of the "chronic painters' syndrome" began to appear from Scandinavia (Arlien-Søborg et al., 1979). Since then, many authoritiies have addressed this condition, also called chronic toxic encephalopathy and the psychoorganic syndrome, and opinions on its existence range from expressions of support (White and Feldman, 1987; Baker, 1994) to skepticism (Rosenberg, 1995; Albers et al., 2000).

At present, low-level exposure to organic solvents including toluene in the workplace cannot be regarded as hazardous to white matter. Neuropsychological testing offers a sensitive approach to the detection of deficits, but whether observed deficits are specific for leukotoxicity is often unknown (Rosenberg, 1995; Albers et al., 2000). Neuroimaging with CT has not been helpful, as CT studies of solvent-exposed workers typically fail to show cerebral atrophy (Treibig and Lang, 1993), and white matter is not well seen with this technique. One MRI study was able to show diffuse white matter hyperintensity in individuals exposed to industrial solvents when compared to age-matched control subjects (Thuomas et al., 1996), but many similarly exposed individuals have normal MRI (Rosenberg, 1995). Perhaps most convincing is an autopsy study of 98 individuals who had been exposed to organic solvents in the workplace; results showed no difference in brain weight compared to control brains and no specific neuropathology that could be attributable to solvent intoxication (Klinken and Arlien-Søborg, 1993). It thus remains true that accurate diagnosis of individuals in this setting is not straightforward, and many cases of alleged cognitive impairment after occupational solvent exposure remain unconvincing after detailed neurobehavioral evaluation. Whereas the leukoencephalopathy of toluene abuse remains the best example of solvent-induced neurobehavioral dysfunction and one of the most instructive types of white matter dementia, similar but less severe effects from low-level exposure to toluene or other solvents remain to be substantiated. Prospective, controlled studies will be necessary to establish whether toxicity occurs in this setting, the threshold of exposure above which the toxicity can be expected, and whether white matter injury is significant.

Radiation

Radiation delivered to the brain as a therapeutic modality for neoplasia is well established in the treatment of many primary and metastatic tumors. As with other modalities for treating cancer, however, radiation confers a substantial potential for toxicity. In the brain, this neurotoxic effect was formerly assumed to fall most heavily on the hippocampus, but recent years have witnessed increasing recognition of the leukotoxic effects of radiation. Thus the problem of radiation leukoencephalopathy has come to be appreciated as one of the major limitations of cranial irradiation (Dietrich et al., 2008; Perry and Schmidt, 2006; Greene-Schloesser and Robbins, 2012).

This idea of a leukotoxic effect of radiation first appeared more than three decades ago with the work of Sheline and colleagues, which established that three types of radiation injury can occur in the brain, all of which primarily affect the cerebral white matter (Sheline, Wara, and Smith, 1980). First, an acute reaction may occur during treatment and is characterized by a confusional state or a worsening of preexisting neurologic signs. This mild syndrome is typically self-limited, and is thought to result from cerebral white matter edema. Next comes the early delayed reaction, which develops as a so-called somnolence syndrome weeks to months after irradiation. This syndrome has been ascribed to cerebral demyelination, and slow recovery takes place after the cessation of radiation. The most severe radiation-induced white matter injury is the late delayed reaction, which appears months to years after therapy and presents as a progressive, often-fatal dementia resulting from widespread demyelination and necrosis. As the acute reaction typically subsides spontaneously, most information on radiation leukoencephalopathy has been gathered from study of the early and late delayed effects.

The most prominent clinical sequelae of any form of radiation leukoencephalopathy are neurobehavioral. In adults, mental status disruptions such as confusion, personality change, apathy, memory loss, and dementia have been often noted (Vigliani et al., 1999; Filley and Kleinschmidt-DeMasters, 2001; Greene-Schloesser and Robbins, 2012), and focal neurobehavioral signs may appear in association with localized neuroradiological abnormalities (Valk and Dillon, 1991). Learning disabilities have been described in children (Constine et al., 1988), and those under 5 years of age may fare worse than older children (Fletcher and Copeland, 1988). The incidence of cognitive impairment after radiation for brain tumors has been reported to be a high as 50% to 90% (Greene-Schloesser and Robbins, 2012), but this figure likely depends to a large extent on age, cumulative dose, concomitant chemotherapy, and comorbid vascular risk factors such as diabetes mellitus (Dietrich et al., 2008). Patients have been described with radiation-induced dementia and prominent white matter neuropathology on neuroimaging, cerebral biopsy, or autopsy; qualitatively, the dementia was similar to that seen with white matter diseases such as BD and normal pressure hydrocephalus (DeAngelis, Delattre, and Posner, 1989; Vigliani et al., 1999; Omuro et al., 2005; Greene-Schloesser and Robbins, 2012). In patients irradiated for tumors located at the base of the skull, neurocognitive deficits correlated with total radiation dose, and the pattern of impairments in cognitive speed, visuospatial skills, and executive function was consistent with injury to the subcortical white matter (Meyers et al., 2000). Learning and memory are also impaired, but, importantly, memory retrieval is affected more than encoding, suggesting primary dysfunction within frontotemporal white matter networks (Dietrich et al., 2008). Long-term follow-up study of patients with glioma treated with radiation has detected deficits in executive function and processing speed in association with white matter lesions (Douw et al., 2009).

The radiation dose thought to induce radiation leukoencephalopathy in adults has generally been reported as greater than 50 Gy, and children are considered vulnerable at lower doses (Schultheiss et al., 1995; Perry and Schmidt, 2006). The safe lower limit of brain irradiation is unknown, although a study of healthy adults who received a dose of 1.2 Gy demonstrated no decrement in attention, a domain quite sensitive to radiation effects (Wenz et al., 1999). Focal irradiation appears to have less neurobehavioral impact than whole brain irradiation (Taphoorn et al., 1994). Significant damage may still occur with focal irradiation, as was found in patients who received focal radiation for nasopharyngeal carcinoma and developed prominent memory and language deficits in association with bilateral temporal lobe white matter necrosis (Cheung et al., 2000).

Evidence acquired since the initial studies of Sheline and colleagues (1980) has confirmed that the cerebral white matter is the major site of radiation injury to the brain (Perry and Schmidt, 2006). Neuropathological abnormalities in radiation leukoencephalopathy may be diffuse or focal, depending on the site(s) of irradiation. In general, a spectrum of changes reflects the range of severity that can develop – from edema to demyelination and ultimately necrosis (Vigliani et al., 1999; Filley and Kleinschmidt-DeMasters, 2001). Radiation does not produce significant damage to the cerebral cortex, and the often-diagnosed cortical atrophy in irradiated patients more likely reflects diminution of white matter volume (Valk and Dillon, 1991; Rogers et al., 2011). Hypothesized causes of radiation leukoencephalopathy include direct oligodendrocyte injury with secondary disturbance in myelin metabolism, damage to vascular endothelium resulting in breakdown of the blood–brain barrier and subsequent edema and demyelination, neuroinflammation, and oxidative stress (Sheline, Wara, and Smith, 1980; Vigliani et al., 1999; Greene-Schloesser and Robbins, 2012). Recent studies have underscored the potential importance of damage to oligodendrocyte progenitor cells (Dietrich et al., 2008).

Neuroimaging studies reflect the spectrum of neuropathological injury from radiation, and MRI findings become more severe with early delayed and particularly late delayed injury. MRI studies have supported an association between greater cognitive impairment and more extensive radiation-induced white matter disease (Corn et al., 1994; Armstrong et al., 1995; Mulhern et al., 1999; Schuitema et al., 2013). A study of medulloblastoma survivors demonstrated a direct correlation between decreased white matter volume due to radiation and a lower mean intelligence quotient (Mulhern et al., 1999). Armstrong and colleagues conducted longitudinal studies of the effects of radiotherapy, and found a decline in cognitive function between 1.5 and 4.5 months after radiation followed first by improvement and then later by a decline again at 2 years; these results were thought to be consistent with the time course of early delayed and late delayed radiation leukoencephalopathy (Armstrong et al., 1995). These investigators also provided evidence that memory retrieval deficits were particularly prominent and may represent a sensitive clinical marker of white matter neuropathology (Armstrong et al., 1995; Armstrong et al., 2000; Armstrong, Stern, and Corn, 2001).

Cancer chemotherapy

Many drugs used for cancer treatment may produce leukoencephalopathy that is clinically, neuropathologically, and neuroradiologically similar to that produced by radiation (Perry and Schmidt, 2006; Deitrich et al., 2008). The clinical effects of these drugs closely resemble those of radiation leukoencephalopathy, and reflect disruption of neurobehavioral function in a similar pattern, with lassitude, drowsiness, confusion, memory loss, and dementia (Lee, Nauert, and Glass, 1986; Moore-Maxwell, Datto, and Hulette, 2004). In clinical practice, radiation and chemotherapy are often administered together, so the toxic effects on the brain are compounded (Perry and Schmidt, 2006). Similarly, the neuroimaging appearance of cancer drug neurotoxicity can closely mimic that of cerebral radiation. Combined treatment typically produces more severe leukoencephalopathy, particularly if the chemotherapy is given by the intrathecal or intraventricular routes (Lee, Nauert, and Glass, 1986; Perry and Schmidt, 2006). However, the capacity of chemotherapeutic drugs alone to be specifically toxic to myelin has been emphasized (Deitrich et al., 2008; Meyers, 2008).

A particularly fulminant form of chemotherapy-related white matter injury is diffuse necrotizing leukoencephalopathy, in which progressive dementia leading to death is thought to result from axonopathy in addition to myelin damage (Rubinstein et al., 1975; Perry and Schmidt, 2006). This unusual disorder illustrates the general principle that axonal loss typically worsens the prognosis after white matter damage of any kind is sustained (Medana and Esiri, 2003).

The first antineoplastic drug recognized to produce leukoencephalopathy was methotrexate, which can be associated with the syndrome when given intrathecally or intravenously (Gilbert, 1998) or even orally in exceptional cases (Worthley and McNeil, 1995). High-dose intravenous methotrexate may cause leukoencephalopathy that manifests clinically as personality change, progressive dementia, and stupor (Allen et al., 1980). Another agent, BCNU (1,3-bis(2-chloroethyl)-1-nitrosourea), may also cause drug-induced leukoencephalopathy, whether given intravenously (Burger et al., 1981) or intra-arterially (Kleinschmidt-DeMasters and Geier, 1989). Progessive dementia and a fatal outcome may ensue (Kleinschmidt-DeMasters and Geier, 1989).

A number of other antineoplastic drugs may produce this syndrome. Cytosine arabinoside, 5-fluorouracil, levamisole, fludarabine, cisplatin, thiotepa, interleukin-2, and interferon-alpha are on this list (Filley and Kleinschmidt-DeMasters, 2001), and more can be expected. In general, these drugs share similar clinical features of toxic leukoencephalopathy, and their effects are typically well seen on MRI scans. The neuropathology of these intoxications, when available, documents variable degrees of

BOX 6.2 Etiologies of brain trauma

- Traumatic brain injury
- Shaken baby syndrome
- Corpus callosotomy
- Frontal lobotomy

cerebral demyelination and necrosis. Many cases show some reversibility, but more intense exposure seems to be associated with more severe leukoencephalopathy and a worse prognosis (Filley and Kleinschmidt-DeMasters, 2001). As with radiation, recent studies have suggested that damage to oligodendrocyte progenitor cells may be involved in more severe cases (Deitrich et al., 2008).

Traumatic disorders

Trauma to the brain can occur because of accidents, falls, assaults, military combat, sporting contests, or therapeutic interventions (Box 6.2). By far the most important form of brain trauma is the category known as traumatic brain injury (TBI), which includes closed or penetrating head injuries that impact brain structure and function among individuals engaged in many civilian activities and in military combat. One of the most urgent problems confronting medicine and society, TBI constitutes one of the most prevalent neurologic disorders. The understanding of neuropathological changes in the brain caused by physical trauma, and how they affect clinical presentation and recovery, is challenging because of the multiple adverse consequences of trauma on brain integrity, and there is no single neuropathological lesion of TBI. Whereas gray matter regions of the brain can be affected by trauma, it is clear that the white matter is significantly damaged, and approaching TBI from this perspective offers instructive new insights into the role of white matter in cognition more generally.

Traumatic brain injury

After a long period of relative neglect (Goldstein, 1990), TBI has recently been the object of considerable and well-deserved interest in neurology. TBI is an important source of neurobehavioral disability and death, estimated to affect 3.6 million Americans per year (Coronado et al., 2011), and serves as the primary example of traumatic white matter damage. Severe TBI may of course be an immediately fatal event, and in the United States more than 50,000 indivduals perish from TBI each year (Coronado et al., 2011). Many more individuals survive, and although most concussions resolve fully within weeks or a few months, it is sobering to consider that more than 5 million Americans are living with the chronic neurologic sequelae of TBI (Chauhan, 2014). TBI is especially problematic because of its high incidence in young adulthood, often leaving patients with decades of disability and lost productivity. The recent military conflicts in Iraq and Afghanistan have accentuated the problem, as many combatants return from active duty with blast injury, a new form of TBI distinct from blunt physical impact. Whatever the mechanism of injury, deficits in cognition and emotional status are typically the most problematic after TBI, far outpacing physical disability. The substantial initial recovery of physical function often misleads clinicians and families to anticipate a good neurobehavioral outcome that may never occur.

The terminology of neurobehavioral impairment in TBI has traditionally been separated from that of dementia, as many prefer to use "dementia" in reference mainly to older people with degenerative diseases. However, the presence of long-standing deficits in multiple cognitive domains in moderate to severe TBI patients surely justifies the descriptor "dementia," and given the prominence of white matter neuropathology with head injury, TBI fully merits inclusion in this book. The dementia of TBI can also be referred to as static encephalopathy, another reasonable categorization, but however this condition is described, the lasting cognitive syndrome produced by TBI is part of a multifaceted illness that prohibits usual social and occupational function (Masel and DeWitt, 2010). Our goal at this point is to highlight the role of white matter injury in the pathogenesis of this lifelong disorder. A related and rapidly emerging topic – the relationship of TBI to degenerative dementia – will be considered in Chapters 14 and 15.

The clinical presentation of TBI necessarily includes impairment of mental status. In all cases, TBI involves some compromise of neurobehavioral function, ranging from transient loss of consciousness, confusion, or amnesia from concussion (Kelly et al., 1991) to the vegetative state following severe injury (Adams, Graham, and Jennett, 2000). The immediate severity of TBI is most often classified on the basis of initial Glasgow Coma Scale (GCS) score (Teasdale and Jennett, 1974) as mild (13–15), moderate (9–12), or severe (3–8), but this measurement is frequently unavailable. Most often, clinicians are faced with the task of diagnosing TBI in retrospect, which can be very challenging unless the injury is obvious. Similarly, the neuropathological basis of neurobehavioral impairment in TBI is often unclear. Despite these uncertainties, however, evidence developed over the past half century has steadily supported the notion that the primary origin of neurobehavioral sequelae after TBI is damage to the cerebral white matter.

Among the many lesions head trauma may produce, including cortical contusion, intracerebral hemorrhage, subdural hematoma, epidural hematoma, penetrating wounds, and hypoxic-ischemic damage, the most important TBI lesion is diffuse axonal injury (DAI) within the white matter (Strich, 1970; Adams et al., 1982; Gennarelli et al., 1982; Alexander, 1995; Adams, Graham, and Jennett, 2000; Smith, Meaney, and Shull, 2003; Chauhan, 2014). Also known as traumatic axonal injury (TAI), DAI produces widespread areas of white matter damage (Adams et al., 1982; Alexander, 1995; Kraus et al., 2007), and has been termed the signature neuropathology of TBI (Chauhan, 2014). Figure 6.3 shows a coronal brain section from a young man with severe, fatal TBI who sustained widespread DAI.

A key insight in this field is that DAI is present in all cases of TBI, from the mildest to the most devastating (Alexander, 1995). This lesion is responsible not only for the acute neurobehavioral effects of

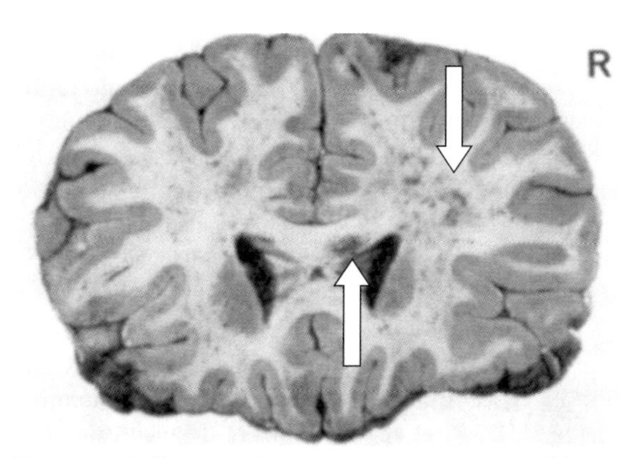

Figure 6.3 Diffuse axonal injury on postmortem coronal brain section of a young man with severe traumatic brain injury (from Strich, 1970). Both cerebral hemispheres are involved, the right more than the left (downward arrow), and the corpus callosum is also injured (upward arrow).

TBI, but also for chronic sequelae, including persistent attentional, executive, comportmental, and memory disturbances (Alexander, 1995), and even the vegetative state (Adams, Graham, and Jennett, 2000). Damage to frontal lobe white matter is particularly detrimental, compromising long-term outcome in many patients by interfering with restoration of normal personality, occupational function, and community reintegration (Filley, 2011).

Clinical and experimental studies of TBI have long supported the prominence of injury to the white matter (Strich, 1956; Adams et al., 1982; Gennarelli et al., 1982; Büki and Povlishock, 2006; Chauhan, 2014). An early term for this lesion in patients with severe posttraumatic dementia was “diffuse degeneration of the cerebral white matter” (Strich, 1956), and later the more specific descriptor “shearing injury” was introduced (Strich, 1961). Subsequently, variable degrees of DAI were demonstrated in both mild TBI (Oppenheimer, 1968) and severe TBI (Adams et al., 1982). The work of Nevin (1967) showed that white matter pathology was present in all individuals who survived more than a week after severe TBI, and the identical pattern of DAI was shown in experimental animals subjected to TBI (Gennarelli et al., 1982). The familiar term DAI was proposed to designate widespread injury to axons within the white matter of the injured brain (Adams et al., 1982), and TAI was used to designate the same process (Büki and Povlishock, 2006). Whereas these terms both point to brain axons as the primary sites of injury, it has now beome clear that myelin is concomittantly damaged (Chauhan, 2014; Mierzwa et al., 2015; Armstrong et al., 2015), and thus DAI serves to designate the white matter damage of TBI that is capable of producing major neurobehavioral sequelae.

Microscopically, DAI was first characterized by the presence of axonal retraction balls, microglial clusters, and Wallerian degeneration in white matter tracts (Gennarelli et al., 1982), and myelin injury is now also recognized (Chauhan, 2014; Mierzwa et al., 2015; Armstrong et al., 2015). Areas most affected by DAI are the dorsal midbrain, the corpus callosum, and the hemispheric white matter (Filley, 2011). The pathophysiology of DAI centers on shearing forces generated in the brain by sudden acceleration and deceleration (Adams et al., 1982; Gennarelli et al., 1982; Alexander, 1995; Büki and Povlishock, 2006; Chauhan, 2014). Rotational forces appear to be most deleterious, often producing instant loss of consciousness by shearing injury of white matter in the brain stem. Long association and commissural fiber tracts are also affected, as they are highly vulnerable to mechanical disruption. Injury to blood vessels producing multiple hemorrhagic foci within the white matter is also common in TBI. Further investigation has elucidated a cascade of cellular events occurring after TBI, including calcium entry into damaged axons, that contribute to additional axonal and myelin disruption (Büki and Povlishock, 2006). The extent of DAI correlates with clinical measures of severity, including the GCS, the length of unconsciousness, and the duration of posttraumatic amnesia (Alexander, 1995; Adams et al., 2011). Taken together, these observations serve to identify the essential difference between mild and more severe forms of TBI as the degree of DAI.

Neuroimaging studies have generally supported neuropathological findings emphasizing the importance of white matter damage in TBI. Most patients with mild TBI have normal conventional MRI, reflecting the microscopic nature of DAI. Early reports using CT in TBI patients demonstrated small focal hemorrhages in the white matter (Zimmerman, Bilaniuk, and Gennarelli, 1978), but CT has since been acknowledged as generally insensitive to the lesions of DAI (Kim and Gean, 2011). The improved sensitivity of MRI was demonstrated by observations that some brain-injured individuals with normal CT scans have white matter lesions on MRI (Mittl et al., 1994). An early prospective MRI study showed that DAI was the most common neuroradiological lesion in TBI, followed by cortical contusions, and that these lesions typically occur in the dorsal brain stem, corpus callosum, and hemispheric white matter, the same sites identified from neuropathological studies (Gentry, Godersky, and Thompson, 1988). With further technical advances, gradient echo (GRE) and susceptibility-weighted images (SWI) became available, and these sequences are now recommended to improve DAI detection because they reveal shearing-related microhemorrhages that accompany traumatic axonal and myelin injury (Kim and Gean, 2011).

The fact that microscopic lesions of DAI are often undetectable with conventional MRI explains why correlations between MRI white matter changes and neuropsychological function have often been modest (Levin et al., 1992). It remains true that one of the major issues with mild TBI is establishing the diagnosis in clinical practice without a sensitive and specific neuroimaging method. GRE and SWI sequences offer some help in this regard, but many DAI lesions still go undetected. As this problem was recognized, more sensitive MRI techniques were sought in the effort to improve white matter–behavior correlations, and the study of NAWM in TBI was initiated. Reduced white matter N-acetyl aspartate (NAA) on MRS was found to correlate with TBI severity (Garnett et al., 2000), and MTI detected white matter abnormalities that correlated with cognitive impairment (Bagley et al., 2000; McGowan et al., 2000). DTI showed similar results, notably in a study of children in whom a composite measure of white matter integrity was related to global outcome and processing speed after TBI (Levin et al., 2008). In longitudinal studies of adults with TBI, DTI disclosed DAI in multiple tracts, and acute abnormalities correlated with impaired learning and memory while lasting abnormalities correlated with slowed processing speed and executive dysfunction (Wang et al., 2011).

The specific neurobehavioral impact of DAI can be difficult to determine in many cases because other neurologic and systemic injuries in TBI also contribute to overall outcome. For example, patients with diffuse injury and superimposed cortical lesions fare worse than those with diffuse injury alone (Filley et al., 1987). However, available data are useful in developing a profile of neurobehavioral deficits that can be ascribed to the effects of DAI. In general, attention, memory, and executive function are most affected in TBI (Wilson and Wyper, 1992), and they also tend to dominate in mild TBI patients who go on to develop the postconcussion syndrome (Alexander, 1995). Sustained attention or concentration may be particularly affected, in contrast to simple attention (Kaufmann et al., 1993). Memory impairment has been associated with ventricular enlargement that is most likely a result of white matter volume loss (Anderson and Bigler, 1995). An intriguing observation is that TBI patients may display relative preservation of procedural memory compared to declarative memory (Ewert et al., 1989). More detailed examination of memory functions also reveals that this sparing of procedural memory may be accompanied by specific difficulty with memory retrieval (Timmerman and Brouwer, 1999). Executive dysfunction has been documented in TBI, and DTI studies have been used to relate this deficit to DAI within frontal lobe connections (Kinnunen et al., 2011). In contrast to these deficit areas, language is relatively preserved after TBI. An early report using Wechsler Adult Intelligence Scale (WAIS) verbal and performance IQ scores after TBI indicated that language is less affected and recovers more quickly than nonverbal skills (Mandleberg and Brooks, 1975). Personality and emotional changes, on the other hand, are frequent. Disinhibition or impaired impulse control may be disabling because of the social disruption that limits or precludes reintegration into society, and depression occurs in nearly half of patients with TBI (van Reekum, Cohen, and Wong, 2000). Cognitive slowing, an emerging feature of white matter dysfunction, has been associated with DAI using MRI volumetric analysis (Levine et al., 2006). A more recent DTI study found that decreased fractional anisotropy (FA) in several cerebral white matter tracts was associated with executive dysfunction among patients with moderate or severe TBI (Spitz et al., 2013). In sum, TBI leads to a wide range of neurobehavioral deficits, and the central role of white matter pathology is supported by the presence of DAI combined with a clinical profile matching that of other white matter disorders.

A discussion of this topic would not be complete without a review of blast injury. Military conflicts in the Middle East in the past decade have brought to attention this new form of TBI, which offers new challenges in terms of understanding pathogenesis and providing treatment (Ling et al., 2009). Many combatants in the Iraq and Afghanistan wars have been subjected to injuries related not to direct head trauma but rather to the impact of high-velocity air, smoke, gas, and debris from a nearby explosion. Symptoms after blast injury are very similar to those following more conventional concussion, leading to the notion that similar mechanisms of brain injury, including DAI, are involved, but the frequent co-occurrence of posttraumatic stress disorder has complicated analysis of these patients. To address this issue, DTI studies are beginning to document multifocal DAI as a mechanism of brain damage associated with blast injuries (Mac Donald et al., 2011; Hetherington et al., 2015).

The question now arises as to the risk of developing dementia after TBI as a result of DAI. There can be no definitive answer to this question, because the term dementia is not often used in the study of TBI outcomes, and the neuropathology of TBI includes but is not confined to DAI. Surely a substantial number of individuals with TBI, in whom DAI is a primary form of injury, must endure lasting intellectual dysfunction that meets criteria for dementia, but specific data on this issue are unavailable. However, some perspective can be achieved by considering the notion of disability, a term used in the TBI literature that serves as a rough equivalent of dementia and may be associated with DAI. The most widely employed measure of outcome after TBI is the Glasgow Outcome Scale (GOS; Jennett and Bond, 1975), which establishes the five outcomes of death, vegetative state, severe disability, moderate disability, and good recovery. TBI outcome data using the GOS, not surprisingly, are quite variable, as many factors influence recovery in any given patient, but lasting cognitive impairment precluding return to normal function has been documented in those who have experienced moderate or severe TBI (Sherer, Madison, and Hannay, 2000; Dikmen et al., 2009). Patients may show improvement over time, but even if they reach good recovery, residual cognitive effects usually preclude normal social and occupational function (Sherer, Madison, and Hannay, 2000). In patients studied neuropsychologically 2 years after moderate and severe TBI, cognitive performance is typically at the 20th percentile compared to matched controls (Schretlein and Shapiro, 2003), and return to work – which rarely assumes pre-injury levels – is possible for only about two-thirds of those with moderate TBI and one-third of those with severe TBI (Sherer, Madison, and Hannay, 2000). Whereas studies are needed to examine correlations between DAI and dementia, the importance of DAI in the pathogenesis of disability after TBI has been emphasized (Medana and Esiri, 2003).

A more recent issue with regard to dementia after TBI is the possibility of degenerative disease developing later in life. It may be that, in addition to the static encephalopathy produced by moderate or severe injury, progressive neurodegeneration may occur as a late sequel in some individuals who have sustained TBI. The two varieties of degenerative dementia most often discussed are AD and chronic traumatic encephalopathy (CTE), with current evidence suggesting an association of AD with moderate or severe TBI, and a link between CTE and multiple episodes of mild TBI (DeKosky, Ikonomovic, and

BOX 6.3 Demyelinative diseases

- Multiple sclerosis
- Neuromyelitis optica
- Acute disseminated encephalomyelitis
- Schilder's disease
- Marburg's disease
- Balò's concentric sclerosis
- Tumefactive multiple sclerosis

Gandy, 2010). This topic warrants close scrutiny from the perspective of white matter neurobiology and will be considered in more detail near the end of this book. At present, the link between TBI and degenerative dementia – either AD or CTE – should be regarded as investigational, but increasing evidence suggests that each disease may result from the very common TBI lesion known as DAI.

Demyelinative diseases

This category of white matter disorders includes multiple sclerosis (MS) and many related but less common inflammatory diseases of myelin (Box 6.3). In terms of higher function, MS has recently been better appreciated as a source of cognitive and emotional impairment, recalling the initial insights of Jean-Martin Charcot in the 1870s (Charcot, 1877). A primary source of cognitive impairment is presumed to be white matter damage, as many studies have found at least modest correlations between extent of MRI white matter lesion burden and the degree of cognitive loss (Filley, 2012). More sophisticated MRI techniques have also documented abnormalities in the NAWM, indicating that subtle white matter pathology may be missed by conventional MRI. Recent studies, however, have also pointed toward cerebral cortical involvement, a form of the disease known as "cortical MS" (Stadelmann et al., 2008). This issue brings up the complexity of MS, and, like other white matter disorders, restriction of the neuropathology to white matter alone is uncommon. Nevertheless, much evidence supports the role of white matter involvement in the pathognesis of cognitive impairment and dementia in MS. This disease will now be discussed as the prototype demyelinative white matter disorder.

Multiple sclerosis

After more than a century of study, MS remains a perplexing disease that attracts the attention of neurologists and neuroscientists because of its clinical variability, uncertain etiology, and ever-improving therapy (Noseworthy, 1999; Hauser and Oksenberg, 2006). Among the many questions with MS requiring continued investigation are the characterization, significance, and treatment of neurobehavioral dysfunction. As recognized by Charcot (1877), both cognitive and emotional disturbances are apparent, but many details of these aspects of MS call out for a more thorough understanding. The wide range of neurobehavioral disturbances that compromise the life of individuals with MS presents a challenge to clinicians and an opportunity for researchers.

Cognitive impairment is an important clinical problem affecting many patients with MS (Rao, 1986; Feinstein, 2007; Langdon, 2011). This disturbance may range from subtle cognitive loss that can easily escape clinical detection to severe dementia that leaves no option except total care. Cognitive impairment can be a problem at all stages of the disease, potentially eroding physical independence, coping skills, driving, employment, medication compliance, and rehabilitation potential (Langdon, 2011). A generally recognized figure for the prevalence of cognitive impairment in MS is 40% to 70% (Langdon, 2011), and dementia, although less common, has been reported in up to 23% of MS patients (Boerner and Kapfhammer, 1999). For most of the history of MS, however, the high prevalence of cognitive impairment was not well appreciated. As late as 1970, for example, the prevalence of cognitive dysfunction of any kind in MS was estimated to be approximately 5% (Kurtzke, 1970). The use of more sensitive neuropsychological tests and improved research design in subsequent studies raised this figure much higher. Peyser and colleagues, for example, found a prevalence of 55% in their series of hospitalized MS patients (Peyser et al., 1980). Later, Heaton and colleagues considered the two major subtypes of relapsing-remitting and chronic-progressive MS, finding that 46% and 72%, respectively, were cognitively impaired (Heaton et al., 1985). A widely cited study of Rao and colleagues (1991) showed that cognitive disturbances are not confined to MS patients referred to university hospital clinics; using a community-based sample, they found a prevalence of 43%. A general consensus has long held that more severe forms of the disease predict more severe cognitive loss.

A key point is that cognitive impairment in MS may not be associated with more obvious features of neurologic disease. While memory and other disturbances may often appear together with elemental neurologic dysfunction in MS, cognitive loss may be isolated and by itself constitute the major source of disability. Clinicians working with MS patients are well advised to be aware of this possibility, as it is often overlooked in those who may be assumed cognitively normal because of the absence of motor and sensory findings on examination. Franklin and colleagues (1989) presented 12 patients with significant cognitive dysfunction, but whose physical disability as measured by the Extended Disability Status Scale (EDSS; Kurtzke, 1983) was minimal. These cases highlight the point that the EDSS, still widely used as a clinical measure of overall disability in MS, is generally insensitive to neurobehavioral dysfunction because of its emphasis on motor disability (Franklin et al., 1990).

Cognitive impairment can even appear as the sole feature of an MS exacerbation. Recent years have witnessed the recognition of the "isolated cognitive relapse" in MS, defined as a transient decline in neuropsychological performance in the absence of other neurologic involvement, and with gadolinium enhancement on brain MRI documenting inflammatory demyelination (Pardini et al., 2014). This newly recognized form of relapse, predictable from the natural history of the disease and now measurable with modern neuroimaging, contributes to gradual cognitive decline over time in patients with relapsing-remitting MS (Pardini et al., 2014).

Clinicians can also be misled by the often-subtle nature of cognitive impairment in MS compared to that of more familiar dementia syndromes such as that caused by AD. The typical pattern of cognitive deficits in AD, for example, features prominent amnesia, aphasia, apraxia, and agnosia, whereas MS patients are more likely to have difficulty with processing speed and sustained attention (Filley et al., 1989b; Rao et al., 1991). These distinctions imply that the use of routine cognitive screening methods may be inadequate. Because the dementia of MS, similar to that of many other white matter disorders, does not significantly disrupt language, heavily language-weighted measures such as the Mini-Mental State Examination (MMSE; Folstein, Folstein, and McHugh, 1975) are not well designed for the detection of cognitive loss (Franklin et al., 1988; Swirsky-Sacchetti et al., 1992).

In view of the inadequacy of both the EDSS and the MMSE for identifying cognitive dysfunction in MS, more detailed office testing or neuropsychological evaluation may be required to confirm a clinical suspicion of cognitive dysfunction. If time permits, a thorough mental status examination can often reveal the critical neurobehavioral deficits in MS patients. In other cases, referral for neuropsychological assessment is appropriate for the documentation of progressive cognitive decline, as in cases with incapacitating executive dysfunction who may otherwise have a benign clinical course (Filley, 2000). Newer approaches to this problem have also been developed by investigators seeking brief cognitive screening batteries. The Brief Repeatable Battery of Neuropsychological Tests for MS (BRB-MS; Rao et al., 1991), the Multiple Sclerosis Functional Composite (MSFC; et al., 1999), and the Minimal Assessment of Cognitive Function in MS (MACFIMS; Benedict et al., 2002) all offer sensitive techniques to detect cognitive impairment in MS.

Understanding the pathogenesis of cognitive impairment in MS begins with the neuropathology of the disease. Some patients have mainly spinal cord disease, but essentially all individuals with MS experience some degree of demyelinative plaque burden in the brain. The distribution of cerebral plaques in MS was studied by Brownell and Hughes (1962), who found that periventricular lesion sites were the most common, that the left and right hemispheres were equally affected, and that plaques were distributed proportionately throughout the white matter. A smaller number of plaques was also noted in cortical and subcortical gray matter regions (Brownell and Hughes, 1962). The classic pattern of white matter disease is well recognized on neuroimaging, with MRI studies of MS typically showing periventricular and callosal hyperintensities on T2-weighted and fluid-attenuated inversion recovery (FLAIR) images (Figure 6.4) consistent with prior neuropathological observations (Brownell and Hughes, 1962).

Neuropathological and neuroimaging advances have clarified the pathophysiology of white matter lesions in MS (Trapp et al., 1998; Simon, 2005). Considering MS as fundamentally an inflammatory disease, the first MRI sign of an acute MS lesion is an area of gadolinium enhancement within the white matter, optimally seen in axial T2-weighted or FLAIR images (Simon, 2005). The enhancement

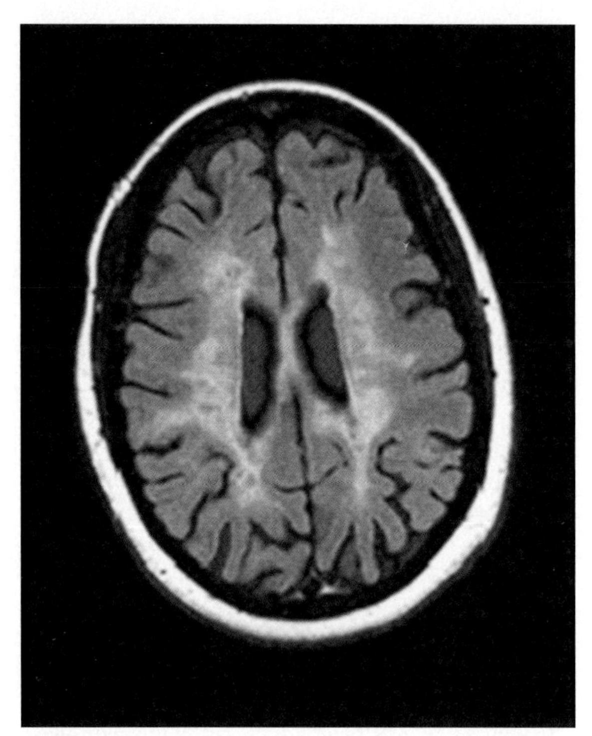

Figure 6.4 Axial fluid-attenuated inversion recovery (FLAIR) MRI scan of an individual with moderately advanced MS. Widespread subcortical demyelination is evident (courtesy of John R. Corboy, MD).

reflects inflammatory demyelination, which lasts for several weeks before it subsides and the lesion becomes either a T2 white matter hyperintensity or, with more extensive damage, a T1 "black hole" (Adams et al., 1999). As T2 hyperintensities reflect an increase in the water content of the affected white matter region, they are nonspecific and can result from other neuropathological processes. T1 lesions in MS, however, typically imply robust demyelination and axonal destruction that often occur in MS. An influential discovery in MS was the finding of axonal transection in many MS lesions, which reflects the intensity of inflammation in affected regions (Trapp et al., 1998). Axonal loss has in fact become widely recognized as a sign of a less favorable prognosis in patients with not only MS but many white matter disorders (Medana and Esiri, 2003). Axonal transection in MS is also one of the features contributing to brain atrophy (Simon, 2005). Atrophy has come to be seen as an important aspect of MS, occurring even early in the disease, measurable over intervals as short as 1 year, and increasingly likely to be a major determinant of disease disability (Trapp et al., 1998; Simon, 2005). The related idea that MS involves neurodegeneration, quite apart from its inflammatory component, has thus been introduced in discussions of MS (Hauser and Oksenberg, 2006). But however the understanding of pathogenesis evolves, MS is increasingly understood as a progressive brain disease affecting myelin, axons, and brain volume even in those with a more benign course.

Brain atrophy in MS clearly has important neurobehavioral implications, but the specific contribution of white matter involvement to atrophy is a crucial question. Atrophy implies diffuse volume loss, but in attempting to define the specific cognitive profile of MS, the regional distribution of white matter lesions assumes more significance. In the study of Brownell and Hughes (1962), the subfrontal white matter was determined to bear the heaviest plaque burden in the brain. This predilection presumably reflects the fact that the frontal lobe is the brain's largest, and because demyelinative lesions occur randomly in the cerebral white matter, the subfrontal white matter logically stands to be the most heavily targeted of the four lobes. Indeed, the similarity of many cognitive deficits in MS to those of other frontal lobe diseases (Filley, 2000) suggests that whereas MS is typically a diffuse brain disease, its neurobehavioral effects may reflect selective interference with frontal systems.

The neuroanatomic basis of cognitive impairment has been extensively investigated with neuroimaging, and substantial evidence over many years has supported the correlation of white matter disease burden with cognitive loss. More than a score of MRI studies have found that white matter lesion burden predicts cognitive impairment as measured neuropsychologically (Medaer et al., 1987; Franklin et al., 1988; Reischies et al., 1988; Rao et al., 1989b; Callanan et al., 1989; Anzola et al., 1990; Pozzilli et al., 1991; Swirsky-Sacchetti et al., 1992; Maurelli et al., 1992; Huber et al., 1992; Feinstein et al., 1992; Comi et al., 1993; Pugnetti et al., 1993; Feinstein, Ron, and Thompson, 1993; Arnett et al., 1994; Möller et al., 1994; Tsolaki et al., 1994; Patti et al., 1995; Ryan et al., 1996; Hohol et al., 1997; Sperling et al., 2001; Penny et al., 2010). In general, cognitive loss becomes more severe as plaques assume a more confluent appearance in the periventricular white matter, and as cerebral atrophy develops. These often-replicated conclusions leave little doubt that cerebral white matter lesions in MS have important neurobehavioral implications.

Correlations between neuropsychological test performance and white matter lesion burden, however, have been generally modest, suggesting that cognitive impairment involves more than these readily identifiable lesions (Filippi et al., 2010). MRI with higher magnet strengths such as 3.0 T improves the detection of MS neuropathology, but conventional MRI is still thought to be able to detect only some of the tissue damage in MS relevant to cognition. Early proposals, such as one suggesting a threshold cerebral white matter disease burden of around 30 cm^2 as the cutoff area above which cognitive impairment is likely (Swirsky-Sacchetti et al., 1992), were soon abandoned after the realization from more advanced MRI techniques that even the NAWM is not invariably normal. Data making this point obvious came from MRS (Sarchielli et al., 1999), MTI (Filippi et al., 2000), and DTI (Filippi et al., 2010) studies of MS that all revealed abnormalities in NAWM correlating with clinical dysfunction. These observations were also confirmed by postmortem studies of MS detecting axonal loss in areas of white matter that appear to be normal (Evangelou et al., 2000). Thus microscopic white matter neuropathology can be found with MRS, MTI, and especially DTI that may add to the clinical assessment and treatment of cognitively impaired MS patients.

Of all the new neuroimaging techniques, DTI has attracted the most attention because of its unequaled capacity to image the details of white matter, including its individual tracts. Studies in MS have used DTI to identify areas of NAWM at risk for degeneration (Simon et al., 2006) or correlated with cognitive dysfunction (Rovaris et al., 2008; Roca et al., 2008; Dineen et al., 2009; Hecke et al., 2010). These studies all support a contribution of white matter damage to cognitive impairment that goes beyond that expected with white matter hyperintensities alone. Advanced neuroimaging of NAWM helps explain why the correlations of lesion volume with cognitive dysfunction in MS have not been more robust.

In spite of the mounting evidence that white matter neuropathology, both from grossly visible plaques and in the NAWM, contributes to cognitive impairment, in recent years the potential contribution of gray matter disease in MS has received much attention (Feinstein, 2007; Stadelmann et al., 2008). This possibility remains alive because of the presence of white matter fascicles in both the cerebral cortex and the subcortical gray matter, where the demyelinative process may also take hold. Most of the recent attention has been devoted to cortical plaques, and the notion of "cortical MS" has been much discussed (Stadelmann et al., 2008). Indeed, as discussed earlier, early neuropathological studies found that MS plaques could occur in the cortex, and were judged to be 5% of the total by Brownell and Hughes (1962). Such a modest disease burden would not be expected to exert a powerful effect on cogntion, and initial studies of cortical plaques with conventional MRI showed that they accounted for just 6% of the total lesion volume and did not correlate with neurocognitive test results (Catalaa et al., 1999). Study of the question has continued, however, as neurologists are attracted to the notion that the effects of MS on cognition may originate in gray matter lesions (Chapter 1).

The contribution of cortical lesions to neurobehavioral dysfunction is uncertain. Both cortical plaques and brain atrophy have been shown to be independent predictors of cognitive dysfunction (Langdon, 2011), but the visualization of cortical plaques with standard MRI field strengths is fraught with difficulty (Filippi et al., 2010). To address this problem, studies with 3.0 and 7.0 T MRI scanners are underway. As this work proceeds, it is worth keeping in mind that not all MS patients have cortical plaques, many of the plaques also involve some adjacent white matter, and gray matter inflammation is generally less extensive than in white matter (Stadelmann et al., 2008).

From a clinical perspective, it is likely that demyelination damages a higher volume of white matter in large fiber tracts than in the cortex, and the close resemblance of cognitive dysfunction in MS to that of other white matter disorders (Filley, 2012) suggests that tract demyelination is likely to be the main determinant of cognitive dysfunction, at least early in the disease. An important variable in this discussion may be the timing of neuropathology, as cortical lesions may postdate white matter lesions in the typical course of MS (Kutzelnigg et al., 2005; DeLuca et al., 2015). The neuropsychological deficits of MS patients have primarily been found in patients in early stages of the disease, and the fact that deficits resemble those of other white matter disorders implies that tract demyelination is the major determining neuropathology. Support for this idea comes from a study of pediatric MS showing that cortical lesions were rare in comparison with white matter plaques (Absinta et al., 2010). Moreover, biopsy studies of adults with early MS showed cortical demyelination in only 38% patients, while white matter lesions were present in 100% (Lucchinetti et al., 2011). In addition, while hippocampal demyelination causing synaptic alterations has been documented, this process was seen only after a mean of 26 years of disease (Dutta et al., 2011).

In general, MS is still considered a disease that predominantly affects white matter, especially early in the course (Simon, 2005; Hauser and Oksenberg, 2006; DeLuca et al., 2015). Although gray matter lesions clearly occur, they may be most significant later in the disease, and only at that time contribute to cognitive dysfunction by producing cortical involvement manifested by aphasia, apraxia, and agnosia (DeLuca et al., 2015). For now, MS surely merits inclusion on the list of diseases that can impair cognition by virtue of damage to the white matter. As the disease progresses, the cortical damage that seems to develop will require further study, and an informative research strategy would involve the longitudinal study of MS to determine if the dementia evolves from a profile of WMD to a cortical dementia as the disease progresses.

Many attempts to characterize the profile of cognitive deficits in MS have been made, and in an influential review Rao (1986) concluded that MS has neuropsychological features that qualify it as one of the subcortical dementias. The prominence of deficits in attention, concentration, memory, executive function, and neuropsychiatric status combined with the absence of significant language disturbance and other cortical deficits were seen as compelling this conclusion (Rao, 1986). Other authorities soon concurred with this opinion (Cummings, 1990). Subsequently, however, additional data were brought forth that invited the possibility that MS might have unique neuropsychological features that separate it not only from cortical diseases but also from subcortical gray matter diseases. To begin, the memory disturbance in MS was reported to involve a retrieval rather than an encoding deficit (Rao, Leo, and Aubin-Flaubert, 1989a; Brassington and Marsh, 1998; Feinstein, 2007). Whereas some evidence suggested a primary memory encoding deficit (DeLuca, Barbieri-Berger, and Johnson, 1994; DeLuca et al., 1998), and other data supported both encoding and retrieval dysfunction (Lafosse et al., 2013), the memory disorder of MS clearly differs from the encoding deficit of cortical dementia (Filley, 2012). Later, another feature that appeared to characterize MS was the sparing of procedural memory (Lafosse et al., 2007), known to be affected in subcortical gray matter diseases (Rao et al., 1993; Feinstein, 2007). These characteristics were postulated to differentiate MS from both the cortical dementias, which involve an encoding deficit, and the traditional subcortical dementias, in which procedural memory is affected; moreover, they make the case that MS may be a prototype for all the white matter dementias (Rao, 1996; Filley, 2012). Most recently, slowing of information processing speed has been emphasized and for many authorities has become a dominant feature of MS-related cognitive impairment (Feinstein, 2007; Chiaravalloti and DeLuca, 2008; Langdon, 2011). These distinctions remain the subject of systematic investigation, and further refinements will no doubt be established.

Inflammatory diseases

White matter can be the target of a diverse group of noninfectious inflammatory diseases (Box 6.4). These diseases share the common feature of autoimmune pathogenesis, and all produce systemic manifestations in addition to those in the nervous system. In the brain, widespread lesions are typical, usually related to vascular inflammation, and in many cases the clinical and neuropathological features of these diseases indicate primary damage to white matter. Many neurologic and neuroradiological similarities exist between inflammatory and demyelinative diseases (Theodoridou and Settas, 2006), and

BOX 6.4 Inflammatory white matter diseases

- Systemic lupus erythematosus
- Behçet's disease
- Sjögren's syndrome
- Wegener's granulomatosis
- Temporal arteritis
- Polyarteritis nodosa
- Scleroderma
- Primary angiitis of the central nervous system
- Sarcoidosis

clinicians often encounter patients whose symptoms and signs invoke the possibility of differential diagnoses within both categories. Recent findings have also underscored neuropsychological commonalities in these two categories that focus on the role of white matter tract dysfunction as the source of cognitive impairment (Benedict et al., 2008). Many areas of uncertainty, however, complicate the interpretation of brain–behavior relationships in the inflammatory autoimmune brain diseases. For the purposes of this book, systemic lupus erythematosus (SLE) proves most illustrative as an inflammatory disease that often attacks white matter.

Systemic lupus erythematosus

SLE is the autoimmune connective tissue disease best known to affect the nervous system. The CNS is affected in up to two-thirds of SLE patients (West, 1994, 1996), and the PNS system may also be involved. The closely related antiphospholipid syndrome is often present in patients with SLE, and the two disorders cannot always be distinguished (Tincani et al., 2009). When SLE involves the brain, the term "lupus cerebritis" was commonly used until the more general descriptor "neuropsychiatric lupus" gained favor (West, 1994). Whereas this latter designation is useful, it includes the entire range of elemental and higher neurologic deficits, and is thus not capable of capturing the range of specific mental status alterations to which SLE patients are susceptible. To address this problem, more specific nomenclature was proposed to clarify the neurobehavioral features of neuropsychiatric lupus (ACR Ad Hoc Committee on Neuropsychiatric Lupus Nomenclature, 1999). A total of 19 neuropsychiatric syndromes were recognized, 12 of which involve the CNS; the most relevant for this account are acute confusional state, cognitive dysfunction, anxiety disorder, mood disorder, psychosis, and a demyelinating syndrome (ACR Ad Hoc Committee on Neuropsychiatric Lupus Nomenclature, 1999). As clinicians have long known, some of these syndromes can be induced by treatment of SLE, most notably with corticosteroids, but it is clear that neuropsychiatric syndromes can often develop when patients are taking small doses of corticosteroids, or none at all (Feinglass et al., 1976), pointing to cerebral involvement rather than iatrogenesis.

On the basis of autopsy data, the CNS neuropathology of SLE has been thought to be dominated by a vasculopathy with hyalinization of vessel walls and perivascular inflammation; a true vasculitis is uncommon (Johnson and Richardson, 1968). Multiple ischemic and hemorrhagic lesions in both gray and white matter result from this process (Brooks et al., 2010). However, because postmortem findings from SLE patients are usually obtained from those with severe disease, the neuropathology of more typical SLE is less well understood. Neuroradiological investigation has thus provided the main body of data on patients with milder SLE affecting the brain. Neuroimaging findings include cerebral atrophy, seen on both CT and MRI scans, but treatment with corticosteroids may confound this common finding because it is possible that atrophy may result from therapy (Jacobs et al., 1988). White matter changes, however, are also prominent, especially on MRI, and these small, multifocal lesions are the most common neuroradiological finding (Sibbitt, Sibbitt, and Brooks, 1999; Benedict et al., 2008; Toledano et al., 2013). These lesions can be distinguished from those of MS in that they display no periventricular predilection, and gadolinium enhancement is uncommon (Miller et al., 1987; Theodoridou and Settas, 2006).

The pathogenesis of neuropsychiatric dysfunction in SLE remains incompletely understood, but a variety of neuropathological processes appear to be involved. Both parenchymal damage from vascular occlusion and neuronal injury from antineuronal antibodies and cytokines have been invoked as causative factors (West, 1994, 1996; Kozora et al., 2008; Hanly et al., 2011). Neuropsychological testing has amply documented that cognitive deficits exist in some SLE patients, including both those with and those without features of neuropsychiatric lupus (Carbotte, Denburg, and Denburg, 1986; Kozora et al., 2008), and a pathogenetic role for white matter involvement has substantial support. Leukoencephalopathy seen on MRI can be associated with dementia in SLE (Kirk, Kertesz, and Polk, 1991), and fulminant, fatal leukoencephalopathy has been reported as the only feature of neuropsychiatric lupus (Prabhakaran et al., 2005).

Neuropsychological study of the profile of cognitive dysfunction in SLE generally indicates that, despite considerable clinical heterogeneity, deficits in attention, concentration, visuospatial skills, and cognitive speed without major language involvement are typical (Ginsburg et al., 1992; Kozora et al., 1996; Denburg,

Carbotte, and Denburg, 1997; Kozora et al., 2008). These deficits can be seen in patients with and without other neurologic signs (Kozora et al., 1996). Fatigue, a common complaint in many patients with cerebral white matter disorders, has been correlated with MRI white matter lesion burden in SLE (Harboe et al., 2008). A study of SLE patients with the lupus anticoagulant described a profile of impairment consistent with subcortical dementia, with the most robust deficit emerging in information processing speed (Denburg et al., 1997). The usual sparing of language means that language-based screening measures such as the MMSE (Folstein, Folstein, and McHugh, 1975) are relatively insensitive to the cognitive impairments of SLE patients (ACR Ad Hoc Committee on Neuropsychiatric Lupus Nomenclature, 1999). Overall, the cognitive deficits of SLE have been interpreted as consistent with subcortical neuropathology (Denburg et al., 1997), but the pattern is also reminiscent of that produced by other white matter disorders (Filley, 2012). Consistent with this idea, a detailed neuropsychological review comparing SLE and MS found the cognitive dysfunction to be remarkably similar in the two diseases (Benedict et al., 2008).

Whereas the presence of scattered white matter lesions on conventional MRI is well known in SLE, a certain threshold burden of disease on MRI may be required to produce cognitive impairment (Kozora et al., 1998; Kozora et al., 2008). This concept implies that more subtle disease in NAWM may also contribute to cognitive loss in some patients. Thus recent research has turned to examining the microstructure of white matter to assess potential damage that cannot be detected by conventional MRI. MRS and DTI have both offered useful insights. Brooks and colleagues (1999) reported that MRS measures of neuronal dysfunction in NAWM strongly correlated with cognitive impairment: Reduced NAA implied axonal damage, and increased choline suggested inflammation and demyelination. A subsequent study of SLE patients with no prior neuropsychiatric involvement found that, in frontal white matter with no hyperintense lesions, elevated choline correlated with impaired processing speed, executive function, and sustained attention, while NAA was unaffected (Filley et al., 2009). These findings suggest that subtle myelinopathy is an early feature of the pathogenesis of cognitive dysfunction in SLE, occurring before neuropsychiatric events or white matter hyperintensities develop (Filley et al., 2009). DTI studies have shown similar findings, identifiying microstructural abnormalities in frontal and other white matter regions among SLE patients both with and without neuropsychiatric dysfunction (Zhang et al., 2007; Schmidt-Wilcke et al., 2014). An informative DTI study showed that decreased FA in a variety of normal-appearing tracts correlated with neuropsychological impairment; this relationship was more apparent for patients with neuropsychiatric SLE, and slowed processing speed was the deficit most strongly correlated with changes in FA (Jung et al., 2012). Thus early myelinopathy, likely involving immune and possibly other factors, may explain subtle neuropsychiatric dysfunction in SLE that is manifested by cognitive slowing, executive dysfunction, and impaired sustained attention (Kozora and Filley, 2011). To illustrate the complex neuropathology of this disease, MRS has also disclosed evidence of hippocampal involvement in early SLE (Kozora et al., 2011), and thus cortical involvement cannot be discounted. However, the opportunity to examine the cerebral white matter before overt neurobehavioral dysfunction begins or conventional MRI findings become apparent represents an important approach to the investigation of cognitive and emotional dysfunction in SLE. The early involvement of white matter in SLE has also been the principal impetus to work on the syndrome of mild cognitive dysfunction, which will be taken up in Chapter 8.

Infectious diseases

Infections of the brain cannot be characterized as strictly confined to the cortical, subcortical gray, or white matter, but a number of infectious diseases display a predilection for white matter (Vargas et al., 2009). These infections are caused by viruses (Box 6.5), and many clinical and immunopathological similarities to demyelinative diseases have been found when these infections are compared

BOX 6.5 Infectious diseases of white matter

- Human immunodeficiency virus infection
- Progressive multifocal leukoencephalopathy
- Subacute sclerosing panencephalitis
- Progressive rubella panencephalitis
- Varicella zoster encephalopathy
- Cytomegalovirus encephalitis

to MS and related disorders. As discussed with MS and SLE, infectious diseases of the white matter also have neurobehavioral consequences.

Human immunodeficiency virus infection

Infection with the human immunodeficiency virus type 1 (HIV-1), commonly known as HIV, has been one of the most publicized medical problems of the past three decades. Since their recognition in 1981, the acquired immunodeficiency syndrome (AIDS) and other forms of HIV infection have become major public health problems worldwide. Despite rapid progress in elucidating its etiology, prevention, and treatment, HIV infection continues to be an incurable disease.

One of the more prominent manifestations of this systemic retroviral infection is brain involvement, which was recognized soon after the AIDS epidemic was identified (Price et al., 1988). The term first employed for this disorder was the AIDS dementia complex (ADC), which emphasized the various cognitive, motor, and behavioral changes that occur (Navia, Jordan, and Price, 1986), and other names have been subacute HIV encephalitis, AIDS-related dementia, and AIDS encephalopathy. As experience with AIDS expanded, a spectrum of cognitive impairment was appreciated, from mild cognitive dysfunction detected on neuropsychological testing (Wilkie et al., 1990) to dementia as the presenting syndrome of patients with a poor prognosis (Navia and Price, 1987; Brew, 1999). The current terminology of cognitive impairment, recognizing the wide range of dysfunction that can be seen (Antinori et al., 2007), uses the overarching term HIV-associated neurocognitive disorder (HAND), within which are included asymptomatic neurocognitive impairment (ANI), HIV-associated mild neurocognitive disorder (MND), and HIV-associated dementia (HAD).

In early studies, the ADC was found to affect approximately 30% of AIDS patients at some point in the disease (McArthur, Sacktor, and Selnes, 1998). With the introduction of antiretroviral therapy (ART) in the 1990s, impressive advances in treating cognitive dysfunction were gradually achieved (Manji, Jäger, and Winston, 2013), so that the prevalence of HAD has recently been cited as just 2% (Heaton et al., 2010). Optimism should be tempered, however, by the continued high prevalence of HAND, which is now slightly over 50% of HIV-infected individuals (Heaton et al., 2010). Whereas much progress in treatment has been made to reduce the burden of dementia, HIV infection often persists in the brain to produce some form of cognitive impairment (Gannon, Khan, and Kolson, 2011).

When first identified in the 1980s, the ADC was observed to manifest diffuse myelin pallor in the cerebral white matter as its most common neuropathological feature (Navia et al., 1986). Cases of HIV infection were reported in which white matter was severely and selectively involved, and in which fulminant fatal leukoencephalopathy was the only clinical manifestation (Jones et al., 1988; Silver et al., 1997). As is now recognized, HIV acts as a Trojan horse, entering the CNS from the bloodstream via infected monocytes to infect glial cells but not neurons (Anthony and Bell, 2008; Gannon et al., 2011). After reaching the brain, the virus is more concentrated in the white matter and basal ganglia than in the cortex (McArthur, Sacktor, and Selnes, 1999; Anthony and Bell, 2008). In typical cases of ADC, pallor of the white matter is accompanied by gliosis, multinucleated giant cells, microglial nodules, and increased numbers of perivascular macrophages (Sharer, 1992). Demyelination is not seen, and white matter pallor is thought to be due to breakdown of the blood–brain barrier and development of vasogenic edema (Power et al., 1993), or to an indirect effect of the host immune response to the virus (Anthony and Bell, 2008). Studies of the cortex in HIV infection have found either no cortical neuronal loss in ADC patients (Seilhean et al., 1993) or that the loss of cortical neurons has no correlation with dementia severity (Weis, Haug, and Budka, 1993; Everall et al., 1994). Cortical neuronal loss may occur late in the course of the disease, but white matter pallor and gliosis are more prominent initially (Gray et al., 1996; Anthony and Bell, 2008). In the ART era, white matter continues to attract neuropathological study (Everall, Hansen, and Masliah, 2005), and a recent autopsy study of HIV-infected brains showed decreased corpus callosum volume (Wohlschlaeger et al., 2009).

Neuroimaging also supports the prominence of white matter changes in HIV infection. Head CT shows some white matter involvement, and brain MRI can disclose patchy or diffuse hyperintensity on T2-weighted images along with with cerebral atrophy (Bencherif and Rottenberg, 1998). The subcortical and cortical gray matter is not affected as early or as significantly as the white matter on neuroimaging scans. MRS studies of patients with ADC suggested that frontal white matter is affected earliest, followed by the basal ganglia and then the frontal gray matter (Chang et al., 1999). Subsequent investigation in HIV patients has found that neuropsychological dysfunction is associated with abnormal MRS findings only within the white matter and not the deep gray matter (Mohamed et al., 2010).

DTI studies in HIV have extended these findings. Early work disclosed abnormalities in NAWM of HIV patients that correlated with disease severity as measured by viral load (Filippi et al., 2000). Later, microstructural damage within association tracts was found in HIV patients who were not demented (Pfefferbaum et al., 2009), and DTI changes in the corpus callosum were found to correlate with cognitive dysfunction (Wu et al., 2006). Moreover, NAWM abnormalities on DTI were found to be more severe in HAD than in nondemented HIV patients (Chen et al., 2009), and DTI global tractography metrics correlated with processing speed and executive function (Tate et al., 2010). Most recently, pervasive white matter dysfunction was found among patients early in the course of AIDS (Xuan et al., 2013), and in older adults with HIV, white matter changes correlated with summary scores of neuropsychological impairment (Nir et al., 2014).

The cognitive profile of HIV brain infection has been steadily clarified. The ADC was initially characterized as a subcortical dementia (Navia, Jordan, and Price, 1986; Tross et al., 1988), based on observations that patients typically had impairments in attention, concentration, memory, and personality, with often striking loss of cognitive speed and mental flexibility (Grant et al., 1987). Tests of choice reaction time showed marked impairment in AIDS patients (Perdices and Cooper, 1989), with usually normal language (McArthur, Sacktor, and Selnes, 1999) but impaired visuospatial function (Tross et al., 1988). Memory was uniformly affected, with a pattern of memory dysfunction rendering ADC a close fit with the hypothesized profile of WMD (Filley, 1998) because of a characteristic retrieval deficit in declarative memory (White et al., 1997) while procedural memory was spared (Jones and Tranel, 1991; Gonzalez et al., 2008). Psychomotor slowing, apathy, and withdrawal were also commonly found (Navia, Jordan, and Price, 1986). An overall relationship between the extent of white matter pallor and degree of cognitive impairment was observed in early studies (Navia et al., 1986; Grant et al., 1987; Price et al., 1988; Bencherif and Rottenberg, 1998). This association was most apparent in ADC with severe dementia, but milder cognitive impairment was also associated with changes in white matter (Post, Berger, and Quencer, 1991). Early and selective involvement of frontal white matter was suggested by a profile of neuropsychological deficits consistent with attentional impairment and executive dysfunction in mildly affected ADC patients (Krikorian and Wrobel, 1991). These observations portrayed a general trend for early white matter involvement producing subtle neurobehavioral features preceding more obvious dysfunction later on. Subsequent studies focused on cognitive slowing as a hallmark feature of HIV cognitive impairment, and the explanation for this problem was postulated to be white matter involvement (Woods et al., 2009).

Whereas the neuropathology of HIV infection has steadily implicated white matter (Navia et al., 1986), and, with further study after the introduction of ART, white matter pathology continues to be recognized (Langford et al., 2002; Langford et al., 2003), this infection does not spare the gray matter (Navia et al., 1986). Indeed, some have regarded changes in the gray matter of the basal ganglia, thalamus, and brain stem as equal to or more prominent than those in the cerebral white matter (Brew, 1999). In light of this complexity, it is problematic to determine precisely what proportion of the neurobehavioral syndrome of ADC can be attributed to white versus gray matter involvement. Some authors have dealt with this conundrum by describing the locus of HIV cognitive impairment with terms such as "frontodiencephalic" (Perdices and Cooper, 1990) and "frontostriatal" (Sahakian et al., 1995), implying that a combination of subcortical white and gray matter pathology may explain the dementia of HIV infection. Cortical involvement has also been proposed in HIV patients (Everall, Hansen, and Masliah, 2005), although one explanation is likely to be AD neuropathology given that HIV-infected persons survive longer with ART and acquire a higher risk for this disease (Brousseau et al., 2009). In view of the neuropathological heterogeneity of HIV infection, a need exists for careful studies correlating clinical features with neuroimaging and neuropathological data to improve the understanding of the origin of neurobehavioral dysfunction in these patients.

Despite the still uncertain clinical-pathological correlation in the HIV infection, further evidence of white matter dysfunction can be found in studies of ART and its effects. As discussed previously, a most welcome development in the 1990s was the marked reduction in the incidence of ADC that accompanied the widespread use of ART (Clifford et al., 2000; Manji, Jäger, and Winston, 2013). This benefit may in part have occurred through the prevention of initial cerebral white matter involvement. The antiretroviral drug zidovudine (AZT), for example, was an early mainstay of AIDS pharmacotherapy, and was shown to improve cognitive function in ADC (Sidtis et al., 1993) in parallel with an improvement accompanied by reduction in MRI white matter lesion burden (Tozzi et al., 1993; Hoogland and Portegies, 2014). Use of the protease inhibitors in the ADC was also associated with improvement in both cognitive function and the extent of white matter involvement on MRI (Filippi et al., 1998; Thurnher et al., 2000). Similarly, a recent case of acutely altered mental status with pontine demyelination in HIV infection was noted to improve both clinically and radiologically after treatment with ART (Tanioka et al., 2007). Whereas this area of inquiry has recently become complicated by concerns that newer forms of ART may be toxic to white matter (Gannon et al., 2011), it is nonetheless encouraging that recent DTI studies have shown that ART can improve white matter structural integrity after the initiation of therapy (Wright et al., 2012).

Available information, therefore, provides considerable support for the hypothesis that the neurobehavioral features of HAND, MND, and particularly HAD may be substantially related to cerebral white matter involvement. This conclusion does not preclude a contribution of changes in gray matter, subcortical and perhaps even cortical, to the clinical presentation. Moreover, the complexity of diffuse metabolic dysfunction in HIV infection, most likely involving a variety of neurotoxic inflammatory mediators (McArthur, Sacktor, and Selnes, 1999; Gannon et al., 2011), should also be considered. Among the factors involved in the pathogenesis of cognitive dysfunction in HIV brain infection, however, white matter dysfunction must be included.

Metabolic disorders

Several disorders in the general category of metabolic dysfunction can result in white matter disease of the brain (Box 6.6). Although considerable overlap exists between metabolic and toxic disorders (Hinchey et al., 1996), the conditions in Box 6.6 can be seen as stemming from a metabolic derangement in which clinical, neuroimaging, or neuropathological evidence of leukoencephalopathy has been observed. The pathophysiology of these diverse disorders is incompletely understood in most cases, but a disturbance of brain metabolism is present in each. Returning to a theme common in the white matter disorders, many of these disorders are reversible if the metabolic derangement is corrected before irreversible damage develops. Neurobehavioral aspects of these disorders have been gradually characterized and consistent findings have emerged, although more study is warranted in the pursuit of specific correlations between well-defined white matter lesions and neurobehavioral features.

BOX 6.6 Metabolic disorders of white matter

- Cobalamin (vitamin B_{12}) deficiency
- Folate deficiency
- Central pontine myelinolysis
- Hypoxia
- Hypertensive encephalopathy
- Eclampsia
- High-altitude cerebral edema

Cobalamin deficiency

For our purposes, the most useful example of this category is dementia related to cobalamin (vitamin B_{12}) deficiency. Cobalamin, routinely measured in the evaluation of neurologic patients, is important in the maintenance of normal myelin, and its deficiency results in the well-known spinal cord syndrome known as subacute combined degeneration (Stabler, 2013). Far less well recognized is that cobalamin deficiency may also cause perivascular degeneration of myelinated fibers in the cerebrum that is identical to the spinal cord pathology in subacute combined degeneration, and these brain lesions have been postulated to account for dementia (Adams and Kubik, 1944). Cobalamin deficiency has been noted in up to 40% of older individuals, and in those who are deficient, as many as 50% may have symptoms referable to cerebral involvement (Goebels and Soyka, 2000). Classically associated with pernicious anemia, it has become clear that neurologically significant cobalamin deficiency can occur in patients with neither anemia nor macrocytosis (Lindenbaum et al., 1988). Thus the routine screening of serum vitamin B_{12} levels in older persons has been recommended (Pennypacker et al., 1992). Some uncertainty exists, however, about the level of cobalamin that indicates significant tissue depletion. Levels below 100 pg/ml are widely thought to produce neurologic mainfestations, and those above 300 pg/ml are regarded by most authorities as normal. B_{12} levels that fall within the 100–300 pg/ml range are intermediate, and many recommend the measurement of serum homocysteine and methlymalonic acid in these patients; if one or both of these metabolites are elevated above the normal range, clinically significant cobalamin deficiency can be assumed (Pennypacker et al., 1992; Stabler, 2013). In patients who are found to be cobalamin deficient, peripheral neuropathy is the most common neurologic syndrome, affecting 70% of those with neurologic complaints (Healton et al., 1991). Clinicians are also well aware of the myelopathy of subacute combined degeneration, but the specific cerebral manifestations of vitamin B_{12} deficiency are not as familiar.

The neurobehavioral manifestations of cobalamin deficiency are generally considered to be protean. Neuropsychiatric dysfunction has often been described (Shorvon et al., 1980), and psychosis appears to be especially common (Hutto, 1997). A study of community-dwelling older women found that metabolically significant cobalamin deficiency increased the risk of severe depression twofold (Penninx et al., 2000). Cognitive loss and dementia have both been documented (Meadows, Kaplan, and Bromfield, 1994; Larner et al., 1999), and the profile of deficits in these syndromes, which may often include cognitive slowing and confusion along with depression, has been interpreted as consistent with subcortical dementia (Tenuisse et al., 1996; Larner et al., 1999). Consistent with this conclusion, Osimani and colleagues (2005) found that B_{12} deficiency produced a reversible dementia characterized by early psychosis and impaired concentration, visuospatial performance, and executive function without language disturbance.

Neuropathological observations of the brain in cobalamin deficiency have long been available (Woltman, 1918; Adams and Kubik 1944), but many clinicians may not associate this disorder with cerebral white matter involvement. The brain lesions usually develop later in the course than spinal cord lesions, and are characterized by perivascular degeneration of myelinated fibers with sparing of cortical and subcortical gray matter (Adams and Kubik, 1944). Laboratory experiments have shown that monkeys deprived of cobalamin have white matter changes in the cerebrum identical to those seen in B_{12}-deficient humans (Agamanolis et al., 1976). The underlying pathophysiology of cobalamin deficiency is thought to involve a disturbance of fatty acid synthesis leading to abnormal myelination (Shevell and Rosenblatt, 1992; Smith and Refsum, 2009). More recently, vascular mechanisms of injury have also been implicated (Tangney et al., 2011).

In the mid-twentieth century, the cerebral white matter lesions seen neuropathologically were proposed to be responsible for the mental status changes in patients with cobalamin deficiency (Adams and Kubik, 1944), and MRI studies have consistently supported this claim. Low cobalamin levels are associated with the severity of MRI white matter lesions (de Lau et al., 2009; Tangney et al., 2011), and several case studies have noted clinical and neuroradiological improvement of leukoencephalopathy occurring in parallel with cobalamin replacement (Chatterjee et al., 1996; Stojsavljević et al., 1997; Vry et al., 2005). A 2-year follow-up study showed that low B_{12} levels were associated with progression of periventricular white matter hyperintensities in lacunar stroke patients (van Overbeek, Staals, and van Oostenbrugge, 2013). A recent literature review concluded that cobalamin deficiency is associated with cognitive impairment, white matter damage, and brain atrophy (Smith and Refsum, 2009).

A variety of pathogenic disturbances occur in the brain and may contribute to the neurobehavioral aspects of this disorder (Penninx et al., 2000). The biochemistry of cobalamin metabolism is complex, and many factors may contribute to the development of dementia. One that has attracted much recent attention is the effect of hyperhomocysteinemia, which is strongly associated with clinically significant cobalamin deficiency (Lindenbaum et al., 1988). Homocysteine has been recognized as an independent risk factor for cerebrovascular disease (Fassbender et al., 1999), and white matter lesions related to elevated homocysteine have been documented (Wright et al., 2005). These considerations further suggest that vascular as well as nonvascular mechanisms are involved in the pathogenesis of cobalamin deficiency (Tangney et al., 2011).

Cobalamin replacement has been observed to benefit neurobehavioral syndromes in some individuals with vitamin B_{12} deficiency. The extent of true reversibility has been debated, as some authorities describe very few responders (Clarfield, 1988), whereas others report a substantial number (Lindenbaum et al., 1988). It is also not entirely clear how significant is the recovery that actually takes place in patients who are reportedly improved. Nevertheless, well-documented examples of meaningful cognitive and neuroimaging recovery with cobalamin treatment (Meadows, Kaplan, and Bromfield, 1994; Chatterjee et al., 1996; Stojsavljević et al., 1997; Vry et al., 2005) suggest that reversible dementia results from white matter involvement in some patients with cobalamin deficiency. Further studies using clinical and neuroimaging measures with larger numbers of subjects will be necessary to expand on these findings. In this regard, encouraging data were recently presented from a community-based European study of older people demonstrating that regular intake of B_{12} reduced the conversion of mild cognitive impairment to dementia, and produced lower grades of MRI white matter hyperintensity (Blasko et al., 2012). The evidence to date thus favors a salutary effect of cobalamin on white matter, and maintenance of at least adequate dietary cobalamin intake has been recommended, especially for older individuals (Smith and Refsum, 2009).

Hydrocephalus

Hydrocephalus refers to the accumulation of excessive water in the cranium (Box 6.7). This added volume is associated with ventricular enlargement, particularly involving the lateral ventricles, and the effects on adjacent brain structures may be relevant for neurobehavioral function. Normally the total volume of cerebrospinal fluid (CSF) within the neuraxis is about 140 cm^3, of which about 25 cm^3 are found in the four ventricles (Fishman, 1992). Higher ventricular volumes of CSF can develop either because additional CSF occupies intracranial space and compresses brain tissue or because the CSF replaces the parenchyma lost through brain atrophy (hydrocephalus ex vacuo). The cerebral white matter is implicated in both of these situations, because either an excessive volume of CSF may injure the periventricular regions, or changes in white matter contribute to cerebral atrophy.

BOX 6.7 Varieties of hydrocephalus

- Early hydrocephalus
- Hydrocephalus ex vacuo
- Normal pressure hydrocephalus

Hydrocephalus can be symptomatic at any age, and its most prominent neuropathological effects are exerted on cerebral white matter (Di Rocco et al., 1977; Akai et al., 1987; Del Bigio, 1993; Del Bigio et al., 1994; Leinonen et al., 2012). Cortical damage is uncommon, occurring only late in the disease course, and involvement of the deep gray matter is also less marked than white matter injury, indicating that the cognitive effects of hydrocephalus are mainly related to tract damage, at least when diagnostic and treatment issues are most crucial. Hydrocephalus occurring acutely in the context of mass lesions, trauma, infarction, and the like will not be reviewed here, because of methodological difficulties in studying the impact of specific white matter neuropathology in these settings. Much useful information, however, has been gained from study of hydrocephalus that arises chronically. In those with chronic sequelae of hydrocephalus, the medical and economic impact can be substantial, and the problem of hydrocephalus in older people represents an especially challenging diagnostic and therapeutic problem in behavioral neurology (Del Bigio, 1998; Shprecher, Schwalb, and Kurlan, 2008; Wilson and Williams, 2010).

Normal pressure hydrocephalus

Few conditions in clinical neurology produce such diagnostic, pathophysiological, and therapeutic perplexity as normal pressure hydrocephalus (NPH). Since the first description of this disease in the 1960s (Adams et al., 1965), NPH has alternately been heralded as an often-overlooked reversible dementia and a questionable entity that may not even exist. While neurologists generally agree that NPH is a diagnosable disease, and the opportunity to effectively treat a dementia syndrome is of course appealing, the vagaries of diagnosis and the risks of surgical treatment are not insubstantial. When patients present with symptoms and signs suggesting NPH, the neurologist is thus challenged to decide upon which individuals actually have the disease and, of these, which ones are likely to benefit from surgical treatment. Such patients are not infrequently seen in neurologic practice, and it has been estimated that 1% to 5% of older people with dementia may have NPH (Wilson and Williams, 2010). The continuing clinical conundrum of this disease will be discussed here in light of evidence that it can be interpreted as a disorder of cerebral white matter.

NPH classically presents with the clinical triad of dementia, gait disorder, and urinary incontinence (Adams et al., 1965). All of these problems were related to frontal lobe damage in the original description of the disease, and cognitive slowing and apathy were called out as prominent features of the dementia (Adams et al., 1965). More recent investigations have led to a consensus that the neuroanatomic alterations of NPH involve the periventricular white matter and disrupt frontal-subcortical circuits (Del Bigio, 2010; Wilson and Williams, 2010). Some cases are thought to follow meningitis, traumatic brain injury, or subarachnoid hemorrhage, but many remain idiopathic despite thorough investigation (Graff-Radford, 1999). CT scans show enlarged ventricles and relatively normal cortical gyri without sulcal enlargement, findings that offer some help but are often difficult to distinguish from other neuropathological states and normal aging.

MRI may reveal additional high signal lesions in the periventricular white matter, and it has been proposed that transpendymal CSF flow is a clue to a good outcome with shunting (Jack et al., 1987). Other investigations have not been consistent in supporting this claim (Graff-Radford, 1999). At present, it is thought that no neuroimaging finding can be used to predict outcome after shunt surgery (Wilson and Williams, 2010). MTI studies have shown a low MTR in the NAWM of patients with NPH (Hähnel et al., 2000), and recent DTI studies have demonstrated improvement in corona radiata FA after shunt surgery or ventriculostomy (Assaf et al., 2006). Data such as these may assist in demonstrating white matter damage in NPH, and its restitution after treatment.

The diagnosis is currently made by identifying the clinical triad, finding a consistent neuroimaging pattern, and ruling out other etiologic possibilities; many clinicians also perform a high-volume CSF "tap test" because a temporary improvement in gait and sometimes cognition may help predict a good surgical outcome (Fisher, 1978). Among patients accurately diagnosed with NPH, 46% to 64% may have a favorable response to shunt surgery, and the gait disorder usually responds better than dementia and urinary dysfunction (Wilson and Williams, 2010). The favorable response to shunt surgery suggests that damaged white matter in NPH may exhibit some degree of plasticity, especially if the disease is treated at an early stage.

The pathophysiology of NPH continues to be a puzzle. Adams and colleagues (1965) offered the first and still most familiar theory, proposing that obstruction of CSF outflow causes ventricular enlargement without cortical atrophy; the assumption here is that the outflow obstruction is at the level of the arachnoid villi. The CSF pressure remains normal because of Pascal's law (Force = Pressure × Area), which predicts that with an increased ventricular wall area, the force applied to the brain parenchyma can be high while pressure is still normal (Adams et al., 1965). This explanation, however, has been questioned by some. Symon and colleagues (Symon, Dorsch, and Stephens, 1972) found episodes of raised intracranial pressure throughout the night in patients with NPH, and suggested that a better term for the condition might be "episodically raised pressure hydrocephalus." Geschwind (1968) questioned the theory of Adams and colleagues on physical grounds, pointing out that the properties of the ventricular wall structure pertain to the pathogenesis of NPH. These ideas helped lead to an alternative hypothesis, which is that ischemia and infarction in the cerebral white matter may lead to ventriculomegaly, and the reduced tensile strength of the white matter could cause further ventricular enlargement under the stress of intraventricular pulse pressure (Earnest et al., 1974). In support of this notion is the finding of reduced cerebral blood flow in the white matter of NPH patients, most notably in the periventricular regions (Momjian et al., 2004). This theory thus suggests a possible overlap of NPH with BD (Wilson and Williams, 2010).

Most authorities, however, still favor the existence of NPH as a discrete entity, recognizing that it may coexist with other neuropathologies. The major comorbid neuropathology of NPH within the white matter is BD, but the two diseases can be distinguished at the microstructural level. CSF sulfatide is markedly increased in BD, consistent with ischemic demyelination (Tullberg et al., 2000), and white matter axons are damaged in BD but relatively intact in NPH, helping explain why BD has a worse prognosis (Tullberg et al., 2009). Moreover, whereas MRI white matter lesions in NPH may be very similar to those of BD (Tullberg et al., 2002), NPH patients without comorbid vascular white matter disease have a better outcome after shunt surgery (Boon et al., 1999;

Tullberg et al., 2000). Clinically, the beneficial response to surgery seen in many NPH patients seems to justify the conclusion that the disease may exist in isolation, but that white matter ischemia and infarction can often be present in addition and limit its reversibility.

Regardless of the pathogenetic mechanism of NPH, neuropathological findings are generally consistent with primary involvement of white matter. Details of the neuropathology have been clarified over many years of investigation, and the cerebral white matter bears the brunt of the damage (Di Rocco et al., 1977; Akai et al., 1987; Del Bigio, 1993; Del Bigio et al., 1994; Del Bigio, 1998; Del Bigio, Wilson, and Enno, 2003; Del Bigio and Enno, 2008; Del Bigio, 2010; Leinonen et al., 2012). The corpus callosum is affected, and its effacement can be seen well on sagittal MRI images (Wilson and Williams, 2010). In the periventricular white matter, evidence exists for direct mechanical compression (Di Rocco et al., 1977; Del Bigio, 2010) as well as ischemic demyelination and infarction (Akai et al., 1987). Gray matter, meanwhile, both of the subcortical nuclear structures and of the cerebral cortex, is less affected, although with severe and prolonged hydrocephalus there may be some neuronal damage in these regions (Del Bigio, 1993; Del Bigio, Wilson, and Enno, 2003; Del Bigio, 2010; Leinonen et al., 2012). As is true of other white matter disorders, however, unrelated neuropathology in the cortex can be found in patients with NPH. One group addressed this issue, and found that 10 of 38 patients thought clinically to have NPH actually had biopsy-proven AD (Bech et al., 1997). BD may also be present in the white matter and compromise recovery after shunting procedures (Wilson and Williams 2010).

The neurobehavioral profile of NPH has been studied in increasing detail. Comprehensive literature reviews have concluded that NPH exhibits neuropsychological features typical of subcortical dementia (Derix, 1994; Devito et al., 2005). Prominent frontal manifestations are seen, including cognitive slowing, inattention, and perseveration, and while memory loss occurs, aphasia, apraxia, and agnosia are not observed (Derix, 1994; Devito et al., 2005). Cognitive slowing, executive dysfunction, impaired attention, poor memory, apathy, and depression have all been noted in NPH patients (Gustafson and Hagberg, 1978; Ogino et al., 2006; Chaudhry et al., 2007; Hellström et al., 2008). Gallassi and colleagues (1991) compared NPH with BD patients and found these groups to have similar cognitive impairment in comparison to control subjects. Later, Iddon and colleagues (1999) demonstrated selective executive function deficits in patients with NPH that were not present in AD patients with comparable dementia severity. A recent DTI study of NPH found that scores on the Frontal Assessment Battery – a measure sensitive to executive dysfunction (Dubois et al., 2000) – correlated with microstructural abnormalities in the frontal and parietal white matter (Kanno et al., 2011). Summarizing the existing literature, Wilson and Williams (2010) concluded that frontal and subcortical systems are primarily involved in this disease. Thus, in light of demonstrable white matter involvement and the similarity of cognitive deficits with those produced by other white matter disorders, NPH merits classification as a white matter disorder capable of causing dementia (Filley, 2012).

The treatment of NPH is surgical, and involves placement of a diversionary shunt in the brain to reduce ventricular volume. These shunts are rubber tubes with one-way valves that can be positioned to provide ventriculoperitoneal, ventriculoatrial, or lumboperitoneal CSF drainage. The critical clinical issue revolves around the decision as to which patients are most likely to benefit from a shunting procedure. This determination is not trivial, particularly in older patients, because of the high incidence of shunt surgery complications such as anesthesia reactions, intracranial hemorrhage, and infection (Vanneste et al., 1992). Although clinicians have individual preferences, it is reasonable to refer for surgery only those patients who have the full clinical triad, neuroimaging studies consistent with NPH, a positive tap test, no evidence of other cerebral diseases, and no prohibitive surgical risk. Graff-Radford (1999) has suggested that additional favorable prognostic signs are the presence of dementia for less than 2 years, a known cause of NPH, and the gait abnormality preceding the dementia.

Gait disorder is viewed by most authorities as the feature of NPH most responsive to surgical treatment (Wilson and Williams, 2010; Klassen and Ahlskog, 2011). A recent controlled trial of shunted NPH patients, however, demonstrated improvements in cognitive speed and sustained attention as well as gait (Katzen et al., 2011). The improvement in cognition may result from restoration of white matter integrity, as both MRI (Tullberg et al., 2002) and DTI (Akiguchi et al., 2008) studies have suggested.

BOX 6.8 **Neoplasms of white matter**

- Gliomas
- Gliomatosis cerebri
- Primary central nervous system lymphoma
- Focal white matter tumor

Another study found that neurologic improvement after the tap test occurred in association with higher white matter integrity as assessed by DTI (Demura et al., 2012), indicating that even temporary CSF drainage may improve the structure of white matter. Last, an intriguing preliminary study of a medical treatment for NPH found that acetazolamide reduced periventricular white matter hyperintensity burden and even improved gait in some subjects (Alperin et al., 2014). These observations add further support to the contention that dementia in NPH is a result of cerebral white matter damage.

Neoplasms

A number of brain neoplasms affect the brain white matter (Box 6.8). In a discussion of brain tumors and neurobehavioral sequelae, the first issue to be dealt with is whether there is any meaningful connection at all. The more salient clinical features of these mass lesions – headache, focal neurologic signs, seizures, and the like – often so dominate the picture that cognitive loss and emotional dysfunction are seen as less critical. Moreover, as discussed earlier, treatment-related cognitive impairment from radiation and cancer chemotherapy is well recognized. Yet neurobehavioral features are also appreciated as clinical aspects of brain tumors, particularly those involving the frontal and temporal lobes (Filley and Kleinschmidt-DeMasters, 1995). A setting in which this issue is highly relevant is the psychiatric clinic, as it is well known that brain tumors can present with such problems as depression, mania, personality change, abulia, visual or auditory hallucinations, or panic attacks, in some cases even when the neoplasm has no neurologic manifestations (Madhusoodanan et al., 2004). A large, population-based study conducted over a decade demonstrated that patients with new-onset psychiatric disorder had a 19-fold increase in brain tumor incidence within the first month after the diagnosis (Benros et al., 2009).

Cognitive dysfunction has also been described in brain tumor patients that appears to be directly related to the disease and its cerebral localization. In contrast to traditional neurologic thinking that cognitive dysfunction in brain tumor patients is usually related to radiation and chemotherapy, the importance of cognitive deficits in tumor patients before any treatment has recently been better appreciated (Taphoorn and Klein, 2004; Klein, Duffau, and De Witt Hamer, 2012). In a neuropsychological study of patients with frontal and temporal lobe neoplasms who were examined before any treatment to obliterate the neoplasm was offered, more than 90% had cognitive deficits in at least one domain, with the most common impairment – 78% – involving executive function (Tucha et al., 2000). No neuroimaging or neuropathological data were provided in this study, but nevertheless the findings are not surprising in that a brain neoplasm involving the frontal and temporal lobes can almost certainly be expected to impact structures that subserve cognition and emotion (Filley and Kleinschmidt-DeMasters, 1995).

A discussion of brain tumors that selectively damage white matter of the brain, however, may appear to be very limited. Brain tumors may not affect one discrete region, and instead may involve widespread areas of both gray and white matter. This characteristic, together with the associated edema and mass effect that so often occur, may render correlations of tumor location with neurobehavioral status problematic. Even early in the clinical course, when the more limited growth and extent of the tumor might predict a more focal location, the full extent of the neoplasm may not be evident, and correlations of lesion site with clinical status are tentative at best. The leukotoxic effects of radiation and chemotherapy can also complicate the understanding of neurobehavioral impairments in individuals with brain tumors.

An underappreciated aspect of primary brain malignancies, however, is their decided proclivity to involve white matter as an initial event. Parenchymal brain neoplasms typically arise from white matter structures throughout the brain (Adams and Graham, 1989; Canoll and Goldman, 2008; Bohman et al., 2010), and disseminate along myelinated tracts (Giese and Westphal, 1996; Geer and Grossman, 1997); major effects on white matter are thus apparent throughout the clinical course. The conventional understanding of how such tumors present clinically emphasizes familiar problems such as headache, focal signs such as hemiparesis and aphasia, and seizures

(DeAngelis, 2001), and these presentations are indeed very important. But the earliest neuropathology does not typically involve the cerebral cortex or produce increased intracranial pressure, and is instead the presence of microscopic collections of malignant cells deep within the cerebral white matter. Hence the initial clinical manifestations of such tumors, if they could be reliably detected, might in fact be much different, and actually implicate subtle neurobehavioral dysfunction related to white matter involvement. Moreover, white matter neuropathology may continue to produce prominent neurobehavioral effects throughout the course of the disease. The proposition that neoplastic white matter involvement can be an important source of neurobehavioral dysfunction, including dementia, is now considered, using gliomatosis cerebri as a prototype malignancy.

Gliomatosis cerebri

Gliomas are malignant neoplasms that arise from glial cells in the brain or spinal cord. The three major gliomas that develop in the brain are the astrocytoma, the oligodendroglioma, and the ependymoma, with the great majority of gliomas classified as one of the first two of these varieties. An unusual type of glioma is gliomatosis cerebri, a diffusely infiltrative glial cell neoplasm of the brain that stands out as a particularly illustrative example of white matter–cognition relationships in neoplasia. Although this disease has infrequently been reported (Ponce et al., 1998), it serves our purposes well because it is a neoplastic disorder confined mainly to the cerebral white matter throughout most of its course (Filley et al., 2003). Because the diagnosis has usually been made at autopsy, the incidence and prevalence of the disease may be underestimated, and advanced neuroimaging techniques may increase its clinical recognition during life (Keene, Jimenez, and Hsu, 1999).

Gliomatosis cerebri usually appears in adults, although it may arise in children as well (Pal et al., 2008). The insidious onset of behavioral and mental status changes is the most frequent manifestation, but headache, motor dysfunction, and seizures may occur as alternate presentations (Couch and Weiss, 1974; Artigas et al., 1985; Taipa et al., 2011). Diagnosis in life is challenging because the clinical presentation can be consistent with a wide range of disorders featuring diffuse white matter involvement, and even with brain biopsy there may be confusion about the accurate classification of this lesion. The clinical course is highly variable, with survival durations reported from weeks to many years (Couch and Weiss, 1974; Artigas et al., 1985), but a fatal outcome has been most common. A recent review concluded that the median survival in this disease is only 18.5 months (Chen et al., 2013). Surgery, chemotherapy, and radiotherapy may be partially effective, but no curative treatment has been discovered. Exceptional cases have shown a dramatic, if unexplained, response to radiotherapy (Shintani, Tsuruoka, and Shiigai, 2000; Mattox, Lark, and Adamson, 2012).

As opposed to gliomas that tend to be single or multicentric in location, gliomatosis cerebri involves infiltration of contiguous areas of the cerebrum. The disease is often bilateral because of extension across the corpus callosum. Although gray matter of the deep subcortical nuclei and cerebral cortex may be infiltrated, the major neuropathological burden falls on the white matter, where there is destruction of the myelin sheath with suprisingly little damage to axons (Artigas et al., 1985). Thus gliomatosis cerebri features widespread white matter infiltration with relatively preserved cerebral architecture. Periventricular white matter often undergoes additional damage because of hydrocephalus and increased intracranial pressure that can follow malignant aqueductal stenosis or tumor overgrowth (Couch and Weiss, 1974).

The origin of the abnormal cells in gliomatosis cerebri has been controversial, and the small number of cases thus far has hindered thorough investigation. Nevin (1938), the first to describe the disease, believed it to represent a blastomatous malformation of glial cells. Many investigators, however, believe that gliomatosis cerebri represents a true neoplasm. Microscopic examination and immunohistochemistry have disclosed that the lesion is a glial cell tumor usually composed of neoplastic astrocytes (Duffy et al., 1980), but occasionally made up of oligodendrocytes (Balko, Blisard, and Samaha, 1992) or cells transitional between the two (Artigas et al., 1985). More recently, strong TP53 immunostaining has been found in gliomatosis cerebri, suggesting a commonality with diffuse fibrillary astrocytomas that may also display this feature (Filley et al., 2003). In any case, the cells are malignant and the clinical outcome is usually poor.

Modern neuroimaging has greatly improved the detection and diagnosis of gliomatosis cerebri, although no pathognomonic neuroradiological features exist.

CT can reveal low-density white matter changes reminiscent of either demyelination or dysmyelination (Geremia, Wollman, and Foust, 1988), and there may be lesion enhancement late in the course (Hayek and Valvanis, 1982). MRI has generally proven more sensitive than CT in detecting white matter changes in this disease (del Carpio-O'Donovan et al., 1996; Filley et al., 2003). An early MRI study found poor gray matter–white matter demarcation as one sign of neoplastic invasion (Koslow et al., 1992), and more recent work revealed widespread high signal in the white matter on T2-weighted images, prominently involving the frontal lobes and the corpus callosum (Keene, Jimenez, and Hsu, 1999). MRS of gliomatosis cerebri disclosed neurometabolic features similar to those of gliomas, but no specific MR spectra were identified (Pyhtinen, 2000). In contrast, DTI may offer more to the evaluation of gliomatosis cerebri by virtue of its potential to distinguish the tumor from normal white matter tracts, to detect neoplastic tract deformation, and to assist in operative planning (Lee, 2012). Most recently, the technique of diffusion kurtosis imaging (DKI) has been applied to neoplastic white matter disease, and this technique appears to differentiate tissue characteristics of the involved regions that can be associated with treatment response (Baek et al., 2012). Functional neuroimaging with positron emission tomography has disclosed hypometabolism in the cerebral cortex consistent with disconnection from subcortical structures (Plowman, Saunders, and Maisey, 1998).

The neurobehavioral alterations of patients with gliomatosis cerebri have been only partially characterized, and no systematic neuropsychological study is available. This paucity of information is in large part due to the rarity of the disease; a review published in 1985 could locate only 58 cases in the literature (Artigas et al., 1985). Moreover, as is often the case in studies of neoplasia, few reports contain substantial detail on neurobehavioral aspects of this disease. Despite these shortcomings, however, personality and mental status changes are repeatedly stated to be the most striking presenting and persistent findings in these patients, whether in the initial or in later stages of the disease (Sarhaddi, Bravo, and Cyrus, 1973; Couch and Weiss, 1974; Artigas et al., 1985; Filley et al., 2003). The mental changes are typically described as confusion, disorientation, and memory loss that proceed on to dementia, and focal cortical signs such as aphasia are infrequent (Filley et al., 2003). Neuropsychiatric dysfunction, usually described as personality change, apathy, or fatigue, is also frequently cited as an initial or early manifestation, and can plausibly be associated with involvement of frontal white matter (Filley et al., 2003). One intriguing case report described a man with autopsy-proven gliomatosis cerebri who had developed depression and then schizophrenia-like psychosis for nearly 2 years before progressive dementia appeared (Vassallo and Allen, 1995). As has been observed in other white matter disorders (Filley and Gross, 1992; Filley, 2012), psychosis can precede dementia in gliomatosis cerebri.

Thus, whereas the presence of gray matter involvement must be considered, the clinical features of this disease are consistent with those expected from diffuse white matter infiltration. Indeed, the localization of the neoplasm strongly indicates that damage to cerebral white matter plays a prominent role in the syndromes produced: The centrum semiovale is involved in 76% of cases, whereas the cerebral cortex is affected in only 19%; and the thalamus and basal ganglia are infiltrated in 43% and 34% of cases, respectively (Lantos and Bruner, 2000). In light of these findings, the classification of gliomatosis cerebri as a neoplastic form of white matter disease causing dementia seems justified (Filley et al., 2003). Study of other neoplasms with early clinical, neuropsychological, and MRI assessment may reveal that they behave similarly.

Genetic diseases

The last category of white matter disorder to be discussed is the large and expanding group of genetic diseases (Box 6.9). White matter can be affected by a

BOX 6.9 Genetic white matter diseases

- Cerebral autosomal-dominant arteriopathy with subcortical infarcts and leukoencephalopathy (CADASIL)
- Leukodystrophies
- Fragile X tremor ataxia syndrome
- Aminoacidurias
- Phakomatosis
- Mucopolysaccharidosis
- Muscular dystrophy
- Callosal agenesis

wide range of genetic diseases, and dementia can be the result. These diseases are thought to be rare and are incompletely understood; many, such as vanishing white matter disease (van der Knaap et al., 1997), are being regularly discovered by combined MRI and genetic analyses. Patients with these diseases typically come to the attention of child neurologists, but occasional individuals develop initial clinical features as adults (Sedel et al., 2008). At any age, however, neurobehavioral manifestations are prominent. Genetic white matter disorders highlight the importance of myelinated tracts in the ontogeny of behavior because they demonstrate how defective white matter can profoundly disrupt the development of cognition and emotion.

The understanding of inherited neurologic disorders continues to evolve, and many unanswered questions remain about their pathogenesis and classification. Among the white matter disorders, a number of familial leukoencephalopathies are defined by their genetic origin, whereas many others have an unknown etiology. Although a genetic cause can generally be assumed in these diseases, it has been estimated that at least half of the childhood leukoencephalopathies seen clinically remain idiopathic and unclassified (van der Knaap et al., 1999). Neuropathologically, the classic distinction between dysmyelination – seen in leukodystrophies – and demyelination – characteristic of MS and other inflammatory white matter diseases – is still generally useful as one way to conceptualize the leukoencephalopathies. Many genetic diseases show a predilection for the cerebral white matter, and the impact of widespread dysmyelination can be clinically devastating. The goal of this section is to consider the impact of genetic white matter disease on cognition, specifically with respect to the propensity of these diseases to cause dementia in adulthood.

Cadasil

The discovery of cerebral autosomal-dominant arteriopathy with subcortical infarcts and leukoencephalopathy (CADASIL) (Tournier-Lasserve et al., 1993; Chabriat et al., 2009) has strongly supported the idea that ischemic white matter disease can lead to dementia. CADASIL is the most common genetic white matter disease to be seen by adult neurologists, and can be classified as both a genetic and a vascular disorder. The disease is in essence a genetic form of vascular dementia, and even though its etiology is entirely distinct from that of vascular dementia, the pathogenesis of dementia is quite similar. CADASIL bears a close clinical resemblance to BD but is due to genetic mutation, and hypertension and related vascular risk factors are typically absent. Credit for the first clinical recognition of CADASIL goes to Van Bogaert (1955), who described a disease similar to BD in two sisters. Several large pedigrees gathered from around the world have confirmed that CADASIL maps to the NOTCH3 region of chromosome 19q12 (Tournier-Lasserve et al., 1993; Chabriat et al., 2009; Hervé and Chabriat, 2010), and several different mutations at this locus appear to be responsible.

Patients with CADASIL resemble those with BD in many clinical and neuroimaging respects, but the usual absence of hypertension and earlier age of onset are distinctive. The disease typically begins in middle to late adulthood, with onset at a mean age of 45 (Hervé and Chabriat, 2010). Stroke, dementia, mood disorders, and migraine with aura have been noted to be the most frequent clinical features (Chabriat et al., 1995; Hervé and Chabriat, 2010). White matter disease resembling LA is regularly encountered on MRI, even in presymptomatic persons, and takes the form of scattered subcortical lesions that progress over many years into confluent leukoencephalopathy (Harris and Filley, 2001). Neurobehavioral dysfunction without significant elemental neurologic deficits may dominate the clinical course, and early neuropsychiatric dysfunction has been observed to antedate the gradual appearance of cognitive decline and dementia (Filley et al., 1999a). The profile of cognitive dysfunction often features abulia, sustained attention deficit, impaired memory retrieval, sparing of language, and perseveration (Filley et al., 1999a; Harris and Filley, 2001; Chabriat et al., 2009).

The diagnosis of CADASIL can be challenging, and similarities with MS and other white matter disorders are numerous. Many patients are in fact first seen by neurologists for the possibility of MS after a brain MRI has been noted to disclose extensive white matter disease in a young adult. The disease should be considered in normotensive adults with significant leukoencephalopathy and clinical features that include stroke, cognitive disturbance, depression, and migraine with aura; a family history consistent with autosomal-dominant inheritance is also useful. Definitive diagnosis requires blood testing to confirm a NOTCH3 mutation (Tournier-Lasserve et al., 1993; Chabriat et al., 2009). Skin biopsy can also be performed, and the characteristic ultrastructural changes of granular osmiophilic inclusions in the vascular smooth muscle of small arteries can be seen using electron microscopy (Chabriat et al., 2009).

The pathogenesis of neurobehavioral dysfunction in CADASIL is being better elucidated. Although many patients have a mixture of subcortical white and gray matter disease, a careful reading of published reports shows that dementia can be seen in those with white matter involvement alone (Hedera and Friedland, 1997). Studies using conventional MRI in CADASIL have demonstrated that cognitive decline can be correlated with white matter lesion burden (Dichgans et al., 1999). As in SIVD, both infarction and ischemia appear to contribute to cognitive dysfunction (Chabriat et al., 2009). Whereas conventional MRI often shows extensive white matter disease, the neuropathology of CADASIL appears to extend beyond these areas of involvement, as studies with MTI (Iannucci et al., 2001), MRS (Akhvlediani et al., 2010), and DTI (Chabriat et al., 1999) have disclosed microstructural damage within NAWM. Cortical pathology involving neuronal apoptosis develops only late in the disease (Chabriat et al., 2009), and likely exerts little impact on the neurobehavioral profile.

CADASIL has a unique neuroradiological pattern of white matter involvement as determined by MRI. Specific regions are known from neuropathological studies to be particularly vulnerable in patients with CADASIL, with the frontal and temporal lobes most affected (Craggs et al., 2014). MRI also demonstrates this localization, and a particularly helpful neuroradiological sign is the extention of white matter changes into the anterior temporal regions, areas usually spared in most white matter disorders (O'Sullivan et al., 2001). The corpus callosum, commonly damaged in MS, is less affected in CADASIL, and this neuroradiological distinction is also helpful (O'Sullivan et al., 2001). Damage in the temporal and frontal lobes correlates with attentional, memory, visuospatial, and conceptual dysfunction (Yousry et al., 1999), and has been interpreted in terms of cerebral disconnection (Craggs et al., 2014). The predilection for frontal and particularly temporal lobe involvement also helps explain the early neuropsychiatric dysfunction that may occur in CADASIL (Filley et al., 1999; Harris and Filley, 2001). Depression is an especially troublesome issue that may find explanation in this neuropathological localization. As in other white matter disorders (Filley and Gross, 1992; Filley, 2012), the tendency for cognitive loss to follow psychiatric dysfunction has been encountered in CADASIL. Longitudinal study of individuals with CADASIL will be needed to establish this sequence more securely.

Metachromatic leukodystrophy

Metachromatic leukodystrophy (MLD) is the best recognized of the leukodystrophies, and the most likely to develop in adulthood, followed by globoid cell leukodystrophy and adrenoleukodystrophy. The usual age of onset is in the second or third year of life, but later presentations have permitted the study of MLD well into adolescence and adulthood. Initial manifestations in infants and children include developmental delay, intellectual deterioration, gait disorder, strabismus, and spasticity, and dysmyelination in peripheral nerves also leads to neuropathy with hyporeflexia. Steady deterioration progresses, and inexorably leads to a vegetative state and death within a few years. A later age of onset confers a less severe prognosis, although diagnosis of this disease always confers a poor outcome. Of the adult cases of leukodystrophy, MLD has received the most neurobehavioral study (Hyde, Ziegler, and Weinberger, 1992; Filley and Gross, 1992; Shapiro et al., 1994; Black, Taber, and Hurley, 2003).

The neuropathology of MLD is well established as diffuse cerebral dysmyelination, implying that normal myelination has not occurred (Köhler, 2010; Orchard and Tolar, 2010; Gieselmann and Krägeloh-Mann, 2010). The leukodystrophies as a group share many neuropathological features, including reduced brain weight, ventriculomegaly, thinning of the corpus callosum, reduced myelin staining, loss of oligodendrocytes, and sparing of axons until late in the course (Lyon, Fattal-Valevski, and Kolodny, 2006). As reviewed in Chapter 3, myelin is laid down in an orderly sequence that begins in utero and continues until decades later. Dysmyelination, closely related to hypomyelination (Schiffmann and van der Knaap, 2009) and vaculoating myelinopathy (Lyon, Fattal-Valevski, and Kolodny, 2006), implies the abnormal development of myelin because of a metabolic error preventing the normal events leading to the establishment and maintenance of the myelin sheath. Although some abnormalities of white matter can also be observed in primary neuronal diseases such as Tay-Sachs disease and Niemann-Pick disease, these effects occur secondarily because of neuronal dysfunction and metabolic effects on oligodendrocytes (Folkerth, 2000). Long myelinated pathways are mainly affected, while U-fibers are spared in most of the leukodystrophies, including MLD (Lyon, Fattal-Valevski, and Kolodny, 2006). Loss of myelin is a major contributor to cognitive impairment, and it has recently become clear that axonal destruction is still more critical (Mar and Noetzel, 2010).

MLD is an autosomal recessive disease caused by a deficiency of arylsulfatase A, an enzyme that converts sulfatide to cerebroside, a major constituent of myelin (Austin et al., 1968). Sulfatide accumulates in myelin and the lysosomes of oligodendrocytes, and is visible microscopically as metachromatically staining granules, a characteristic microscopic feature of MLD. The clinical diagnosis is confirmed by the finding of reduced arylsulfatase A activity in leukocytes. Diffuse dysmyelination occurs in the cerebrum, cerebellum, spinal cord, and peripheral nerves. In the brain, the eventual death of oligodendrocytes precludes the possibility of any remyelination as the disease worsens.

Neuroimaging studies are useful in demonstrating the dysmyelination of MLD. Head CT shows symmetric low-density white matter lesions and ventriculomegaly (Skomer, Stears, and Austin, 1983), and MRI, particularly with the use of T2-weighted images, provides a more detailed depiction of diffuse and symmetric cerebral white matter involvement (Filley and Gross, 1992). In contrast to adrenoleukodystrophy, which shows a posterior cerebral distribution of white matter disease, MLD features early frontal involvement that soon advances to widespread cerebral dysmyelination (Schiffmann and van der Knaap, 2009).

In older children and adults with MLD, the longer disease course has permitted detailed study of neurobehavioral features. Dementia is the major syndrome, typically dominated by frontal lobe dysfunction with disinhibition, impulsivity, and poor attention span. Neuropsychological testing has revealed a pattern of deficits that include inattention, poor vigilance, impaired memory, relatively intact language, impaired visuospatial function, and executive dysfunction (Shapiro et al., 1994). These observations are consistent with a frontal predominance of dysmyelination (Shapiro et al., 1994; Schiffmann and van der Knaap, 2009). In addition, a tendency for psychosis to herald the onset of the disease has been noted (Hyde, Ziegler, and Weinberger, 1992; Filley and Gross, 1992; Black, Taber, and Hurley, 2003; Kumperscak et al., 2007). In a thorough literature review, Hyde and colleagues (1992) reported that 53% of published cases of adolescent and early-adult onset MLD had psychosis as an early clinical feature. It has been proposed that psychosis occurs because of disrupted corticocortical connections between frontal and temporal lobes (Hyde, Ziegler, and Weinberger, 1992), and that dementia follows as more extensive dysmyelination proceeds to disrupt other connections and hence result in more widespread cerebral dysfunction (Filley and Gross, 1992). More recent studies have examined genotypic differences in adult MLD, finding that the genotype associated with psychosis and dementia tends to manifest frontally predominant leukodystrophy (Rauschka et al., 2006).

The treatment of MLD has been limited to only supportive therapy, but newer possibilities include enzyme replacement, stem cell transplantation, and gene therapy (Gieselmann and Krägeloh-Mann, 2010). These approaches shed some light on the possibility that repairing white matter may have a beneficial effect on cognition. The study of bone marrow transplantation has been instructive with regard to whether restoration of normal arylsulfatase A activity can lead to clinical benefit (Krivit et al., 1990). This procedure entails the engraftment of hematopoietic stem cells from healthy donors, which results in normal monocytes entering the recipient brain to correct the deficient enzymatic activity (Krivit, Peters, and Shapiro, 1999). Early treatment presumably takes advantage of oligodendrocytes that are still viable so that myelination can be normalized. The procedure can restore the activity of the enzyme, and in some cases stabilize cognitive deterioration in MLD, both in children (Shapiro, Lipton, and Krivit, 1992) and in adults (Navarro et al., 1996). The beneficial effects on cognition may be a result of improved structure of cerebral white matter as shown on MRI (Krivit et al., 1990). Most recently, a small controlled study of young adults with MLD showed that hematopoietic stem cell transplantation was associated with stability of neuropsychological function and

MRI-determined myelin integrity and cerebral atrophy (Solders et al., 2014). While the phenotypic variability of MLD patients and disease severity both impact treatment efficacy (Orchard and Tolar, 2010), bone marrow tranplantation offers some evidence for the neurobehavioral importance of white matter in that cognitive improvement can occur in parallel with restoration of myelinated tracts.

Fragile X tremor ataxia syndrome

As mentioned at the beginning of this chapter, neurodegeneration has not been listed as a potential cause of WMD, but this view may require revision. In the past decade, knowledge has rapidly accumulated regarding the inherited neurodegenerative disease fragile X tremor ataxia syndrome (FXTAS) (Leehey, 2009). Typically seen in older men, FXTAS is due to a cytosine-guanine-guanine (CGG) repeat expansion in the premutation range of the fragile X mental retardation 1 (*fMR1*) gene (Leehey, 2009). The CGG repeat expansion of FXTAS is in the 55–200 range, in contrast to the fragile X syndrome, the most common heritable form of mental retardation and autism, in which CGG repeats of > 200 occur (Leehey, 2009). While intention tremor and gait ataxia are characteristic, individuals with FXTAS also develop cognitive impairment that can often progress to dementia, characterized by executive dysfunction and slowed processing speed in the absence of language disturbance (Grigsby et al., 2008). In addition, mood, anxiety, and other psychiatric disorders are often encountered in patients with FXTAS (Bourgeois et al., 2009).

Widespread neuronal pathology is found in FXTAS (Hagerman and Hagerman, 2004), but evidence is accumulating that white matter is significantly involved in the pathogenesis of dementia. MRI scans disclose scattered cerebral white matter hyperintensities and atrophy, and the unusual finding of hyperintensity in the middle cerebellar peduncle – the "MCP sign" – occurs in about 60% of affected men (Leehey, 2009; Figure 6.5). Moreover, in a thorough postmortem study of 11 older adults with FXTAS, the most prominent neuropathological finding was widely distributed cerebral and cerebellar white matter disease (Greco et al., 2006). The neuropathological changes ranged from subtle white matter pallor to severe white matter degeneration, most notably in subcortical regions; in a pattern differing from that of atherosclerotic vascular disease, CADASIL, demyelination, and inflammatory disease, the periventricular white matter was spared while arcuate fibers were affected (Greco et al., 2006). Axons within white matter were also damaged, but cerebral cortical thickness and neuronal counts were similar to controls (Greco et al., 2006). In the MCP, the major afferent pathway into the cerebellum, spongiosis was typically observed along with the white matter changes (Greco et al., 2006).

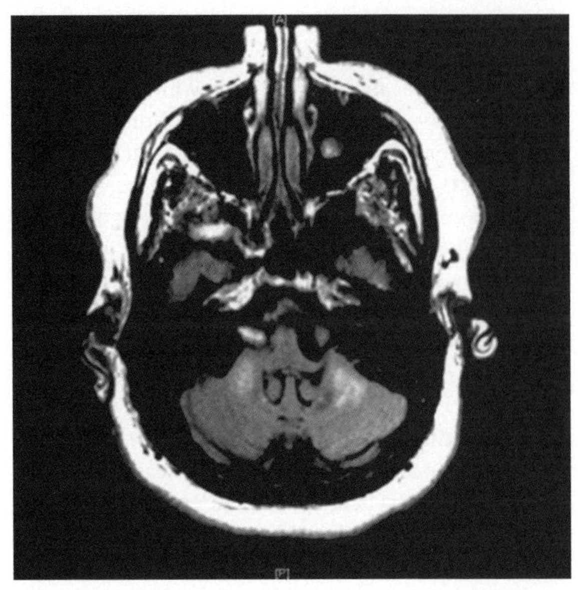

Figure 6.5 Axial fluid-attenuated inversion recovery (FLAIR) MRI scan of an older man with fragile X tremor ataxia syndrome. This image shows hyperintensity in the middle cerebellar peduncle, the "MCP sign."

Recent findings have also brought to attention the high prevalence of corpus callosum hyperintensity, which may be seen as commonly as the MCP sign (Apartis et al., 2012). Moreover, FXTAS may present with a dysexecutive syndrome and prominent frontal lobe white matter hyperintensity on MRI (Kasuga et al., 2011). The combination of cognitive deficits and MRI findings qualifies FXTAS for discussion in this book, and studies are underway with advanced neuroimaging to assess the role of white matter neuropathology in the dementia associated with FXTAS (Grigsby et al., 2014). Recent MRS and DTI data from individuals with the *fMR1* premutation have in fact documented microstructural disease in the MCP and corpus callosum genu consistent with both axonal loss and dysmyelination, and these neuroimaging changes have been correlated with executive dysfunction and slowed processing speed (Filley et al., 2015).

References

ACR Ad Hoc Committee on Neuropsychiatric Lupus Nomenclature. The American College of Rheumatology nomenclature and case definitions for neuropsychiatric lupus syndromes. Arthritis Rheum 1999; 42: 599–608.

Adams HP, Wagner S, Sobel DF, et al. Hypointense and hyperintense lesions on magnetic resonance imaging in secondary-progressive MS patients. Eur Neurol 1999; 42: 52–63.

Adams JH, Graham DI, Murray LS, Scott G. Diffuse axonal injury due to nonmissile head injury: an analysis of 45 cases. Ann Neurol 1982; 12: 557–563.

Adams JH, Graham DI, Jennett B. The neuropathology of the vegetative state after an acute brain insult. Brain 2000; 123: 1327–1338.

Adams JH, Jennett B, Murray LS, et al. Neuropathological findings in disabled survivors of a head injury. J Neurotrauma 2011; 28: 701–709.

Adams RD, Fisher CM, Hakim S, et al. Symptomatic occult hydrocephalus with "normal" cerebrospinal-fluid pressure. N Engl J Med 1965; 273: 117–126.

Adams RD, Kubik CS. Subacute degeneration of the brain in pernicious anemia. N Engl J Med 1944; 231: 1–9.

Agamanolis DP, Chester EM, Victor M, et al. Neuropathology of experimental vitamin B_{12} deficiency in monkeys. Neurology 1976; 26: 905–914.

Akai K, Uchigasaki S, Tanaka U, Komatsu A. Normal pressure hydrocephalus: neuropathological study. Acta Pathol Jpn 1987; 37: 97–110.

Akhvlediani T, Henning A, Sándor PS, et al. Adaptive metabolic changes in CADASIL white matter. J Neurol 2010; 257: 171–177.

Akiguchi I, Ishii M, Watanabe Y, et al. Shunt-responsive parkinsonism and reversible white matter lesions in patients with idiopathic NPH. J Neurol 2008; 255: 1392–1399.

Albers JW, Wald JJ, Garabrant DH, et al. Neurologic evaluation of workers previously diagnosed with solvent-induced toxic encephalopathy. J Occup Env Med 2000; 42: 410–423.

Alexander MP. Mild traumatic brain injury: pathophysiology, natural history, and clinical management. Neurology 1995; 45: 1252–1260.

Al-Hajri Z, Del Bigio MR. Brain damage in a large cohort of solvent abusers. Acta Neuropathol 2010; 119: 435–445.

Allen JC, Rosen G, Mehta BM, Horten B. Leukoencephalopathy following high-dose IV methotrexate chemotherapy with leukovorin rescue. Cancer Treat Rep 1980; 64: 1261–1273.

Alperin N, Oliu CJ, Bagci AM, et al. Low-dose acetazolamide reverses periventricular white matter hyperintensities in iNPH. Neurology 2014; 82: 1347–1351.

Alzheimer A (1902). Mental disturbances of arteriosclerotic origin (trans. Förstl H, Howard R, Levy R). Neuropsychiatry Neuropsychiatry Behav Neurol 1992; 5: 1–6.

Anderson CV, Bigler ED. Ventricular dilation, cortical atrophy, and neuropsychological outcome following traumatic brain injury. J Neuropsychiatry Clin Neurosci 1995; 7: 42–48.

Anthony IC, Bell JE. The neuropathology of HIV/AIDS. Int Rev Psychiatry 2008; 20: 15–24.

Antinori A, Arendt G, Becker JT, et al. Updated research nosology for HIV-associated neurocognitive disorders. Neurology 2007; 69: 1789–1799.

Anzola GP, Bevilacqua L, Cappa SF, et al. Neuropsychological assessment in patients with relapsing-remitting multiple sclerosis and mild functional impairment: correlation with magnetic resonance imaging. J Neurol Neurosurg Psychiatry 1990; 53: 142–145.

Apartis E, Blancher A, Meissner WG, et al. FXTAS: new insights and the need for revised diagnostic criteria. Neurology 2012; 79: 1898–1907.

Arlien-Søborg P, Bruhn P, Glydensted C, Melgaard B. Chronic painters' syndrome: chronic toxic encephalopathy in house painters. Acta Neurol Scand 1979; 60: 149–156.

Armstrong C, Ruffer J, Corn B, et al. Biphasic patterns of memory deficits following moderate-dose partial brain irradiation: neuropsychologic outcome and proposed mechanisms. J Clin Oncol 1995; 13: 2263–2271.

Armstrong CL, Corn BW, Ruffer JE, et al. Radiotherapeutic effects on brain function: double dissociation of memory systems. Neuropsychiatry Neuropsychol Behav Neurol 2000; 13: 101–111.

Armstrong CL, Stern CH, Corn BW. Memory performance used to detect radiation effects on cognitive function. Appl Neuropsychol 2001; 8: 129–139.

Armstrong RC, Mierzwa AJ, Marion CM, Sullivan GM. White matter involvement after TBI: clues to axon and myelin repair capacity. Exp Neurol 2015 Feb 16. [Epub ahead of print]

Arnett PA, Rao SM, Bernardin L, et al. Relationship between frontal lobe lesions and Wisconsin Card Sorting Test performance in patients with multiple sclerosis. Neurology 1994; 44: 420–425.

Artigas J, Cervos-Navarro J, Iglesias JR, Ebhardt G. Gliomatosis cerebri: clinical and histological findings. Clin Neuropathol 1985; 4: 135–148.

Assaf Y, Ben-Sira L, Constantini S, et al. Diffusion tensor imaging in hydrocephalus: initial experience. AJNR 2006; 27: 1717–1724.

Au R, Massaro JM, Wolf PA, et al. Association of white matter hyperintensity volume with decreased cognitive functioning: the Framingham Heart Study. Arch Neurol 2006; 63: 246–250.

Austin J, Armstrong D, Fouch S, et al. Metachromatic leukodystrophy (MLD): VIII. MLD in adults: diagnosis and pathogenesis. Arch Neurol 1968; 18: 225–240.

Babikian V, Ropper AH. Binswanger's disease: a review. Stroke 1987; 18: 2–12.

Baek HJ, Kim HS, Kim N, et al. Percent change of perfusion skewness and kurtosis: a potential imaging biomarker for early treatment response in patients with newly diagnosed glioblastomas. Radiology 2012; 264: 834–843.

Bagley LJ, McGowan JC, Grossman RI, et al. Magnetization transfer imaging of traumatic brain injury. J Magn Res Imaging 2000; 11: 1–8.

Baker EL. A review of recent research on health effects of human occupational exposure to organic solvents. J Occup Med 1994; 36: 1079–1092.

Balko MG, Blisard KS, Samaha FJ. Oligodendroglial gliomatosis cerebri. Hum Pathol 1992; 23: 706–707.

Barkhof F, Scheltens P. Imaging of white matter lesions. Cerebrovasc Dis 2002; 13 Suppl 2: 21–30.

Bech RA, Juhler M, Waldemar G, et al. Frontal brain and leptomeningeal biopsy specimens correlated with cerebrospinal fluid outflow resistance and B-wave activity in patients suspected of normal-pressure hydrocephalus. Neurosurgery 1997; 40: 497–502.

Bencherif B, Rottenberg DA. Neuroimaging of the AIDS dementia complex. AIDS 1998; 12: 233–244.

Benedict RH, Fischer JS, Archibald CJ, et al. Minimal neuropsychological assessment of MS patients: a consensus approach. Clin Neuropsychol 2002; 16: 381–397.

Benedict RH, Shucard JL, Zivadinov R, Shucard DW. Neuropsychological impairment in systemic lupus erythematosus: a comparison with multiple sclerosis. Neuropsychol Rev 2008; 18: 149–166.

Bennett DA, Wilson RS, Gilley DW, Fox JH. Clinical diagnosis of Binswanger's disease. J Neurol Neurosurg Psychiatry 1990; 53: 961–965.

Benros ME, Laursen TM, Dalton SO, Mortensen PB. Psychiatric disorder as a first manifestation of cancer: a 10-year population-based study. Int J Cancer 2009; 124: 2917–2922.

Black DN, Taber KH, Hurley RA. Metachromatic leukodystrophy: a model for the study of psychosis. J Neuropsychiatry Clin Neurosci 2003; 15: 289–293.

Blahak C, Baezner H, Pantoni L, et al. Deep frontal and periventricular age related white matter changes but not basal ganglia and infratentorial hyperintensities are associated with falls: cross sectional results from the LADIS study. J Neurol Neurosurg Psychiatry 2009; 80: 608–613.

Blasko I, Hinterberger M, Kemmler G, et al. Conversion from mild cognitive impairment to dementia: influence of folic acid and vitamin B12 use in the VITA cohort. J Nutr Health Aging 2012; 16: 687–694.

Blass JP, Hoyer S, Nitsch R. A translation of Otto Binswanger's article, "The delineation of the generalized progressive paralyses." Arch Neurol 1991; 48: 961–972.

Boerner RJ, Kapfhammer HP. Psychopathological changes and cognitive impairment in encephalomyelitis disseminata. Eur Arch Psychiatry Clin Neurosci 1999; 249: 96–102.

Bogucki A, Janczewska E, Koszewska I, et al. Evaluation of dementia in subcortical arteriosclerotic encephalopathy (Binswanger's Disease). Eur Arch Psychiatry Clin Neurosci 1991; 241: 91–97.

Bohman LE, Swanson KR, Moore JL, et al. Magnetic resonance imaging characteristics of glioblastoma multiforme: implications for understanding glioma ontogeny. Neurosurgery 2010; 67: 1319–1327.

Boon AJ, Tans JT, Delwel EJ, et al. Dutch normal-pressure hydrocephalus study: the role of cerebrovascular disease. J Neurosurg 1999; 90: 221–226.

Boone KB, Miller BL, Lesser IM, et al. Neuropsychological correlates of white-matter lesions in healthy elderly subjects: a threshold effect. Arch Neurol 1992; 49: 549–554.

Bourgeois JA, Coffey SM, Rivera SM, et al. A review of fragile X premutation disorders: expanding the psychiatric perspective. J Clin Psychiatry 2009; 70: 852–862.

Brassington JC, Marsh NV. Neuropsychological aspects of multiple sclerosis. Neuropsychol Rev 1998; 8: 43–77.

Brew BJ. AIDS dementia complex. Neurol Clin 1999; 17: 861–881.

Briley DP, Haroon S, Sergent SM, Thomas S. Does leukoaraiosis predict morbidity and mortality? Neurology 2000; 54: 90–94.

Brooks WM, Jung RE, Ford CC, et al. Relationship between neurometabolite derangement and neurocognitive dysfunction in systemic lupus erythematosus. J Rheumatol 1999; 26: 81–85.

Brooks WM, Sibbitt WL Jr, Kornfeld M, et al. The histopathologic associates of neurometabolite abnormalities in fatal neuropsychiatric systemic lupus erythematosus. Arthritis Rheum 2010; 62: 2055–2063.

Brousseau KM, Filley CM, Kaye K, et al. Dementia with features of Alzheimer's disease and HIV-associated dementia in an elderly man with AIDS. AIDS 2009; 23: 1029–1031.

Brown WR, Thore CR. Review: cerebral microvascular pathology in ageing and neurodegeneration. Neuropathol Appl Neurobiol 2011; 37: 56–74.

Brownell B, Hughes JT. The distribution of plaques in the cerebrum in multiple sclerosis. J Neurol Neurosurg Psychiatry 1962; 25: 315–320.

Büki A, Povlishock JT. All roads lead to disconnection? – Traumatic axonal injury revisited. Acta Neurochir (Wien). 2006; 148: 181–193.

Burger PC, Kamenar E, Schold SC, et al. Encephalomyelopathy following high-dose BCNU therapy. Cancer 1981; 48: 1318–1327.

Büttner A. Review: the neuropathology of drug abuse. Neuropathol Appl Neurobiol 2011; 37: 118–134.

Caldemeyer KS, Pascuzzi RM, Moran CC, Smith RS. Toluene abuse causing reduced MR signal intensity in the brain. AJR 1993; 161: 1259–1261.

Callanan MM, Logsdail SJ, Ron MA, Warrington EK. Cognitive impairment in patients with clinically isolated lesions of the type seen in multiple sclerosis: a psychometric and MRI study. Brain 1989; 112: 361–374.

Canoll P, Goldman JE. The interface between glial progenitors and gliomas. Acta Neuropathol 2008; 116: 465–477.

Caplan LR. Binswanger's disease – revisited. Neurology 1995; 45: 626–633.

Caplan LR, Gomes JA. Binswanger disease – an update. J Neurol Sci 2010; 299: 9–10.

Carbotte RM, Denburg SD, Denburg JA. Prevalence of cognitive impairment in systemic lupus erythematosus. J Nerv Ment Dis 1986; 174: 357–364.

Catalaa I, Fulton JC, Zhang X, et al. MR imaging quantitation of gray matter involvement in multiple sclerosis and its correlation with disability measures and neurocognitive testing. AJNR 1999; 20: 1613–1618.

Chabriat H, Vahedi K, Iba-Zizen MT, et al. Clinical spectrum of CADASIL: a study of 7 families. Lancet 1995; 346: 934–939.

Chabriat H, Pappata S, Poupon C, et al. Clinical severity in CADASIL related to ultrastructural damage in white matter: in vivo study with diffusion tensor MRI. Neurology 1999; 30: 2637–2643.

Chabriat H, Joutel A, Dichgans M, et al. Cadasil. Lancet Neurol 2009; 8: 643–653.

Chang L, Ernst T, Leonido-Yee M, et al. Cerebral metabolic abnormalities correlate with clinical severity of HIV-1 cognitive motor complex. Neurology 1999; 52: 100–108.

Charcot JM. *Lectures on the diseases of the nervous system delivered at La Salpêtrière.* London: New Sydenham Society, 1877.

Charlton RA, Barrick TR, McIntyre DJ, et al. White matter damage on diffusion tensor imaging correlates with age-related cognitive decline. Neurology 2006; 66: 217–222.

Charlton RA, Schiavone F, Barrick TR, et al. Diffusion tensor imaging detects age related white matter change over a 2 year follow-up which is associated with working memory decline. J Neurol Neurosurg Psychiatry 2010; 81: 13–19.

Chatterjee A, Yapundich R, Palmer CA, et al. Leukoencephalopathy associated with cobalamin deficiency. Neurology 1996; 46: 832–834.

Chaudhry P, Kharkar S, Heidler-Gary J, et al. Characteristics and reversibility of dementia in normal pressure hydrocephalus. Behav Neurol 2007; 18: 149–158.

Chauhan NB. Chronic neurodegenerative consequences of traumatic brain injury. Restor Neurol Neurosci 2014; 32: 337–365.

Chen S, Tanaka S, Giannini C, et al. Gliomatosis cerebri: clinical characteristics, management, and outcomes. J Neurooncol 2013; 112: 267–275.

Chen Y, An H, Zhu H, et al. White matter abnormalities revealed by diffusion tensor imaging in non-demented and demented HIV+ patients. Neuroimage 2009; 47: 1154–1162.

Cheung M, Chan AS, Law SC, et al. Cognitive function of patients with nasopharyngeal carcinoma with and without temporal lobe radionecrosis. Arch Neurol 2000; 57: 1347–1352.

Chiaravalloti ND, DeLuca J. Cognitive impairment in multiple sclerosis. Lancet Neurol 2008; 7: 1139–1151.

Clarfield AM. The reversible dementias: do they reverse? Ann Int Med 1988; 109: 476–486.

Clifford DB, Cohen IJ, Stark B, Kaplinsky C, et al. Human immunodeficiency virus–associated dementia. Arch Neurol 2000; 57: 321–324.

Comi G, Filippi M, Martinelli V, et al. Brain magnetic resonance imaging correlates of cognitive impairment in multiple sclerosis. J Neurol Sci 1993; 115 (Suppl): S66–S73.

Constine LS, Knoski A, Ekholm S, et al. Adverse effects of brain irradiation correlated with MR and CT imaging. Int J Radiation Oncology Biol Phys 1988; 15: 319–330.

Corn BW, Yousem DM, Scott DB, et al. White matter changes are correlated significantly with radiation dose. Cancer 1994; 10: 2828–2835.

Coronado VG, Xu L, Basavaraju SV, et al. Surveillance for traumatic brain injury–related deaths – United States, 1997–2007. MMWR Surveill 2011; 60: 1–32.

Couch JR, Weiss SA. Gliomatosis cerebri: report of four cases and review of the literature. Neurology 1974; 24: 504–511.

Craggs LJ, Yamamoto Y, Ihara M, et al. White matter pathology and disconnection in the frontal lobe in CADASIL. Neuropathol Appl Neurobiol 2014; 40: 591–602.

Cummings JL. *Subcortical dementia*. New York: Oxford University Press, 1990.

DeAngelis LM. Brain tumors. N Engl J Med 2001; 344: 114–123.

DeAngelis LM, Delattre J-Y, Posner JB. Radiation-induced dementia in patients cured of brain metastases. Neurology 1989; 39: 789–796.

Debette S, Markus HS. The clinical importance of white matter hyperintensities on brain magnetic resonance imaging: systematic review and meta-analysis. BMJ 2010; 341: c3666.

DeCarli C, Fletcher E, Ramey V, et al. Anatomical mapping of white matter hyperintensities (WMH): exploring the relationships between periventricular WMH, deep WMH, and total WMH burden. Stroke 2005; 36: 50–55.

De Groot JC, de Leeuw F-E, Oudkerk M, et al. Cerebral white matter lesions and cognitive function: the Rotterdam Scan study. Ann Neurol 2000; 47: 145–151.

DeKosky ST, Ikonomovic MD, Gandy S. Traumatic brain injury – football, warfare, and long-term effects. N Engl J Med 2010; 363: 1293–1296.

de Lau LM, Smith AD, Refsum H, et al. Plasma vitamin B12 status and cerebral white-matter lesions. J Neurol Neurosurg Psychiatry 2009; 80: 149–157.

Del Bigio MR. Neuropathological changes caused by hydrocephalus. Acta Neuropathol 1993; 85: 573–585.

Del Bigio MR. Epidemiology and direct economic impact of hydrocephalus: a community based study. Can J Neurol Sci 1998; 25: 123–126.

Del Bigio MR. Neuropathology and structural changes in hydrocephalus. Dev Disabil Res Rev 2010; 16: 16–22.

Del Bigio MR, da Silva MC, Drake JM, Tuor UI. Acute and chronic cerebral white matter damage in neonatal hydrocephalus. Can J Neurol Sci 1994; 21: 299–305.

Del Bigio MR, Wilson MJ, Enno T. Chronic hydrocephalus in rats and humans: white matter loss and behavior changes. Ann Neurol 2003; 53: 337–346.

Del Bigio MR, Enno TL. Effect of hydrocephalus on rat brain extracellular compartment. Cerebrospinal Fluid Res 2008; 10: 5–12.

del Carpio-O'Donovan R, Korah I, Salazar A, Melançon D. Gliomatosis cerebri. Radiology 1996; 198: 831–835.

DeLuca GC, Yates RL, Beale H, Morrow SA. Cognitive impairment in multiple sclerosis: clinical, radiologic and pathologic insights. Brain Pathol 2015; 25: 79–98.

DeLuca J, Barbieri-Berger S, Johnson SK. The nature of memory acquisition in multiple sclerosis: acquisition versus retrieval. J Clin Exp Neuropsychol 1994; 16: 183–189.

DeLuca J, Gaudino EA, Diamond BJ, et al. Acquisition and storage deficits in multiple sclerosis. J Clin Exp Neuropsychol 1998; 20: 376–390.

Demura K, Mase M, Miyati T, et al. Changes of fractional anisotropy and apparent diffusion coefficient in patients with idiopathic normal pressure hydrocephalus. Acta Neurochir Suppl 2012; 113: 29–32.

Denburg SD, Carbotte RM, Denburg JA. Cognition and mood in systemic lupus eythematosus: evaluation and pathogenesis. Ann NY Acad Sci 1997; 823: 44–59.

Denburg SD, Carbotte RM, Ginsberg JS, Denburg JA. The relationship of antiphospholipid antibodies to cognitive function in patients with systemic lupus erythematosus. J Int Neuropsychol Soc 1997; 3: 377–386.

Derix MMA. *Neuropsychological differentiation of dementia syndromes*. Lisse: Swets and Zeitlinger, 1994.

Desmond DW. Cognition and white matter lesions. Cerebrovasc Dis 2002; 13 Suppl 2: 53–57.

Devito EE, Pickard JD, Salmond CH, et al. The neuropsychology of normal pressure hydrocephalus (NPH). Br J Neurosurg 2005; 19: 217–224.

Dichgans M, Filippi M, Brüning R, et al. Quantitative MRI in CADASIL: correlation with disability and cognitive performance. Neurology 1999; 52: 1361–1367.

Dietrich J, Monje M, Wefel J, Meyers C. Clinical patterns and biological correlates of cognitive dysfunction associated with cancer therapy. Oncologist 2008; 13: 1285–1295.

Dikmen SS, Corrigan JD, Levin HS, et al. Cognitive outcome following traumatic brain injury. J Head Trauma Rehabil 2009; 24: 430–438.

Dineen RA, Vilisaar J, Hlinka J, et al. Disconnection as a mechanism for cognitive dysfunction in multiple sclerosis. Brain 2009; 132: 239–249.

Di Rocco C, Di Trapani G, Maira G, et al. Anatomo-clinical correlations in normotensive hydrocephalus. J Neurol Sci 1977; 33: 437–452.

Douw L, Klein M, Fagel SS, et al. Cognitive and radiological effects of radiotherapy in patients with low-grade glioma: long-term follow-up. Lancet Neurol 2009; 8: 810–818.

Dubois B, Slachevsky A, Litvan I, Pillon B. The FAB: a Frontal Assessment Battery at bedside. Neurology 2000; 55: 1621–1626.

Duffy PE, Huang YY, Rapport MM, Graf L. Glial fibrillary acidic protein in giant cell tumors of brain and other gliomas. A possible relationship to malignancy, differentiation, and pleomorphism of glia. Acta Neuropathol 1980; 52: 51–57.

Dufouil C, Alpérovitch A, Tzourio C. Influence of education on the relationship between white matter lesions and cognition. Neurology 2003; 60: 831–936.

Dutta R, Chang A, Doud MK, et al. Demyelination causes synaptic alterations in hippocampi from multiple sclerosis patients. Ann Neurol 2011; 69: 445–454.

Earnest MP, Fahn S, Karp JH, Rowland LP. Normal pressure hydrocephalus and hypertensive cerebrovascular disease. Arch Neurol 1974; 31: 262–266.

Evangelou N, Esiri MM, Smith S, et al. Quantitative pathological evidence for axonal loss in normal appearing white matter in multiple sclerosis. Ann Neurol 2000; 47: 392–395.

Everall IP, Glass JD, McArthur J, et al. Neuronal density in the superior frontal and temporal gyri does not correlate with the degree of human immunodeficiency virus-associated dementia. Acta Neuropathol 1994; 88: 538–544.

Everall IP, Hansen LA, Masliah E. The shifting patterns of HIV encephalitis neuropathology. Neurotox Res 2005; 8: 51–61.

Ewert L, Levin HS, Watson MG, Kalisky Z. Procedural memory during posttraumatic amnesia in survivors of severe closed head injury: implications for rehabilitation. Arch Neurol 1989; 46: 911–916.

Fassbender K, Mielke O, Bertsch T, et al. Homocysteine in cerebral macroangiopathy and microangiopathy. Lancet 1999; 353: 1586–1587.

Fazekas F, Kleinert R, Offenbacher H, et al. Pathologic correlates of incidental MRI white matter signal hyperintensities. Neurology 1993; 43: 1683–1689.

Feinglass EJ, Arnett FC, Dorsch CA, et al. Neuropsychiatric manifestations of systemic lupus erythematosus: diagnosis, clinical spectrum, and relationship to other features of the disease. Medicine 1976; 55: 323–339.

Feinstein A. *The clinical neuropsychiatry of multiple sclerosis*. 2nd ed. Cambridge: Cambridge University Press, 2007.

Feinstein A, Kartsounis LD, Miller DH, et al. Clinically isolated lesions of the type seen in multiple sclerosis: a cognitive, psychiatric, and MRI follow up study. J Neurol Neurosurg Psychiatry 1992; 55: 869–876.

Feinstein A, Ron MA, Thompson A. A serial study of psychometric and magnetic resonance imaging changes in multiple sclerosis. Brain 1993; 116: 569–602.

Filippi CG, Sze G, Farber SJ, et al. Regression of HIV encephalopathy and basal ganglia signal intensity abnormality at MR imaging in patient with AIDS after the initiation of protease inhibitor therapy. Radiology 1998; 206: 491–498.

Filippi M, Tortorella C, Rovaris M, et al. Changes in the normal appearing brain tissue and cognitive impairment in multiple sclerosis. J Neurol Neurosurg Psychiatry 2000; 68: 157–161.

Filippi M, Rocca MA, Benedict RH, et al. The contribution of MRI in assessing cognitive impairment in multiple sclerosis. Neurology 2010; 75: 2121–2128.

Filley CM. The behavioral neurology of cerebral white matter. Neurology 1998; 50: 1535–1540.

Filley CM. Clinical neurology and executive dysfunction. Semin Speech Lang 2000; 21: 95–108.

Filley CM. *Neurobehavioral anatomy*. 3rd ed. Boulder: University Press of Colorado, 2011.

Filley CM. *The behavioral neurology of white matter*. 2nd ed. New York: Oxford University Press, 2012.

Filley CM. Toluene abuse and white matter: a model of toxic leukoencephalopathy. Psychiatr Clin North Am 2013; 36: 293–302.

Filley CM, Cranberg LD, Alexander MP, Hart EJ. Neurobehavioral outcome after closed head injury in childhood and adolescence. Arch Neurol 1987; 44: 194–198.

Filley CM, Franklin GM, Heaton RK, Rosenberg NL. White matter dementia: clinical disorders and implications. Neuropsychiatry Neuropsychol Behav Neurol 1988; 1: 239–254.

Filley CM, Davis KA, Schmitz SP, et al. Neuropsychological performance and magnetic resonance imaging in Alzheimer's disease and normal aging. Neuropsychiatry Neuropsychol Behav Neurol 1989a; 2: 81–91.

Filley CM, Heaton RK, Nelson LM, et al. A comparison of dementia in Alzheimer's Disease and multiple sclerosis. Arch Neurol 1989b; 46: 157–161.

Filley CM, Heaton RK, Rosenberg NL. White matter dementia in chronic toluene abuse. Neurology 1990; 40: 532–534.

Filley CM, Gross KF. Psychosis with cerebral white matter disease. Neuropsychiatry Neuropsychol Behav Neurol 1992; 5: 119–125.

Filley CM, Kleinschmidt-DeMasters BK. Neurobehavioral presentations of brain neoplasms. West J Med 1995; 163: 19–25.

Filley CM, Thompson LL, Sze C-I, et al. White matter dementia in CADASIL. J Neurol Sci 1999a; 163: 163–167.

Filley CM, Young DA, Reardon MS, Wilkening GN. Frontal lobe lesions and executive dysfunction in children. Neuropsychiatry Neuropsychol Behav Neurol 1999b; 12: 156–160.

Filley CM, Kleinschmidt-DeMasters BK. Toxic leukoencephalopathy. N Engl J Med 2001; 345: 425–432.

Filley CM, Kleinschmidt-DeMasters BK, Lillehei KO, et al. Gliomatosis cerebri: neurobehavioral and neuropathological observations. Cogn Behav Neurol 2003; 16: 149–159.

Filley CM, Halliday W, Kleinschmidt-DeMasters BK. The effects of toluene on the central nervous system. J Neuropathol Exp Neurol 2004; 63: 1–12.

Filley CM, Kozora E, Brown MS, et al. White matter microstructure and cognition in non-neuropsychiatric systemic lupus erythematosus. Cogn Behav Neurol 2009; 22: 38–44.

Filley CM, Brown MS, Onderko K, et al. White matter disease and cognitive impairment in FMR1 premutation carriers. Neurology 2015; 84: 2146–2152.

Firbank MJ, Minett T, O'Brien JT. Changes in DWI and MRS associated with white matter hyperintensities in elderly subjects. Neurology 2003; 61: 950–954.

Fischer JS, Rudick RA, Cutter GR, Reingold SC. The Multiple Sclerosis Functional Composite Measure (MSFC): an integrated approach to MS clinical outcome assessment. National MS Society Clinical Outcomes Assessment Task Force. Mult Scler 1999; 5: 244–250.

Fisher CM. Communicating hydrocephalus. Lancet 1978; 1 (8054): 37.

Fisher CM. Binswanger's encephalopathy. J Neurol 1989; 236: 65–79.

Fishman RA. *Cerebrospinal fluid in diseases of the nervous system*. 2nd ed. Philadelphia: W.B. Saunders, 1992.

Fletcher JM, Copeland DR. Neurobehavioral effects of central nervous system prophylactic treatment of cancer in children. J Clin Exp Neuropsychol 1988; 10: 495–538.

Folkerth RD. Abnormalities of developing white matter in lysosomal storage diseases. J Neuropathol Exp Neurol 2000; 58: 887–902.

Folstein MF, Folstein SE, McHugh PR. "Mini-Mental State": A practical method of grading the cognitive state of patients for the clinician. J Psychiat Res 1975; 12: 189–198.

Fornage M, Debette S, Bis JC, et al. Genome-wide association studies of cerebral white matter lesion burden: the CHARGE consortium. Ann Neurol 2011; 69: 928–939.

Fornazzari L, Pollanen MS, Myers V, Wolf A. Solvent abuse-related toluene leukoencephalopathy. J Clin Forensic Med 2003; 10: 93–95.

Franklin GM, Heaton RK, Nelson LM, et al. Correlation of neuropsychological and magnetic resonance imaging findings in chronic/progressive multiple sclerosis. Neurology 1988; 38: 1826–1829.

Franklin GM, Nelson LM, Filley CM, Heaton RK. Cognitive loss in multiple sclerosis: case reports and review of the literature. Arch Neurol 1989; 46: 162–167.

Franklin GM, Nelson LM, Heaton RK, Filley CM. Clinical perspectives in the identification of cognitive impairment. In: Rao SM, ed. *Neurobehavioral aspects of multiple sclerosis*. New York: Oxford University Press, 1990: 161–174.

Fukuda H, Kitani M. Cigarette smoking is correlated with the periventricular hyperintensity grade of brain magnetic resonance imaging. Stroke 1996; 27: 645–649.

Gallassi R, Morreale A, Montagna P, et al. Binswanger's Disease and normal-pressure hydrocephalus: clinical and neuropsychological comparison. Arch Neurol 1991; 48: 1156–1159.

Gannon P, Khan MZ, Kolson DL. Current understanding of HIV-associated neurocognitive disorders pathogenesis. Curr Opin Neurol 2011; 24: 275–283.

Garnett MR, Blamire AM, Rajagopalan B, et al. Evidence for cellular damage in normal-appearing white matter correlates with injury severity in patients following traumatic brain injury: a magnetic resonance spectroscopy study. Brain 2000; 123: 1403–1409.

Geer CP, Grossman SA. Interstitial flow along white matter tracts: a potentially important mechanism for the dissemination of primary brain tumors. J Neurooncol 1997; 32: 193–201.

Gennarelli TA, Thibault LE, Adams JH, et al. Diffuse axonal injury and traumatic coma in the primate. Ann Neurol 1982; 12: 564–574.

Gentry LR, Godersky JC, Thompson B. MR imaging of head trauma: review of the distribution and radiopathologic features of traumatic lesions. AJNR 1988; 150: 663–672.

Gerard G, Weisberg LA. MRI periventricular lesions in adults. Neurology 1986; 36: 998–1001.

Geremia GK, Wollman R, Foust R. Computed tomography of gliomatosis cerebri. J Comput Assist Tomogr 1988; 12: 698–701.

Geschwind N. The mechanism of normal pressure hydrocephalus. J Neurol Sci 1968; 7: 481–493.

Giese A, Westphal M. Glioma invasion in the central nervous system. Neurosurgery 1996; 39: 235–250.

Gieselmann V, Krägeloh-Mann I. Metachromatic leukodystrophy – an update. Neuropediatrics 2010; 41: 1–6.

Gilbert MR. The neurotoxicity of cancer chemotherapy. Neurologist 1998; 4: 43–53.

Ginsburg KS, Wright EA, Larsen MG, et al. A controlled study of the prevalence of cognitive impairment in randomly selected patients with systemic lupus erythematosus. Arthritis Rheum 1992; 35: 776–782.

Godin O, Tzourio C, Maillard P, et al. Apolipoprotein E genotype is related to progression of white matter lesion load. Stroke 2009; 40: 3186–3190.

Goebels N, Soyka M. Dementia associated with vitamin B_{12} deficiency: presentation of two cases and review of the literature. J Neuropsychiatry Clin Neurosci 2000; 12: 389–394.

Goldstein M. Traumatic brain injury: a silent epidemic. Ann Neurol 1990; 27: 327.

Gonzalez R, Jacobus J, Amatya AK, et al. Deficits in complex motor functions, despite no evidence of procedural learning deficits, among HIV+ individuals with history of substance dependence. Neuropsychology 2008; 22: 776–786.

Graff-Radford NR. Normal pressure hydrocephalus. Neurologist 1999; 5: 194–204.

Grant I, Atkinson JH, Hesselink JR, et al. Evidence for early central nervous system involvement in the acquired immunodeficiency syndrome (AIDS) and other human immunodeficiency virus (HIV) infections. Ann Int Med 1987; 107: 828–836.

Gray F, Scaravelli F, Everall I, et al. Neuropathology of early HIV-1 infection. Brain Pathol 1996; 6: 1–15.

Greco CM, Berman RF, Martin RM, et al. Neuropathology of fragile X–associated tremor/ataxia syndrome (FXTAS). Brain 2006; 129: 243–255.

Greene-Schloesser D, Robbins ME. Radiation-induced cognitive impairment – from bench to bedside. Neuro Oncol 2012; 14 Suppl 4: iv37–iv44.

Grigsby J, Brega AG, Engle K, et al. Cognitive profile of fragile X premutation carriers with and without fragile X–associated tremor/ataxia syndrome. Neuropsychology 2008; 22: 48–60.

Grigsby J, Cornish K, Hocking D, et al. The cognitive neuropsychological phenotype of carriers of the FMR1 premutation. J Neurodev Disord 2014; 6: 28.

Gustafson L, Hagberg B. Recovery in hydrocephalic dementia after shunt operation. J Neurol Neurosurg Psychiatry 1978; 41: 940–947.

Hachinski VC. Binswanger's disease: neither Binswanger's nor a disease. J Neurol Sci 1991; 103: 1.

Hachinski VC, Potter P, Merskey H. Leuko-araiosis. Arch Neurol 1987; 44: 21–23.

Hagerman PJ, Hagerman RJ. Fragile X–associated tremor/ataxia syndrome (FXTAS). Ment Retard Dev Disabil Res Rev 2004; 10: 25–30.

Hähnel S, Freund M, Münkel K, et al. Magnetisation transfer ratio is low in normal-appearing cerebral white matter in patients with normal pressure hydrocephalus. J Neurol 2000; 42: 174–179.

Hanly J, Urowitz M, Su L, et al. Autoantibodies as biomarkers for the prediction of neuropsychiatric events in systemic lupus erythematosus. Ann Rheum Dis 2011; 70: 1726–1732.

Hanyu H, Asano T, Sakurai H, et al. Magnetization transfer ratio in cerebral white matter lesions of Binswanger's Disease. J Neurol Sci 1999; 166: 85–90.

Harboe E, Greve OJ, Beyer M, et al. Fatigue is associated with cerebral white matter hyperintensities in patients with systemic lupus erythematosus. J Neurol Neurosurg Psychiatry 2008; 79: 199–201.

Harris JG, Filley CM. CADASIL: neuropsychological findings in three generations of an affected family. J Int Neuropsychol Soc 2001; 7: 768–774.

Hauser SL, Oksenberg JR. The neurobiology of multiple sclerosis: genes, inflammation, and neurodegeneration. Neuron 2006; 52: 61–76.

Hayek J, Valvanis A. Computed tomography of gliomatosis cerebri. Comput Radiol 1982; 6: 93–98.

Healton EB, Savage DG, Brust JC, et al. Neurologic aspects of cobalamin deficiency. Medicine 1991; 70: 229–245.

Heaton RK, Clifford DB, Franklin DR Jr, et al. HIV-associated neurocognitive disorders persist in the era of potent antiretroviral therapy: CHARTER Study. Neurology 2010; 75: 2087–2096.

Heaton RK, Nelson LM, Thompson DS, et al. Neuropsychological findings in relapsing-remitting and chronic-progressive multiple sclerosis. J Consul Clin Psychol 1985; 53: 103–110.

Hecke WV, Nagels G, Leemans A, et al. Correlation of cognitive dysfunction and diffusion tensor MRI measures in patients with mild and moderate multiple sclerosis. J Magn Reson Imaging 2010; 31: 1492–1498.

Hedera P, Friedland RP. Cerebral autosomal dominant arteriopathy with subcortical infarcts and leukoencephalopathy: study of two American families with predominant dementia. J Neurol Sci 1997; 146: 27–33.

Hellström P, Edsbagge M, Blomsterwall E, et al. Neuropsychological effects of shunt treatment in idiopathic normal pressure hydrocephalus. Neurosurgery 2008; 63: 527–535.

Hervé D, Chabriat H. CADASIL. J Geriatr Psychiatry Neurol 2010; 23: 269–276.

Hetherington H, Bandak A, Ling G, Bandak FA. Advances in imaging explosive blast mild traumatic brain injury. Handb Clin Neurol 2015; 127: 309–318.

Hinchey J, Chaves C, Appignani B, et al. A reversible posterior leukoencephalopathy syndrome. N Engl J Med 1996; 334: 494–500.

Hohol MJ, Guttmann CRG, Orav J, et al. Serial neuropsychological assessment and magnetic resonance imaging analysis in multiple sclerosis. Arch Neurol 1997; 54: 1018–1025.

Hoogland ICM, Portegies P. HIV-associated dementia: prompt response to zidovudine. Neurol Clin Pract 2014; 4: 264–265.

Hormes JT, Filley CM, Rosenberg NL. Neurologic sequelae of chronic solvent vapor abuse. Neurology 1986; 36: 698–702.

Huber SJ, Bornstein RA, Rammohan KW, et al. Magnetic resonance imaging correlates of neuropsychological impairment in multiple sclerosis. J Neuropsychiatry Clin Neurosci 1992; 4: 152–158.

Huisa BN, Rosenberg GA. Binswanger's disease: toward a diagnosis agreement and therapeutic approach. Expert Rev Neurother 2014; 14: 1203–1213.

Hurley RA, Tomimoto H, Akiguchi I, et al. Binswanger's Disease: an ongoing controversy. J Neuropsychiatry Clin Neurosci 2000; 12: 301–304.

Hutto BR. Folate and cobalamin in psychiatric illness. Comp Psychiatry 1997; 38: 305–314.

Hyde TM, Ziegler JC, Weinberger DR. Psychiatric disturbances in metachromatic leukodystrophy: insights into the neurobiology of psychosis. Arch Neurol 1992; 49: 401–406.

Iannucci G, Dichgans M, Rovaris M, et al. Correlations between clinical findings and magnetization transfer imaging metrics of tissue damage in individuals with cerebral autosomal dominant arteriopathy with subcortical infarcts and leukoencephalopathy. Stroke 2001; 32: 643–648.

Iddon JL, Pickard JD, Cross JJL, et al. Specific patterns of cognitive impairment in patients with idiopathic normal pressure hydrocephalus and Alzheimer's disease: a pilot study. J Neurol Neurosurg Psychiatry 1999; 67: 723–732.

Inzitari D, Diaz F, Fox A, et al. Vascular risk factors and leuko-araiosis. Arch Neurol 1987; 44: 42–47.

Inzitari D, Simoni M, Pracucci G, et al. Risk of rapid global functional decline in elderly patients with severe cerebral age-related white matter changes: the LADIS study. Arch Intern Med 2007; 167: 81–88.

Jack CR, Mokri B, Laws ER, et al. MR findings in normal-pressure hydrocephalus: significance and comparison with other forms of dementia. J Comput Assist Tomogr 1987; 11: 923–931.

Jacobs L, Kinkel PR, Costello PB, et al. Central nervous system lupus erythematosus: the value of magnetic resonance imaging. J Rheumatol 1988; 15: 601–606.

Jagust W, Harvey D, Mungas D, Haan M. Central obesity and the aging brain. Arch Neurol 2005; 62: 1545–1548.

Jennett B, Bond M. Assessment of outcome after severe brain damage. Lancet 1975; 1: 480–484.

Johnson RT, Richardson EP. The neurological manifestations of systemic lupus erythematosus. Medicine 1968; 47: 337–369.

Jones DK, Lythgoe D, Horsfield MA, et al. Characterization of white matter damage in ischemic leukoaraiosis with diffusion tensor MRI. Stroke 1999; 30: 393–397.

Jones HR, Ho DD, Forgacs P, et al. Acute fulminating fatal leukoencephalopathy as the only manifestation of human immunodeficiency virus infection. Ann Neurol 1988; 23: 519–522.

Jones RD, Tranel D. Preservation of procedural memory in HIV-positive patients with subcortical dementia. J Clin Exp Neuropsychol 1991; 13: 74.

Jones RS, Waldman AD. 1H-MRS evaluation of metabolism in Alzheimer's disease and vascular dementia. Neurol Res 2004; 26: 488–495.

Jung RE, Chavez RS, Flores RA, et al. White matter correlates of neuropsychological dysfunction in systemic lupus erythematosus. PLoS One 2012; 7: e28373.

Junqué C, Pujol J, Vendrell P, et al. Leuko-araiosis on magnetic resonance imaging and speed of mental processing. Arch Neurol 1990; 47: 151–156.

Kanno S, Abe N, Saito M, et al. White matter involvement in idiopathic normal pressure hydrocephalus: a voxel-based diffusion tensor imaging study. J Neurol 2011; 258: 1949–1957.

Kasuga, K, Ikeuchi, T, Arakawa K., et al. A patient with fragile x–associated tremor/ataxia syndrome presenting with executive cognitive deficits and cerebral white matter lesions. Case Rep Neurol 2011; 3: 118–123.

Katzen H, Ravdin LD, Assuras S, et al. Postshunt cognitive and functional improvement in idiopathic normal pressure hydrocephalus. Neurosurgery 2011; 68: 416–419.

Kaufmann PM, Fletcher JM, Levin HS, et al. Attentional disturbance after pediatric closed head injury. J Child Neurol 1993; 8: 348–353.

Keene DL, Jimenez C, Hsu E. MRI diagnosis of gliomatosis cerebri. Pediatr Neurol 1999; 20: 148–151.

Kelly JP, Nichols JS, Filley CM, et al. Concussion in sports: guidelines for the prevention of catastrophic outcome. JAMA 1991; 266: 2867–2869.

Kim JJ, Gean AD. Imaging for the diagnosis and management of traumatic brain injury. Neurotherapeutics 2011; 8: 39–53.

Kinkel WR, Jacobs L, Polachini I, et al. Subcortical arteriosclerotic encephalopathy (Binswanger's Disease). Arch Neurol 1985; 42: 951–959.

Kinnunen KM, Greenwood R, Powell JH, et al. White matter damage and cognitive impairment after traumatic brain injury. Brain 2011; 134: 449–563.

Kirk A, Kertesz A, Polk MJ. Dementia with leukoencephalopathy in systemic lupus erythematosus. Can J Neurol Sci 1991; 18: 344–348.

Klassen BT, Ahlskog JE. Normal pressure hydrocephalus: how often does the diagnosis hold water? Neurology 2011; 77: 1119–1125.

Klein M, Duffau H, De Witt Hamer PC. Cognition and resective surgery for diffuse infiltrative glioma: an overview. J Neurooncol 2012; 108: 309–318.

Kleinschmidt-DeMasters BK, Geier JM. Pathology of high-dose intraarterial BCNU. Surg Neurol 1989; 31: 435–443.

Klinken L, Arlien-Søborg P. Brain autopsy in organic solvent syndrome. Acta Neurol Scand 1993; 87: 371–375.

Köhler W. Leukodystrophies with late disease onset: an update. Curr Opin Neurol 2010; 23: 234–241.

Kornfeld M, Moser AB, Moser HW, et al. Solvent vapor abuse leukoencephalopathy: comparison to adrenoleukodystrophy. J Neuropathol Exp Neurol 1994; 53: 389–398.

Koslow SA, Claassen D, Hirsch WL, Jungreis CA. Gliomatosis cerebri: a case report with autopsy correlation. Neuroradiology 1992; 34: 331–333.

Kozora E, Thompson LL, West SG, Kotzin BL. Analysis of cognitive and psychological deficits in systemic lupus erythematosus patients without overt central nervous system disease. Arthritis Rheum 1996; 39: 2035–2045.

Kozora E, West SG, Kotzin BL, et al. Magnetic resonance imaging abnormalities and cognitive deficits in systemic lupus erythematosus patients without overt central nervous system disease. Arthritis Rheum 1998; 41: 41–47.

Kozora E, Hanly JG, Lapteva L, Filley CM. Cognitive dysfunction in systemic lupus erythematosus: past, present, and future. Arthritis Rheum 2008; 58: 3286–3298.

Kozora E, Brown MS, Filley CM, et al. Memory impairment associated with neurometabolic abnormalities of the hippocampus in patients with non-neuropsychiatric systemic lupus erythematosus. Lupus 2011; 20: 598–606.

Kozora E, Filley CM. Cognitive dysfunction and white matter abnormalities in systemic lupus erythematosus. J Int Neuropsychol Soc 2011; 17: 1–8.

Kraus MF, Susmaras T, Caughlin BP, et al. White matter integrity and cognition in chronic traumatic brain injury: a diffusion tensor imaging study. *Brain* 2007 Oct; 130(Pt 10): 2508–2519.

Krikorian R, Wrobel AJ. Cognitive impairment in HIV infection. AIDS 1991; 5: 1501–1507.

Krivit W, Shapiro E, Kennedy W, et al. Treatment of late infantile metachromatic leukodystrophy by bone marrow transplantation. N Engl J Med 1990; 322: 28–32.

Krivit W, Peters C, Shapiro EG. Bone marrow transplantation as effective treatment of central nervous system disease in globoid cell leukodystrophy, metachromatic leukodystrophy, adrenoleukodystrophy, mannosidosis, fucosidosis, aspartylglucosaminuria, Hurler, Maroteaux-Lamy, and Sly syndromes, and Gaucher disease type III. Curr Opin Neurol 1999; 12: 167–176.

Kumperscak HG, Plesnicar BK, Zalar B, et al. Adult metachromatic leukodystrophy: a new mutation in the schizophrenia-like phenotype with early neurological signs. Psychiatr Genet 2007; 17: 85–91.

Kurtzke JF. Neurologic impairment in multiple sclerosis and the Disability Status Scale. Acta Neurol Scand 1970; 46: 493–512.

Kurtzke JF. Rating neurologic impairment in multiple sclerosis: an expanded disability scale. Neurology 1983; 33: 1444–1452.

Kutzelnigg A, Lucchinetti CF, Stadelmann C, et al. Cortical demyelination and diffuse white matter injury in multiple sclerosis. Brain 2005; 128: 2705–2712.

Lafosse JM, Corboy JR, et al. MS vs. HD: can white matter and subcortical gray matter pathology be distinguished neuropsychologically? J Clin Exp Neuropsychol 2007; 29: 142–154.

Lafosse JM, Mitchell SM, Corboy JR, Filley CM. The nature of verbal memory impairment in multiple sclerosis: a list-learning and meta-analytic study. J Int Neuropsychol Soc 2013; 19: 995–1008.

Langdon DW. Cognition in multiple sclerosis. Curr Opin Neurol 2011; 24: 244–249.

Langford TD, Letendre SL, Marcotte TD, et al. Severe, demyelinating leukoencephalopathy in AIDS patients on antiretroviral therapy. AIDS 2002; 16: 1019–1029.

Langford TD, Letendre SL, Larrea GJ, Masliah E. Changing patterns in the neuropathogenesis of HIV during the HAART era. Brain Pathol 2003; 13: 195–210.

Lantos PL, Bruner JM. Gliomatosis cerebri. In: Kleihues P, Cavenee WK, eds. *World Health Organization classification of tumours: pathology and genetics of tumours of the central nervous system.* Lyon: IARC Press, 2000: 92–93.

Larner AJ, Janssen JC, Cipolotti L, Rossor MN. Cognitive profile in dementia associated with B_{12} deficiency due to pernicious anaemia. J Neurol 1999; 246: 317–319.

Lawrence RM, Hillam JC. Psychiatric symptomatology in early-onset Binswanger's disease: two case reports. Behav Neurol 1995; 8: 43–46.

Lee A, Yu YL, Tsoi M, et al. Subcortical arteriosclerotic encephalopathy – a controlled psychometric study. Clin Neurol Neurosurg 1989; 91: 235–241.

Lee JH, Kim SH, Kim GH, et al. Identification of pure subcortical vascular dementia using 11C-Pittsburgh compound B. Neurology 2011; 77: 18–25.

Lee SK. Diffusion tensor and perfusion imaging of brain tumors in high-field MR imaging. Neuroimaging Clin N Am 2012; 22: 123–134.

Lee Y-Y, Nauert C, Glass JP. Treatment-related white matter changes in cancer patients. Cancer 1986; 57: 1473–1482.

Leehey MA. Fragile X-associated tremor/ataxia syndrome: clinical phenotype, diagnosis, and treatment. J Investig Med 2009; 57: 830–836.

Leifer D, Buonanno FS, Richardson EP. Clinicopathologic correlates of cranial magnetic resonance imaging of periventricular white matter. Neurology 1990; 40: 911–918.

Leinonen V, Koivisto AM, Savolainen S, et al. Post-mortem findings in 10 patients with presumed normal-pressure hydrocephalus and review of the literature. Neuropathol Appl Neurobiol 2012; 38: 72–86.

Levin HS, Williams DH, Eisenberg HM, et al. Serial MRI and neurobehavioral findings after mild to moderate closed head injury. J Neurol Neurosurg Psychiatry 1992; 55: 255–262.

Levin HS, Wilde EA, Chu Z, et al. Diffusion tensor imaging in relation to cognitive and functional outcome of traumatic brain injury in children. J Head Trauma Rehabil 2008; 23: 197–208.

Levine B, Fujiwara E, O'Connor C, et al. In vivo characterization of traumatic brain injury neuropathology with structural and functional neuroimaging. J Neurotrauma 2006; 23: 1396–1411.

Libon DJ, Price CC, Davis Garrett K, Giovannetti T. From Binswanger's disease to leuokoaraiosis: what we have learned about subcortical vascular dementia. Clin Neuropsychol 2004; 18: 83–100.

Libon DJ, Price CC, Giovannetti T, et al. Linking MRI hyperintensities with patterns of neuropsychological impairment: evidence for a threshold effect. Stroke 2008; 39: 806–813.

Lindenbaum J, Healton EB, Savage DG, et al. Neuropsychiatric disorders caused by cobalamin deficiency in the absence of anemia or macrocytosis. N Engl J Med 1988; 318: 1720–1728.

Ling G, Bandak F, Armonda R, et al. Explosive blast neurotrauma. J Neurotrauma 2009; 26: 815–825.

Liu CK, Miller BL, Cummings JL, et al. A quantitative MRI study of vascular dementia. Neurology 1992; 42: 138–143.

Loizou LA, Kendall BE, Marshall J. Subcortical arteriosclerotic encephalopathy: a clinical and radiological investigation. J Neurol Neurosurg Psychiatry 1981; 44: 294–304.

Longstreth WT, Manolio TA, Arnold A, et al. Clinical correlates of white matter findings on cranial magnetic resonance imaging of 3301 elderly people: the Cardiovascular Health Study. Stroke 1996; 27: 1274–1282.

Lucchinetti CF, Popescu BF, Bunyan RF, et al. Inflammatory cortical demyelination in early multiple sclerosis. N Engl J Med 2011 365: 2188–2197.

Lyon G, Fattal-Valevski A, Kolodny EH. Leukodystrophies: clinical and genetic aspects. Top Magn Reson Imaging 2006; 17: 219–242.

Mac Donald CL, Johnson AM, Cooper D, et al. Detection of blast-related traumatic brain injury in U.S. military personnel. N Engl J Med 2011; 364: 2091–2100.

Madhusoodanan S, Danan D, Brenner R, Bogunovic O. Brain tumor and psychiatric manifestations: a case report and brief review. Ann Clin Psychiatry 2004; 16: 111–113.

Mandleberg IA, Brooks DN. Cognitive recovery after severe head injury. 1. Serial testing on the Wechsler Adult Intelligence Scale. J Neurol Neurosurg Psychiatry 1975; 38: 1121–1126.

Manji H, Jäger HR, Winston A. HIV, dementia and antiretroviral drugs: 30 years of an epidemic. J Neurol Neurosurg Psychiatry 2013; 84: 1126–1137.

Mar S, Noetzel M. Axonal damage in leukodystrophies. Pediatr Neurol 2010; 42: 239–242.

Markus HS, Lythgoe DJ, Ostegaard L, et al. Reduced cerebral blood flow in white matter in ischaemic leukoaraiosis demonstrated using quantitative exogenous contrast based perfusion MRI. J Neurol Neurosurg Psychiatry 2000; 69: 48–53.

Masel BE, DeWitt DS. Traumatic brain injury: a disease process, not an event. J Neurotrauma 2010; 27: 1529–1540.

Mattox AK, Lark AL, Adamson DC. Marked response of gliomatosis cerebri to temozolomide and whole brain radiotherapy. Clin Neurol Neurosurg 2012; 114: 299–306.

Maurelli M, Marchioni E, Cerretano R, et al. Neuropsychological assessment in MS: clinical, neurophysiological and neuroradiological relationships. Acta Neurol Scand 1992; 86: 124–128.

McArthur JC, Sacktor N, Selnes O. Human immunodeficiency virus–associated dementia. Semin Neurol 1999; 19: 129–150.

McGowan JC, Yang JH, Plotkin RC, et al. Magnetization transfer imaging in the detection of injury associated with mild head trauma. AJNR 2000; 21: 875–880.

Meadows M-E, Kaplan RF, Bromfield EB. Cognitive recovery with vitamin B_{12} therapy: a longitudinal neuropsychological assessment. Neurology 1994; 44: 1764–1765.

Medaer R, Nelissen E, Appel B, et al. Magnetic resonance imaging and cognitive functioning in multiple sclerosis. J Neurol 1987; 235: 86–89.

Medana IM, Esiri MM. Axonal damage: a key predictor of outcome in human CNS diseases. Brain 2003; 126: 515–530.

Merino JG, Hachinski V. Leukoaraiosis: reifying rarefaction. Arch Neurol 2000; 57: 925–926.

Meyers CA. How chemotherapy damages the central nervous system. J Biol 2008; 7: 11.

Meyers CA, Geara F, Wong PF, Morrison WH. Neurocognitive effects of therapeutic irradiation for base of skull tumors. Int J Radiation Oncology Biol Phys 2000; 46: 51–55.

Mierzwa AJ, Marion CM, Sullivan GM, et al. Components of myelin damage and repair in the progression of white matter pathology after mild traumatic brain injury. J Neuropathol Exp Neurol 2015; 74: 218–232.

Miller DH, Ormerod IEC, Gibson A, et al. MR brain scanning in patients with vasculitis: differentiation from multiple sclerosis. Neuroradiology 1987; 29: 226–231.

Mittl RL, Grossman RI, Hiehle JF, et al. Prevalence of MR evidence of diffuse axonal injury in patients with mild head injury and normal head CT findings. AJNR 1994; 15: 1583–1589.

Mohamed MA, Lentz MR, Lee V, et al. Factor analysis of proton MR spectroscopic imaging data in HIV infection: metabolite-derived factors help identify infection and dementia. Radiology 2010; 254: 577–586.

Möller A, Wiedemann G, Rhode U, et al. Correlates of cognitive impairment and depressive mood disorder in multiple sclerosis. Acta Psychiatr Scand 1994; 89: 117–121.

Momjian S, Owler BK, Czosnyka Z, et al. Pattern of white matter regional cerebral blood flow and autoregulation in normal pressure hydrocephalus. Brain 2004; 127: 965–972.

Moore-Maxwell CA, Datto MB, Hulette CM. Chemotherapy-induced toxic leukoencephalopathy causes a wide range of symptoms: a series of four autopsies. Mod Pathol 2004; 17: 241–247.

Mulhern RK, Reddick WE, Palmer SL, et al. Neurocognitive deficits in medulloblastoma survivors and white matter loss. Ann Neurol 1999; 46: 834–841.

Murray ME, Senjem ML, Petersen RC, et al. Functional impact of white matter hyperintensities in cognitively normal elderly subjects. Arch Neurol 2010; 67: 1379–1385.

Navarro C, Fernandez JM, Dominguez C, et al. Late juvenile metachromatic leukodystrophy treated with bone marrow transplantation: a 4-year follow-up study. Neurology 1996; 46: 254–256.

Navia BA, Jordan BD, Price RW. The AIDS dementia complex: I. Clinical features. Ann Neurol 1986; 19: 517–524.

Navia BA, Cho E-S, Petito CK, Price RW. The AIDS dementia complex: II. Neuropathology. Ann Neurol 1986; 19: 525–535.

Navia BA, Price RW. The acquired immunodeficiency syndrome dementia complex as the presenting or sole manifestation of human immunodeficiency virus infection. Arch Neurol 1987; 44: 65–69.

Nevin NC. Neuropathological changes in the white matter following head injury. J Neuropathol Exp Neurol 1967; 26: 77–84.

Nevin S. Gliomatosis cerebri. Brain 1938; 61: 170–191.

Nir TM, Jahanshad N, Busovaca E, et al. Mapping white matter integrity in elderly people with HIV. Hum Brain Mapp 2014; 35: 975–992.

Noseworthy JH. Progress in determining the causes and treatment of multiple sclerosis. Nature 1999; 399 (Suppl): A40–A47.

Ogino A, Kazui H, Miyoshi N, et al. Cognitive impairment in patients with idiopathic normal pressure hydrocephalus. Dement Geriatr Cogn Disord 2006; 21: 113–119.

Olszewski J. Subcortical arteriosclerotic encephalopathy: review of the literature on the so-called Binswanger's disease and presentation of two cases. World Neurol 1962; 3: 359–374.

Omuro AM, DeAngelis LM, Yahalom J, Abrey LE. Chemoradiotherapy for primary CNS lymphoma: an intent-to-treat analysis with complete follow-up. Neurology 2005; 64: 69–74.

Oppenheimer DR. Microscopic lesions in the brain following head injury. J Neurol Neurosurg Psychiatry 1968; 31: 299–306.

Orchard PJ, Tolar J. Transplant outcomes in leukodystrophies. Semin Hematol 2010; 47: 70–78.

Osimani A, Berger A, Friedman J, et al. Neuropsychology of vitamin B12 deficiency in elderly dementia patients and control subjects. J Geriatr Psychiatry Neurol 2005; 18: 33–38.

O'Sullivan M. Leukoaraiosis. Pract Neurol 2008; 8: 26–38.

O'Sullivan M, Jarosz JM, Martin RJ, et al. MRI hyperintensities of the temporal lobe and external capsule in patients with CADASIL. Neurology 2001; 56: 628–634.

Pal L, Behari S, Kumar S, et al. Gliomatosis cerebri – an uncommon neuroepithelial tumor in children with oligodendroglial phenotype. Pediatr Neurosurg 2008; 44: 212–215.

Pantoni L, Garcia JH, Gutierrez JA. Cerebral white matter is highly vulnerable to ischemia. Stroke 1996; 27: 1641–1647.

Pantoni L, Garcia JH. Pathogenesis of leukoaraiosis: a review. Stroke 1997; 28: 652–659.

Pantoni L, Poggesi A, Inzitari D. The relation between white-matter lesions and cognition. Curr Opin Neurol 2007; 20: 390–397.

Pardini M, Uccelli A, Grafman J, et al. Isolated cognitive relapses in multiple sclerosis. J Neurol Neurosurg Psychiatry 2014; 85: 1035–1037.

Park K, Yasuda N, Toyonaga S, et al. Significant association between leukoaraiosis and metabolic syndrome in healthy subjects. Neurology 2007; 69: 974–978.

Patti F, Di Stefano M, De Pascalis D, et al. May there exist specific MRI findings predictive of dementia in multiple sclerosis patients? Funct Neurol 1995; 10: 83–90.

Penninx BWJH, Guralnik JM, Ferrucci L, et al. Vitamin B_{12} deficiency and depression in physically disabled older women: epidemiologic evidence from the Women's Health and Aging Study. Am J Psychiatry 2000; 157: 715–721.

Penny S, Khaleeli Z, Cipolotti L, et al. Early imaging predicts later cognitive impairment in primary progressive multiple sclerosis. Neurology 2010; 74: 545–552.

Pennypacker LC, Allen RH, Kelly JP, et al. High prevalence of cobalamin deficiency in elderly outpatients. J Am Geriatr Soc 1992; 40: 1197–1204.

Perdices M, Cooper DA. Simple and choice reaction time in patients with human immunodeficiency virus infection. Ann Neurol 1989; 25: 460–467.

Perdices M, Cooper DA. Neuropsychological investigation of patients with AIDS and ARC. J AIDS 1990; 3: 555–564.

Perry A, Schmidt RE. Cancer therapy-associated CNS neuropathology: an update and review of the literature. Acta Neuropathol 2006; 111: 197–212.

Peyser JM, Edwards KR, Poser CM, Filskov SB. Cognitive function in patients with multiple sclerosis. Arch Neurol 1980; 37: 577–579.

Pfefferbaum A, Rosenbloom MJ, Rohlfing T, et al. Frontostriatal fiber bundle compromise in HIV infection without dementia. AIDS 2009; 23: 1977–1985.

Plowman PN, Saunders CA, Maisey MN. Gliomatosis cerebri: disconnection of the cortical grey matter, demonstrated on PET scan. Br J Neurosurg 1998; 12: 240–244.

Ponce P, Alvarez-Santullano MV, Otermin E, et al. Gliomatosis cerebri: findings with computed tomography and magnetic resonance imaging. Eur J Radiol 1998; 28: 226–229.

Post MJ, Berger JR, Quencer RM. Asymptomatic and neurologically symptomatic HIV-seropositive individuals: prospective evaluation with cranial MR imaging. Radiology 1991; 178: 131–139.

Power C, Kong P-A, Crawford TO, et al. Cerebral white matter changes in acquired immunodeficiency syndrome dementia: alterations of the blood–brain barrier. Ann Neurol 1993; 34: 339–350.

Pozzilli C, Passfiume D, Bernardi S, et al. SPECT, MRI and cognitive functions in multiple sclerosis. J Neurol Neurosurg Psychiatry 1991; 54: 110–115.

Prabhakaran S, Bramlage M, Edgar MA, et al. Overwhelming leukoencephalopathy as the only sign of neuropsychiatric lupus. J Rheumatol 2005; 32: 1843–1845.

Price RW, Brew B, Sidtis J, et al. The brain in AIDS: central nervous system HIV-1 infection and AIDS dementia complex. Science 1988; 239: 586–592.

Pugnetti L, Mendozzi L, Motta A, et al. MRI and cognitive patterns in relapsing-remitting multiple sclerosis. J Neurol Sci 1993; 115 (Suppl): S59–S65.

Pullicino P, Ostrow P, Miller L, et al. Pontine ischemic rarefaction. Ann Neurol 1995; 37: 460–466.

Pyhtinen J. Proton MR spectroscopy in gliomatosis cerebri. Neuroradiology 2000; 42: 612–615.

Rao SM. Neuropsychology of multiple sclerosis: a critical review. J Clin Exp Neuropsychol 1986; 8: 503–542.

Rao SM. White matter disease and dementia. Brain Cogn 1996; 31: 250–268.

Rao SM, Leo GJ, Aubin-Faubert P. On the nature of memory disturbance in multiple sclerosis. J Clin Exp Neuropsycyhol 1989a; 11: 699–712.

Rao SM, Leo GJ, Haughton VM, et al. Correlation of magnetic resonance imaging with neuropsychological testing in multiple sclerosis. Neurology 1989b; 39: 161–166.

Rao SM, Mittenberg W, Bernardin L, et al. Neuropsychological test findings in subjects with leukoaraiosis. Arch Neurol 1989c; 46: 40–44.

Rao SM, Leo GJ, Bernardin L, Unverzagt F. Cognitive dysfunction in multiple sclerosis: I. Frequency, patterns, and prediction. Neurology 1991; 41: 685–691.

Rao SM, Grafman J, DiGiulio D, et al. Memory dysfunction in multiple sclerosis: its relation to working memory, semantic encoding, and implicit learning. Neuropsychology 1993; 7: 364–374.

Rauschka H, Colsch B, Baumann N, et al. Late-onset metachromatic leukodystrophy: genotype strongly influences phenotype. Neurology 2006; 67: 859–863.

Reischies FM, Baum K, Brau H, et al. Cerebral magnetic resonance imaging findings in multiple sclerosis: relation to disturbance of affect, drive and cognition. Arch Neurol 1988; 45: 1114–1116.

Révész T, Hawkins CP, du Boulay EPGH, et al. Pathological findings correlated with magnetic resonance imaging in subcortical arteriosclerotic encephalopathy (Binswanger's disease). J Neurol Neurosurg Psychiatry 1989; 52: 1337–1344.

Roca M, Torralva T, Meli F, et al. Cognitive deficits in multiple sclerosis correlate with changes in fronto-subcortical tracts. Mult Scler 2008; 14: 364–369.

Rogers LR, Gutierrez J, Scarpace L, et al. Morphologic magnetic resonance imaging features of therapy-induced cerebral necrosis. J Neurooncol 2011; 101: 25–32.

Román GC. Senile dementia of the Binswanger type: a vascular form of dementia in the elderly. JAMA 1987; 258: 1782–1788.

Román GC. From UBOs to Binswanger's disease: impact of magnetic resonance imaging on vascular dementia research. Stroke 1996; 27: 1269–1273.

Román GC, Tatemichi TK, Erkinjuntti T, et al. Vascular dementia: diagnostic criteria for research studies; report of the NINDS-AIREN International Workshop. Neurology 1993; 43: 250–260.

Román GC, Erkinjuntti T, Wallin A, et al. Subcortical ischaemic vascular dementia. Lancet Neurol 2002; 1: 426–436.

Ropper AH, Samuels MA, Klein JP. *Adams and Victor's principles of neurology*. 10th ed. New York: McGraw-Hill, 2014.

Rosenberg NL. Neurotoxicity of organic solvents. In: Rosenberg NL, ed. *Occupational and environmental neurology*. Boston: Butterworth-Heinemann, 1995: 71–113.

Rosenberg NL, Spitz MC, Filley CM, et al. Central nervous system effects of chronic toluene abuse – clinical, brainstem evoked response and magnetic resonance imaging studies. Neurotoxicol Teratol 1988a; 10; 489–495.

Rosenberg NL, Kleinschmidt-DeMasters BK, Davis KA, et al. Toluene abuse causes diffuse central nervous system white matter changes. Ann Neurol 1988b; 23: 611–614.

Rovaris M, Riccitelli G, Judica E, et al. Cognitive impairment and structural brain damage in benign multiple sclerosis. Neurology 2008; 71: 1521–1526.

Rubinstein LJ, Herman MM, Long TF, Wilbur JR. Disseminated necrotizing leukoencephalopathy: a complication of treated central nervous system leukemia and lymphoma. Cancer 1975; 35: 291–305.

Ryan L, Clark CM, Klonoff H, et al. Patterns of cognitive impairment in relapsing-remitting multiple sclerosis and their relationship to neuropathology on magnetic resonance images. Neuropsychology 1996; 10: 176–193.

Sacquena T, Guttmann S, Giuliani S, et al. Binswanger's disease: a review of the literature and a personal contribution. Eur Neurol 1989; 29 (suppl 2): 20–22.

Sahakian BJ, Elliott R, Low N, et al. Neuropsychological deficits in tests of executive function in asymptomatic and symptomatic HIV-1 seropositive men. Psychol Med 1995; 25: 1233–1246.

Santamaria Ortiz J, Knight PV. Binswanger's disease, leukoaraiosis and dementia. Age Ageing 1994; 23: 75–81.

Sarchielli P, Presciutti O, Pellicioli G, et al. Absolute quantification of brain metabolites by proton magnetic spectroscopy in normal-appearing white matter of multiple sclerosis patients. Brain 1999; 122: 513–521.

Sarhaddi S, Bravo E, Cyrus AE. Gliomatosis cerebri: a case report and review of the literature. South Med J 1973; 66: 883–888.

Schiffmann R, van der Knaap MS. Invited article: an MRI-based approach to the diagnosis of white matter disorders. Neurology 2009; 72: 750–759.

Schmidt R, Fazekas F, Offenbacher H, et al. Neuropsychologic correlates of MRI white matter hyperintensities: a study of 150 normal volunteers. Neurology 1993; 43: 2490–2494.

Schmidt-Wilcke T, Cagnoli P, Wang P, et al. Diminished white matter integrity in patients with systemic lupus erythematosus. Neuroimage Clin 2014; 5: 291–297.

Schretlein DJ, Shapiro AM. A quantitative review of the effects of traumatic brain injury on cognitive functioning. Int Rev Psychiatry 2003; 15: 341–349.

Schuitema I, Deprez S, Van Hecke W, et al. Accelerated aging, decreased white matter integrity, and associated neuropsychological dysfunction 25 years after pediatric lymphoid malignancies. J Clin Oncol 2013; 31: 3378–3388.

Schultheiss TE, Kun LE, Ang KK, Stephens LC. Radiation response of the central nervous system. Int J Radiation Oncology Biol Phys 1995; 31: 1093–1112.

Sedel F, Tourbah A, Fontaine B, et al. Leukoencephalopathies associated with inborn errors of metabolism in adults. J Inherit Metab Dis 2008; 31: 295–307.

Seilhean D, Duyckaerts C, Vazeux R, et al. HIV-1-associated cognitive/motor complex: absence of neuronal loss in the cerebral neocortex. Neurology 1993; 43: 1492–1499.

Shapiro EG, Lipton ME, Krivit W. White matter dysfunction and its neuropsychological correlates: a longitudinal study of a case of metachromatic leukodystrophy treated with bone marrow transplant. J Clin Exp Neuropsychol 1992; 14: 610–624.

Shapiro EG, Lockman LA, Knopman D, Krivit W. Characteristics of the dementia in late-onset metachromatic leukodystrophy. Neurology 1994; 44: 662–665.

Sharer L. Pathology of HIV-1 infection of the central nervous system: a review. J Neuropathol Exp Neurol 1992; 51: 3–11.

Sheline GE, Wara WM, Smith V. Therapeutic irradiation and brain injury. Int J Radiation Oncology Biol Phys 1980; 6: 1215–1228.

Sherer M, Madison CF, Hannay HJ. A review of outcome after moderate and severe closed head injury with an introduction to life care planning. J Head Trauma Rehabil 2000; 15: 767–782.

Shevell MI, Rosenblatt DS. The neurology of cobalamin. Can J Neurol Sci 1992; 19: 472–486.

Shintani S, Tsuruoka S, Shiigai T. Serial positron emission tomography (PET) in gliomatosis cerebri treated with radiotherapy: a case report. J Neurol Sci 2000; 173: 25–31.

Shorvon SD, Carney MWP, Chanarin I, Reynolds EH. The neuropsychiatry of megaloblastic anaemia. Br Med J 1980; 281: 1036–1038.

Shprecher D, Schwalb J, Kurlan R. Normal pressure hydrocephalus: diagnosis and treatment. Curr Neurol Neurosci Rep 2008; 8: 371–376.

Sibbitt WL Jr, Sibbitt RR, Brooks WM. Neuroimaging in neuropsychiatric systemic lupus erythematosus. Arthritis Rheum 1999; 42: 2026–2038.

Sidtis JJ, Gatsonis C, Price RW, et al. Zidovudine treatment of the AIDS dementia complex: results of a placebo-controlled trial. Ann Neurol 1993; 33: 343–349.

Silver B, McAvoy K, Mikesell S, Smith TW. Fulminating encephalopathy with perivenular demyelination and vacuolar myelopathy as the initial presentation of human immunodeficiency virus infection. Arch Neurol 1997; 54: 647–650.

Simon JH. MRI in multiple sclerosis. Phys Med Rehabil Clin N Am 2005; 16: 383–409.

Simon JH, Zhang S, Laidlaw DH, et al. Identification of fibers at risk for degeneration by diffusion tractography in patients at high risk for MS after a clinically isolated syndrome. J Magn Reson Imaging 2006; 24: 983–988.

Skomer C, Stears J, Austin J. Metachromatic leukodystrophy (MLD): XV. Adult MLD with focal lesions by computed tomography. Arch Neurol 1983; 40: 354–355.

Smith AD, Refsum H. Vitamin B-12 and cognition in the elderly. Am J Clin Nutr 2009; 89 (Suppl): 707S–711S.

Smith DH, Meaney DF, Shull WH. Diffuse axonal injury in head trauma. J Head Trauma Rehabil 2003; 18: 307–316.

Smith EE. Leukoaraiosis and stroke. Stroke 2010; 41 (10 Suppl): S139–S143.

Smith EE, O'Donnell M, Dagenais G, et al. Early cerebral small vessel disease and brain volume, cognition, and gait. Ann Neurol 2015; 77: 251–261.

Solders M, Martin DA, Andersson C, et al. Hematopoietic SCT: a useful treatment for late metachromatic leukodystrophy. Bone Marrow Transplant 2014; 49: 1046–1051.

Soumaré A, Elbaz A, Zhu Y, et al. White matter lesions volume and motor performances in the elderly. Ann Neurol 2009; 65: 706–715.

Sperling RA, Guttmann CR, Hohol MJ, et al. Regional magnetic resonance imaging lesion burden and cognitive function in multiple sclerosis: a longitudinal study. Arch Neurol 2001; 58: 115–121.

Spitz G, Maller JJ, O'Sullivan R, Ponsford JL. White matter integrity following traumatic brain injury: the association with severity of injury and cognitive functioning. Brain Topogr 2013; 26: 648–660.

Stabler SP. Vitamin B12 deficiency. N Engl J Med. 2013; 368: 2041–2042.

Stadelmann C, Albert M, Wegner C, Brück W. Cortical pathology in multiple sclerosis. Curr Opin Neurol 2008; 21: 229–234.

Stojsavljević N, Lević Z, Drulović J, Dragutinović G. A 44-month clinical-brain MRI follow-up in a patient with B_{12} deficiency. Neurology 1997; 49: 878–881.

Strich SJ. Diffuse degeneration of the cerebral white matter in severe dementia following head injury. J Neurol Neurosurg Psychiatry 1956; 19: 163–185.

Strich SJ. Shearing injury of nerve fibres as a cause of brain damage due to head injury. Lancet 1961; 2: 443–448.

Strich SJ. Lesions in the cerebral hemispheres after blunt head injury. J Clin Pathol Suppl (R Coll Pathol) 1970; 4: 166–171.

Stuss DT, Cummings JL. Subcortical vascular dementias. In: Cummings JL, ed. *Subcortical dementia*. New York: Oxford University Press, 1990: 145–163.

Swirsky-Sacchetti T, Mitchell DR, Seward J, et al. Neuropsychological and structural brain lesions in multiple sclerosis: a regional analysis. Neurology 1992; 42: 1291–1295.

Symon L, Dorsch NWC, Stephens RJ. Pressure waves in so-called low-pressure hydrocephalus. Lancet 1972; 2: 1291–1292.

Taipa R, da Silva AM, Santos E, Pinto PS, Melo-Pires M. Gliomatosis cerebri diagnostic challenge: two case reports. Neurologist 2011; 17: 269–272.

Tanabe JL, Ezekiel F, Jagust WJ, et al. Magnetization transfer ratio of white matter hyperintensities in subcortical vascular dementia. AJNR 1999; 20: 839–844.

Tangney CC, Aggarwal NT, Li H, et al. Vitamin B12, cognition, and brain MRI measures: a cross-sectional examination. Neurology 2011; 77: 1276–1282.

Tanioka R, Yamamoto Y, Sakai M, et al. Convalescence of atypical reversible posterior leukoencephalopathy syndrome in human immunodeficiency virus infection. J Med Invest 2007; 54: 191–194.

Taphoorn MJ, Schiphost AK, Snoek FJ, et al. Cognitive functions and quality of life in patients with low-grade gliomas: the impact of radiotherapy. Ann Neurol 1994; 36: 48–54.

Taphoorn MJ, Klein M. Cognitive deficits in adult patients with brain tumours. *Lancet Neurol* 2004; 3: 159–168.

Tate DF, Conley J, Paul RH, et al. Quantitative diffusion tensor imaging tractography metrics are associated with cognitive performance among HIV-infected patients. Brain Imaging Behav 2010; 4: 68–79.

Teasdale G, Jennett B. Assessment of coma and impaired consciousness: a practical scale. Lancet 1974; 2: 81–84.

Tenuisse S, Bollen AE, van Gool WA, Walstra GJM. Dementia and subnormal levels of vitamin B_{12}: effects of replacement therapy on dementia. J Neurol 1996; 243: 522–529.

Theodoridou A, Settas L. Demyelination in rheumatic diseases. J Neurol Neurosurg Psychiatry 2006; 77: 290–205.

Thuomas K-Å, Möller C, Ödkvist LM, et al. MR imaging in solvent-induced chronic toxic encephalopathy. Acta Radiol 1996; 37: 177–179.

Thurnher MM, Schindler EG, Thurnher SA, et al. Highly active antiretroviral therapy for patients with AIDS dementia complex: effect on MR imaging findings and clinical course. AJNR 2000; 21: 670–678.

Timmerman ME, Brouwer WH. Slow information processing after very severe closed head injury: impaired access to declarative knowledge and intact application and acquisition of procedural knowledge. Neuropsychologia 1999; 37: 467–478.

Tincani A, Andreoli L, Chighizola C, Meroni PL. The interplay between the antiphospholipid syndrome and systemic lupus erythematosus. Autoimmunity 2009; 42: 257–259.

Toledano P, Sarbu N, Espinosa G, et al. Neuropsychiatric systemic lupus erythematosus: magnetic resonance imaging findings and correlation with clinical and immunological features. Autoimmun Rev 2013; 12: 1166–1170.

Tournier-Lasserve E, Joutel A, Melki J, et al. Cerebral autosomal dominant arteriopathy with subcortical infarcts and leukoencephalopathy maps to chromosome 19q12. Nature Gen 1993; 3: 256–259.

Tozzi V, Narciso P, Galgani S, et al. Effects of zidovudine in 30 patients with mild to end-stage AIDS dementia complex. AIDS 1993; 7: 683–692.

Trapp BD, Peterson J, Ransohoff RM, et al. Axonal transection in the lesions of multiple sclerosis. N Engl J Med 1998; 338: 278–285.

Triebig G, Lang C. Brain imaging techniques applied to chronically solvent-exposed workers: current results and clinical evaluation. Environ Res 1993; 61: 239–250.

Tross S, Price RW, Navia B, et al. Neuropsychological characterization of the AIDS dementia complex: a preliminary report. AIDS 1988; 2: 81–88.

Tsolaki M, Drevelegas A, Karachristianou S, et al. Correlation of dementia, neuropsychological and MRI findings in multiple sclerosis. Dementia 1994; 5: 48–52.

Tucha O, Smely C, Preier M, Lange KW. Cognitive deficits before treatment among patients with brain tumors. Neurosurgery 2000; 47: 324–333.

Tullberg M, Månsson J-E, Fredman P, et al. CSF sulfatide distinguishes between normal pressure hydrocephalus and subcortical arteriosclerotic encephalopathy. J Neurol Neurosurg Psychiatry 2000; 69: 74–81.

Tullberg M, Hultin L, Ekholm S, et al. White matter changes in normal pressure hydrocephalus and Binswanger disease: specificity, predictive value and correlations to axonal degeneration and demyelination. Acta Neurol Scand 2002; 105: 417–426.

Tullberg M, Fletcher E, DeCarli C, et al. White matter lesions impair frontal lobe function regardless of their location. Neurology 2004; 63: 246–253.

Tullberg M, Ziegelitz D, Ribbelin S, Ekholm S. White matter diffusion is higher in Binswanger disease than in idiopathic normal pressure hydrocephalus. Acta Neurol Scand 2009; 120: 226–234.

Unger E, Alexander A, Fritz T, et al. Toluene abuse: physical basis for hypointensity of the basal ganglia on T2-weighted images. Radiology 1994; 193: 473–476.

Valk PE, Dillon WP. Radiation injury of the brain. AJNR 1991; 12: 45–62.

Van Bogaert L. Encéphalopathie sous corticale progressive (Binswanger) à évolution rapide chez des soeurs. Méd Hellen 1955; 24: 961–972.

van der Knaap MS, Barth PG, Gabreëls FJ, et al. A new leukoencephalopathy with vanishing white matter. Neurology 1997; 48: 845–855.

van der Knaap MS, Breiter SN, Naidu S, et al. Defining and categorizing leukoencephalopathies of unknown origin: MR imaging approach. Radiology 1999; 213: 121–133.

van Gijn J. Leukoaraiosis and vascular dementia. Neurology 1998; 51 (suppl 3): S3–S8.

van Reekum R, Cohen T, Wong J. Can traumatic brain injury cause psychiatric disorders? J Neuropsychiatry Clin Neurosci 2000; 12: 316–327.

Vanneste J, Augustijn P, Dirven C, et al. Shunting normal-pressure hydrocephalus: do the benefits outweigh the risks? A multicenter study and literature review. Neurology 1992; 42: 54–59.

van Norden AG, de Laat KF, van Dijk EJ, et al. Diffusion tensor imaging and cognition in cerebral small vessel disease: the RUN DMC study. Biochim Biophys Acta 2012; 1822: 401–407.

van Overbeek EC, Staals J, van Oostenbrugge RJ. Vitamin B12 and progression of white matter lesions: a 2-year follow-up study in first-ever lacunar stroke patients. PLoS One 2013; 8: e78100.

van Swieten JC, Geyskes GG, Derix MMA, et al. Hypertension in the elderly is associated with white matter lesions and cognitive decline. Ann Neurol 1991; 30: 825–830.

Van Zandvoort MJE, Kapelle LJ, Algra A, De Haan EHF. Decreased capacity for mental effort after single supratentorial lacunar infarct may affect performance in everyday life. J Neurol Neurosurg Psychiatry 1998; 65: 697–702.

Vargas MI, Pereira VM, Haller S, et al. Magnetic resonance imaging of infections of the white matter. Top Magn Reson Imaging 2009; 20: 325–331.

Vassallo M, Allen S. An unusual cause of dementia. Postgrad Med J 1995; 71: 483–484.

Vernooij MW, Ikram MA, Vrooman HA, et al. White matter microstructural integrity and cognitive function in a general elderly population. Arch Gen Psychiatry 2009; 66: 545–553.

Vigliani MC, Duyckaerts C, Hauw JJ, et al. Dementia following treatment of brain tumors with radiotherapy administered alone or in combination with nitrosourea-based chemotherapy: a clinical and pathological study. J Neurooncol 1999; 41: 137–149.

Vry MS, Haerter K, Kastrup O, et al. Vitamine-B12-deficiency causing isolated and partially reversible leukoencephalopathy. J Neurol 2005; 252: 980–982.

Wang JY, Bakhadirov K, Abdi H, et al. Longitudinal changes of structural connectivity in traumatic axonal injury. Neurology 2011; 77: 818–826.

Weis S, Haug H, Budka H. Neuronal damage in the cerebral cortex of AIDS brains: a morphometric study. Acta Neuropathol 1993; 85: 185–189.

Wenz F, Steinvorth S, Lohr F, et al. Acute central nervous system (CNS) toxicity of total body irradiation (TBI) measured using neuropsychological testing of attention functions. Int J Radiation Oncology Biol Phys 1999; 44: 891–894.

West SG. Neuropsychiatric lupus. Rheum Dis Clin N Am 1994; 20: 129–158.

West SG. Lupus and the central nervous system. Curr Opin Rheumatol 1996; 8: 408–414.

White DA, Taylor MJ, Butters N, et al. Memory for verbal information in individuals with HIV-associated dementia complex; HNRC Group. J Clin Exp Neuropsychol 1997; 19: 357–366.

White RF, Feldman RG. Neuropsychological assessment of toxic encephalopathy. Am J Ind Med 1987; 11: 395–398.

Wilkie FL, Eisdorfer C, Morgan R, et al. Cognition in early human immunodeficiency virus infection. Arch Neurol 1990; 47: 433–440.

Wilson RK, Williams MA. The role of the neurologist in the longitudinal management of normal pressure hydrocephalus. Neurologist 2010; 16: 238–248.

Wohlschlaeger J, Wenger E, Mehraein P, Weis S. White matter changes in HIV-1 infected brains: a combined gross anatomical and ultrastructural morphometric investigation of the corpus callosum. Clin Neurol Neurosurg 2009; 111: 422–429.

Woltman HW. Brain changes associated with pernicious anemia. Arch Intern Med 1918; 21: 791–843.

Woods SP, Moore DJ, Weber E, Grant I. Cognitive neuropsychology of HIV-associated neurocognitive disorders. Neuropsychol Rev 2009; 19: 152–168.

Worthley SG, McNeil JD. Leukoencephalopathy in a patient taking low dose oral methotrexate therapy for rheumatoid arthritis. J Rheumatol 1995; 22: 335–337.

Wright CB, Paik MC, Brown TR, et al. Total homocysteine is associated with white matter hyperintensity volume: the Northern Manhattan Study. Stroke 2005; 36: 1207–1211.

Wright PW, Heaps JM, Shimony JS, et al. The effects of HIV and combination antiretroviral therapy on white matter integrity. AIDS 2012; 26: 1501–1508.

Wu Y, Storey P, Cohen BA, et al. Diffusion alterations in corpus callosum of patients with HIV. AJNR 2006; 27: 656–660.

Xiong L, Matthes JD, Li J, Jinkins JR. MR imaging of "spray heads": toluene abuse via aerosol paint inhalation. AJNR 1993; 14: 1195–1199.

Xu Q, Zhou Y, Li YS, et al. Diffusion tensor imaging changes correlate with cognition better than conventional MRI findings in patients with subcortical ischemic vascular disease. Dement Geriatr Cogn Disord 2010; 30: 317–326.

Xuan A, Wang GB, Shi DP, Xu JL, Li YL. Initial study of magnetic resonance diffusion tensor imaging in brain white matter of early AIDS patients. Chin Med J (Engl) 2013; 126: 2720–2724.

Yamanouchi N, Okada S, Kodama K, et al. Effects of MRI abnormalities in WAIS-R performance in solvent abusers. Acta Neurol Scand 1997; 34–39.

Ylikoski R, Ylikoski A, Erkinjuntti T, et al. White matter changes in healthy elderly persons correlate with attention and speed of mental processing. Arch Neurol 1993; 50: 818–824.

Yousry TA, Seelos K, Mayer M, et al. Characteristic MR lesion pattern and correlation of T1 and T2 lesion volume with neurologic and neuropsychological findings in cerebral autosomal dominant arteriopathy with subcortical infarcts and leukoencephalopathy (CADASIL). AJNR 1999; 20: 91–100.

Yücel M, Takagi M, Walterfang M, Lubman DI. Toluene misuse and long-term harms: a systematic review of the neuropsychological and neuroimaging literature. Neurosci Biobehav Rev 2008; 32: 910–926.

Yücel M, Zalesky A, Takagi MJ, et al. White-matter abnormalities in adolescents with long-term inhalant and cannabis use: a diffusion magnetic resonance imaging study. J Psychiatry Neurosci 2010; 35: 409–412.

Zhang L, Harrison M, Heier LA, et al. Diffusion changes in patients with systemic lupus erythematosus. Magn Reson Imaging 2007; 25: 399–405.

Zimmerman RA, Bilaniuk LT, Gennarelli T. Computed tomography of shearing injuries of the white matter. Radiology 1978; 127: 393–396.

Chapter 7

White matter dementia

The long list of disorders that exert prominent or exclusive effects on the white matter of the brain (Filley, 2012), some of which were reviewed in the previous chapter, constitutes a major portion of neurology. Many clinical features of these disorders represent their impact on sensorimotor and autonomic functions, and the problems associated with visual loss, hemiparesis, ataxia, gait disorder, incontinence, and other such manifestations pose important clinical challenges in their own right. Still, the neurobehavioral manifestations of these disorders merit equal attention, as in many cases cognitive or emotional disturbances rival or exceed elemental deficits in clinical significance (Filley, 2012). This chapter focuses on the major cognitive effects of white matter disorders, attempting to collate and summarize a broad and extensive literature supporting the idea of white matter dementia (WMD).

Historical Background

As discussed in Chapter 1, white matter occupies roughly one-half the brain volume, but has received nowhere near the interest of its gray matter counterpart. White matter was not even recognized by anatomists until 1543, when Andreas Vesalius (1514–1564) first depicted the white matter of the cerebrum as distinct from gray matter in the seventh book of his masterful *De Humani Corporis Fabrica* (Saunders and O'Malley, 1973). Vesalius and his assistants, working in the Renaissance when human dissection was permitted after centuries of religious prohibition that restrained medical and scientific progress, produced drawings of the human body as notable for their artistic appeal as for their anatomic accuracy. Like other organs, the brain was beautifully drawn, although Vesalius had no conception of the functional role of white matter.

The function of white matter was addressed in the nineteenth century as investigators came to understand the role of myelinated systems in motor and sensory functions. The corticospinal tract, spinothalamic tract, and visual radiations were among many tracts described as neuroanatomy established the role of major efferent and afferent pathways of the brain. The potential contribution of white matter tracts to higher function was, however, far less straightforward. Exploring this issue in the early nineteenth century, Franz Joseph Gall and Johann Kaspar Spurzheim performed competent neuroanatomic studies and were the first to surmise that white matter fascicles interconnected gray matter regions and were thus related to higher functions. Gall and Spurzheim subsequently became famously ridiculed for their fanciful speculations on phrenology, and although this criticism was justified, the insights on white matter generated by these early neuroanatomists not only deserve credit but were remarkably modern in their anticipation of current thinking with respect to brain connectivity (Schmahmann and Pandya, 2006).

As the nineteenth century advanced, clinical neurologists began to incorporate white matter into their views of how higher functions were organized. A notable idea was advanced by Karl Wernicke in 1874 with the notion that the arcuate fasciculus connected Wernicke's area to Broca's area and had a key role in language repetition. In France, the widely acclaimed neurologist Jean-Martin Charcot appreciated that diseases of white matter might have important neurobehavioral consequences. In patients with multiple sclerosis (MS), Charcot's recognition of an "enfeeblement of memory" and a "foolish laughter without cause" (Charcot, 1877) resonate today with present understanding of the dementia and euphoria that can develop in this disease.

In the twentieth century, the role of white matter in higher functions was further advanced by the introduction of subcortical dementia as a category distinguishable from cortical dementia. As discussed in Chapter 4, the term was first proposed by von Stockert (1932) to describe the effects of subcortical pathology on cognition, and was intended to expand the thinking of the time, expressed notably by Eugen Bleuler (1924), who thought that whereas affective disturbances could accompany subcortical lesions, dementia could result only from diseases of the cerebral cortex. The idea of subcortical dementia initially received little attention, but in the 1970s two nearly simultaneous reports – one on progressive supranuclear palsy (Albert, Feldman, and Willis, 1974) and the other on Huntington's chorea (McHugh and Folstein, 1975) – revived the concept and fostered its development as a foundational principle in the understanding of dementia (Cummings and Benson, 1984). For the first time, the dementias were systematically divided into two major categories, emphasizing that the syndrome could result from pathology in many brain regions, not only the cerebral cortex.

Substantial criticism was soon directed at the cortical-subcortical dichotomy because of considerable clinical and neuropathological overlap between the two categories (Mayeux et al., 1983; Whitehouse, 1986; Tierney et al., 1987; Brown and Marsden, 1988). To use the example of Alzheimer's Disease (AD) as contrasted with Parkinson's Disease (PD), it was pointed out that not only may clinical features fail to distinguish between these diseases, but also that AD may exhibit neuropathological changes in subcortical regions while PD can show cortical abnormalities. Indeed, experience with the dementias does engender a considerable sense of respectful humility when the diversity of neurobehavioral syndromes and the varieties of neuropathology are considered. The classification of a syndrome with clinical-pathological phenomena as protean as those of dementia is of course fraught with difficulty. The topic in question, after all, is essentially the deterioration of the highest human faculties in the context of diseases of the most complex human organ. In this light, it is hardly surprising that a broad division of the sort intended by the cortical-subcortical dichotomy will admit of many subtleties and much overlap.

On the other hand, behavioral neurology must necessarily grapple with often highly indistinct symptoms, signs, syndromes, and neuropathologies, and indeed the great majority of neurology as a whole is beset by a lack or paucity of precise diagnostic differentiation. Symptoms of axonal versus demyelinative peripheral neuropathy are often indistinguishable, for example, and yet the electrical distinction between these categories is uncontroversial. Similarly, a cortical infarct is widely accepted as a gray matter lesion even though there is typically damage to underlying white matter as well. The overlapping aspects of cortical and subcortical dementias cannot be denied, but they need not discredit the entire idea. Rather, the dichotomy can be used as a useful early step toward a broad understanding of the behavioral neurology of dementia.

Over the years, the contrast has served to be steadily if not spectacularly useful. A multi-authored monograph appeared in 1990 that provided a comprehensive account of the topic (Cummings, 1990), and, particularly for neuropsychologists, the cortical-subcortical distinction has quietly continued to inform clinical and research work on the dementias (Huber et al., 1986; Drebing et al., 1994; Darvesh and Freedman, 1996; Bonelli and Cummings, 2008). In 2005, Martin Albert, a principal advocate of the concept of subcortical dementia, acknowledged the controversy engendered by the notion, but concluded that the most important contribution of the idea was that the "dynamic aspects" of cognition and emotion were brought into focus (Albert, 2005). This conclusion proves relevant to the main subject of this book.

With regard to white matter and its disorders, the cortical-subcortical distinction initially had relatively limited direct utility, as the white matter disorders were generally included along with the subcortical dementias (Cummings and Benson, 1984; Cummings, 1990). All brain regions below the thin ribbon of the cerebral cortex were considered as a functional unit, and thus, for example, the subcortical gray matter dementias such as PD were lumped in with white matter diseases such as MS. It is readily apparent that such broad inclusivity is likely to conceal differences that could emerge with study of individual subcortical regions, and the stage was set for further refinements in the idea. At this point the field was poised for a new step forward to improve the understanding of how dementia can arise from the disordered brain.

Toluene leukoencephalopathy: a turning point

The idea that dementia can be solely related to white matter involvement contradicts a long history in neurology and neuroscience more generally dominated by the primacy of the cerebral cortex in higher function. This corticocentric perspective (Parvizi, 2009) is indeed justified to some degree, inasmuch as a wealth of evidence supports the role of cortical structures in the operations of language, memory, attention, executive function, praxis, perception, and visuospatial abilities. But slavish adherence to conventional wisdom, however well entrenched, should always give the critical thinker pause, and clinicians have long suspected that attention to all areas of the brain is germane to the complex manifestations of cognitive dysfunction. To counteract the corticocentric bias, as well as refine the idea that subcortical regions are not passive observers of the cerebral activity around them, a strikingly novel paradigm was apparently necessary, the genesis of which appeared in the early 1980s with the arrival of magnetic resonance imaging (MRI) and its application to a little-known but tragic affliction of adolescents and young adults.

As discussed at many points in this book, MRI has spectacular capacity to visualize the brain white matter, demonstrating as never before the delineation of white and gray matter structures in a noninvasive, safe, and convenient manner. As experience grew with MRI after its introduction, it was quickly realized that this technique far exceeded computed tomography (CT) in the clarification of the neuropathology underlying neurobehavioral syndromes (Tanridag and Kirshner, 1987). This advantage was nowhere more evident than in the white matter disorders, and advances rapidly occurred in MS and many other diseases. This advantage continues today, as known white matter disorders are clarified and new ones routinely discovered when patients have their brains revealed by MRI (Filley, 2012).

In this light, it becomes clear how the clinical disorder that most securely established the legitimacy of WMD as a distinct syndrome was the dementia from intense inhalant abuse known as toluene leukoencephalopathy. This disorder, for a short time known informally as the "painted brain syndrome," was recognized by neurologists at the Denver General Hospital in the early 1980s, as the opportunity arose to examine a substantial number of young, socially disadvantaged inhalant abusers who could be studied with clinical assessment (Hormes, Filley, and Rosenberg, 1986), MRI (Rosenberg et al., 1988a), neuropsychological testing (Filley, Heaton, and Rosenberg, 1990), and, in a small number of cases, autopsy (Rosenberg et al., 1988b; Filley, Halliday, and Kleinschmidt-DeMasters, 2004). The patients who formed the basis for the pivotal observations establishing toluene leukoencephalopathy had adopted a habit of inhaling the fumes emanating from cans of spray paint, a favored substance at the time that was found to contain toluene as the major solvent. As many individuals inhaled, on a daily basis, the toluene contained in one or two cans of paint for periods lasting months to years, the opportunity for examining the range of neurotoxic effects presented itself. Experience with this unique syndrome offered remarkable insights into brain–behavior relationships, and proved to be the inspiration for the idea of WMD.

Inhalant abuse is a common and often catastrophic form of substance abuse, but among all abusable agents, inhalants have been the object of the least formal study (Howard et al., 2011). When neurologists consider substance abuse as a potential cause of clinical symptoms and signs, it is usually in the context of acute intoxication with alcohol or illicit drugs, or in the evaluation of stroke or new-onset seizures in a patient who may have recently abused one of more substances. Inhalant abuse is not typically emphasized in neuroscience curricula or neurology residencies, and physicians in general may have little or no familiarity with this problem. It was with this background that patients with toluene leukoencephalopathy were first encountered by our group in the early 1980s. The initial contact with affected individuals was in the Denver General Hospital Emergency Room, where on-call neurologists were asked to see young, usually Hispanic or African-American men and women with confusion, ataxia, and variable cranial nerve and motor signs. Most tellingly, these patients would often have the odor of paint on their breath, and in some cases flecks of paint around the mouth and nose. Clinical evaluation proceeded, and the diagnosis of inhalant abuse quickly became obvious, with spray paint as the preferred vehicle. The acute intoxication, now known as acute toxic leukoencephalopathy (McKinney et al., 2009), usually resolved with supportive care. However, as patients began to be seen in follow-up, it became apparent that chronic sequelae could also be expected as a major, if not paramount, concern in this underappreciated problem.

Long after the acute confusional state of inhalant abusers had subsided, many of the patients were found to have a distinctive and lasting neurologic syndrome consisting of cognitive, pyramidal, cerebellar, brain stem, and cranial nerve signs (Hormes, Filley, and Rosenberg, 1986). Cognitive impairment was the most common and clinically significant feature of affected patients. As interest grew in the pathogenesis of this unique syndrome, the constituents of the paint were investigated. In the Denver area of the early 1980s, and in many communities today, the spray paint used to achieve euphoria via inhalation was found by gas chromatographic analysis to contain high levels of toluene (Hormes, Filley, and Rosenberg, 1986). With more study, this solvent was securely identified as the hydrocarbon responsible for both the acute syndrome and the chronic neurologic sequelae of inhalant abuse.

The first imaging studies of this syndrome were conducted with CT, disclosing cerebral atrophy in most patients, and there were also frequent electrical abnormalities seen on electroencephalography and brain stem auditory evoked responses (Hormes, Filley, and Rosenberg, 1986). No postmortem or biopsy tissue was available at that time, however, and the neuropathological basis for the syndrome was not readily apparent from these investigations.

As MRI was being rapidly introduced into clinical practice, inhalant abusers were soon studied with this technique. The scanners of that era featured magnet strengths of only 0.35 T, far less powerful than today's magnets, but the findings in chronic impaired inhalant abusers were unmistakable. Not only did MRI confirm the diffuse cerebral atrophy seen on CT, but it also disclosed cerebellar and brain stem atrophy; and, most important, on T2-weighted images a loss of differentiation between the gray and white matter was evident throughout the brain, along with increased periventricular white matter signal intensity (Rosenberg et al., 1988a). Here for the first time was clear in vivo evidence that white matter could be selectively damaged by a systemic intoxication. The high lipophilicity of toluene was presumed responsible for the entry of the solvent into the brain that then enabled the euphoria of inhalant abuse and produced its acute and chronic neurotoxicity. MRI was thus able to show what could not be demonstrated by any other noninvasive technique (Figure 7.1). As one astute observer commented at the time, "toluene is the only imagible neurotoxin" (Herbert H. Schaumburg, personal communication).

The suspicion that brain white matter bore the brunt of injury related to toluene was quickly confirmed by a postmortem study of a long-term inhalant abuser who died as a result of toluene-induced cardiac arrhythmia (Rosenberg et al., 1988a). The autopsy demonstrated diffuse myelin pallor in the cerebral and cerebellar white matter, with perservation of neurons throughout the brain, consistent with selective toxic changes in myelin (Rosenberg et al., 1988a). Later studies showed that this case was typical of toluene abuse (Kornfeld et al., 1994; Fornazzari et al., 2003; Filley, Halliday, and Kleinschmidt-DeMasters, 2004; Al-Hajri and Del Bigio, 2010), and it became increasingly clear that myelin was the principal target of this agent, sparing cell bodies and even axons in all but the most severe cases. The large white matter tracts of the cerebrum and cerebellum were primarily affected, and in the cerebral hemispheres the periventricular white matter was most affected while subcortical U fibers were relatively spared (Rosenberg et al., 1988a; Filley et al., 2004). Of note, when the intracortical white matter was investigated, it was found to be either unaffected (Rosenberg et al., 1988a; Filley et al., 2004) or minimally involved (Kornfeld et al., 1994). Moreover, the importance of cerebral white matter involvement in the pathogenesis of dementia was made clear by a study of toluene abusers showing that the degree of cognitive impairment correlated not only with the duration of toluene abuse but with the severity of white matter change on MRI (Filley, Heaton, and Rosenberg, 1990). These

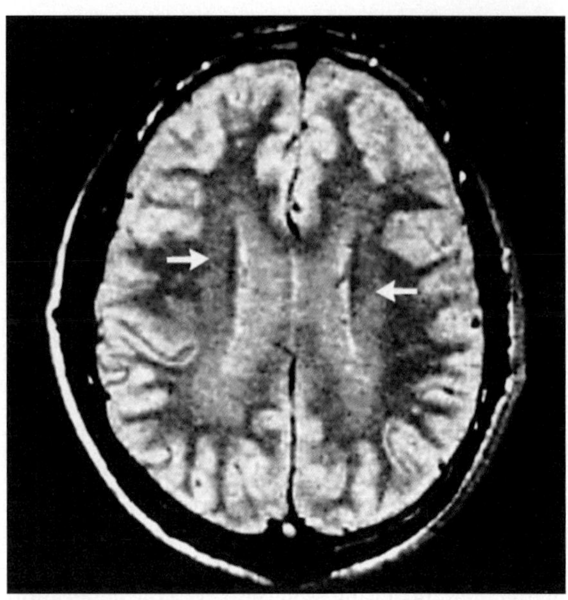

Figure 7.1 Axial T2-weighted MRI scan of a man with chronic toluene abuse and dementia. Arrows point out white matter hyperintensity, and there is also lateral ventricular enlargement (from Filley and Kleinschmidt-DeMasters, 2001).

observations were subsequently confirmed by many similar studies around the world (Yücel et al., 2008).

The chronic sequelae of toluene abuse therefore served to transform the understanding of dementia and its neuropathological basis. White matter was now unequivocally a consideration in the pathogenesis of dementia, and, even in its nascent form, this idea deserved formal designation. So it was that in 1988, based primarily on experience with this syndrome (Hormes, Filley, and Rosenberg, 1986; Filley, Heaton, and Rosenberg, 1990) but also on detailed study of MS (Franklin et al., 1989) and other disorders, the syndrome of WMD was proposed to describe the dementia that can accompany brain white matter involvement (Filley et al., 1988). Implicit in the idea was that white matter disorders typically involve widespread areas, and the disruption of myelinated tracts affects cognition regardless of the specific neuropathology present. Toluene leukoencephalopathy stands out today as the most convincing example of this syndrome, although both the novelty of the WMD concept and the relative invisibility of inhalant abuse continue to hinder the appreciation of this emerging area of behavioral neurology.

Definition and characterization

WMD is defined as a dementia syndrome resulting from diffuse or multifocal cerebral white matter damage (Filley et al., 1988; Filley, 1998; Schmahmann et al., 2008). Implicit in this definition is the assumption, based on experience with all the white matter disorders, that the total amount of white matter damaged determines the nature and severity of the cognitive impairment. That is, if dementia is destined to occur in a white matter disorder, a sufficient amount of cerebral white matter must be rendered dysfunctional. This assumption does not necessarily mean that white matter is equipotential in its mediation of higher functions. Instead, the WMD concept implies that a critical amount of tissue involved in multiple distributed neural networks must be affected before clinical features develop. Much as the extent of cortical disease is thought to accumulate to the point of clinical impairment in cortical dementias such as AD, so too does white matter disease advance in the stages leading to the syndrome of WMD. The notion of WMD should not be taken to imply that focal white matter lesions have no specific neurobehavioral correlates, as indeed a host of focal syndromes are well known to be associated with discrete white matter lesions (Geschwind, 1965; Filley, 2012). Rather, WMD develops when a sufficient lesion burden is present across several parallel networks to reach the point where dementia ensues. As the idea matured, it became clear that all recognized white matter disorders have the potential to produce a similar profile of cognitive impairment. Because these disorders tend to be multifocal or diffuse in their distribution, it was appreciated that multiple tracts are typically affected, and a neurobehavioral profile of multitract involvement began to emerge. The realization of this synthesis was nothing less than astonishing, as an impressive range of seemingly disparate disorders all became united by virtue of their common origin in white matter.

Overview

The clinical profile of WMD has been investigated by considering the wide variety of white matter disorders as a group. Box 7.1 displays the profile of WMD as currently understood, including expected cognitive deficits and areas of preserved function. This profile resembles other, more familiar characterizations of dementia (McKhann et al., 1984; Mendez and Cummings, 2003; American Psychiatric Association, 2013), but emphasizes features that are uniquely relevant to dementia associated with white matter disorders.

In the years after the WMD proposal in 1988, further investigation steadily shed light on the hypothesis (Filley et al., 1989; Merriam, Hegarty, and Miller, 1989, 1990; Filley et al., 1990; Filley and Gross, 1992; Swirsky-Sacchetti et al., 1992; Rao et al., 1993; Filley and Cullum, 1994; Shapiro et al., 1994; Yamanouchi et al., 1997; Filley et al., 1999; Riva, Bova, and Bruzzone, 2000; Mendez, Perryman, and Bronstein, 2000; Harris and Filley, 2001; Price et al.,

BOX 7.1 The profile of white matter dementia

- Cognitive slowing
- Executive dysfunction
- Sustained attention impairment
- Memory retrieval deficit
- Visuospatial impairment
- Psychiatric disturbance
- Relatively preserved language
- Normal extrapyramidal function
- Normal procedural memory

2005; Lafosse et al., 2007; Shibata et al., 2007; Libon et al., 2008; Filley et al., 2009; Grigsby et al., 2014), and several reviews have dealt with conceptual issues (Rao, 1993, 1996; Filley and Kleinschmidt-DeMasters 2001; Feinstein, 2007; Schmahmann et al., 2008; Coltman et al., 2011; Al-Hasani and Smith, 2011; Miyamoto et al., 2013; Kloppenborg et al., 2014; Prins and Scheltens, 2015). Systematic study of the distinctions between these dementia categories has been undertaken to a considerable extent (Filley et al., 1989; Gallassi et al., 1991; Rao et al., 1993; Derix, 1994; Bennett et al., 1994; Doody et al., 1998; Iddon et al., 1999; Aharon-Peretz, Kliot, and Tomer, 2000; Lafosse et al., 2007; Lafosse et al., 2013). These and many other contributions have contributed to ongoing refinement of the idea.

A crucial objective is to distinguish WMD from both cortical and subcortical dementia, and studies comparing MS with AD (Filley et al., 1989) and MS with Huntington's Disease (HD) (Lafosse et al., 2007) were instructive. First, in comparing the dementia of MS with AD – diseases of white and cortical gray matter – it was shown that while MS features processing speed and executive dysfunction, AD manifests memory encoding and language deficits (Filley et al., 1989). Then, comparison of MS with HD – diseases of white and subcortical gray matter – disclosed that while both diseases produce attentional and memory retrieval deficits, MS does not affect procedural memory whereas HD is associated with impairment in this domain (Lafosse et al., 2007). These reports were foundational in establishing that WMD differs from both cortical and subcortical gray matter dementia. WMD was distinguished from cortical dementia by relative normalcy of language and declarative memory encoding while cognitive speed, executive function, and sustained attention are impaired, and from subcortical dementia by sparing of procedural memory and extrapyramidal function (Filley et al., 1988; Filley, 1998, 2011). Core distinctions between the three syndromes are most specifically apparent in aspects of memory and language, differences that are displayed in Table 7.1.

As time progressed and new data emerged, the importance of cognitive slowing also became apparent. Whereas slowed cognition was long associated with the subcortical dementias (Albert et al., 1974; McHugh and Folstein, 1975), and indeed all dementia patients may struggle with slowed processing speed, the advent of advanced neuroimaging allowed detailed study of white matter tracts in vivo to address this issue specifically. When the white matter is specifically queried by diffusion tensor imaging (DTI), for example, cognitive processing speed has been tightly linked with the integrity of myelinated systems (Turken et al., 2008; Penke et al., 2010, Haász et al., 2013). Disorders that impair central impulse conduction thus produce slowed cognition – a reasonable assumption now increasingly supported by neuroimaging evidence – and cognitive slowing has become a distinctive feature of WMD. Thus a patient with entirely normal gray matter of the cerebral cortex and deep nuclei may still experience slowing of cognition from damage to white matter tracts alone. With this important addition to the list of cognitive deficits and areas of relative strength, the clinical profile of WMD now highlights this deficit (Box 7.1).

A clinically helpful point deserving emphasis is the tendency for the differentiating characteristics of dementias to be most evident in the early and middle stages of the disorder. Thus, although typical cognitive deficits associated with diffuse white matter lesions may progress over time (Kloppenborg et al., 2014; Smith et al., 2015), WMD is more easily detected before it becomes severe. This feature is particularly useful in that it assists in the diagnosis of dementia when the greatest opportunity for effective treatment still presents itself. As the dementia progresses, the accumulation of neuropathology usually results in a clinical picture of neurobehavioral and neurologic disability that appears increasingly uniform. In the most severe and terminal stages, little if any distinction between cortical, subcortical gray matter, or white matter dementia can be detected. In short, as neuronal loss in the brain from any cause

Table 7.1 Core distinctions between cortical, white matter, and subcortical dementias

Domain	Cortical dementia	White matter dementia	Subcortical dementia
Declarative memory	Amnesia	Retrieval deficit	Retrieval deficit
Procedural memory	Normal	Normal	Impaired
Language	Aphasia	Normal	Normal

proceeds, all dementias increasingly come to resemble one another. However, the early stages of dementia manifest important differences, as will now be discussed in more detail.

Cognitive slowing

Among the most obvious deficits that might be expected in patients with white matter disorders is cognitive slowing, often known alternatively as slowed speed of information processing or psychomotor slowing. As discussed in Chapter 3, the core neurophysiological function of myelin is the enhancement of axonal conduction velocity, and all white matter disorders discussed in this book share a prominent disturbance of this process. The idea that white matter disorders induce cognitive slowing is disarming in its simplicity, but this clinical phenomenon quite accurately reflects the neurobiology involved. In patient populations as well as normal subjects, recent MRI and DTI observations have shown that the integrity of white matter tracts significantly impacts the speed of cognitive processing (Turken et al., 2008; Bartzokis et al., 2008; Kochunov et al., 2010; Penke et al., 2010; Bendlin et al., 2010; Haász et al., 2013). Thus it is appropriate to conclude that, generally stated, neurons that are slow to conduct impulses contribute to slowed thinking. Other conditions that exert their impact on gray matter may of course also produce slowed cognition, but the primacy of cognitive slowing seems particularly characteristic of white matter disorders.

Cognitive slowing has been emphasized as a cardinal feature of subcortical dementia (Cummings, 1990), and the central role of white matter in frontal-subcortical networks implies that impaired timing and activation of cortical systems can result from diffuse white matter involvement. Slowed information processing has been correlated with vascular white matter disease (Kloppenborg et al., 2014), and has long been observed in MS (Litvan et al., 1988; Demaree et al., 1999), allying white matter disorders with the subcortical gray matter diseases broadly considered. Impaired cognitive speed will most often be apparent in everyday tasks dependent on rapid information processing, and, as a result, patients may complain of being overwhelmed with the burden of multiple tasks present in a work setting. In the clinical encounter, cognitive slowing contributes most importantly to impairments in attention, and memory retrieval is also affected, as will be discussed later. A close relationship exists, for example, between cognitive speed and sustained attention (Weinstein et al., 1999). Evidence can be found to suggest that "cognitive fatigue" contributes to poor performance on tasks requiring sustained attention such as the Paced Auditory Serial Addition Test (PASAT; Krupp and Elkins, 2000; Schwid et al., 2003). In the neuropsychology laboratory, this deficit will be evident on vigilance tests, and an increase in reaction time may coexist with a deficit in sustained attention (Rueckert and Grafman, 1996). Indeed, some have suggested that impairments in vigilance are entirely explained by cognitive slowing (Spikman, van Zomeren, and Deelman, 1996). However its specific mechanisms are delineated, cognitive slowing is a common impairment that often dominates the behavioral repertoire of patients with white matter disorders of any type. In the context of WMD, cognitive slowing is best viewed as a deficit that most obviously becomes manifest in the performance of attentional, memory, and executive function tasks.

Executive dysfunction

The capacity to plan, carry out, monitor, and complete cognitive tasks while avoiding distraction is the essence of what has come to be regarded as executive function. This domain is crucial to normal cognition, and its dissolution can be observed in many brain diseases. Executive dysfunction has steadily risen to the status of a defining deficit in the white matter disorders affecting cognition (Filley, 2010). White matter involvement in Binswanger's Disease (BD), for example, prominently impairs executive dysfunction (Román et al., 1993), and a severe burden of ischemic white matter disease produces selective executive deficits that are not explained by cortical amyloid deposition (Yoon et al., 2013).

Executive dysfunction is a feature of toxic leukoencephalopathies related to toluene and other agents, and results primarily from frontal lobe myelin loss (Filley and Kleinschmidt-DeMasters, 2001; Filley, Halliday, and Kleinschmidt-DeMasters, 2004). Deficits on tests that measure executive function have similarly been noted in MS patients (Feinstein, 2007), and MRI studies have correlated these deficits with demyelinative plaques in the frontal white matter (Arnett et al., 1994). In comparing patients with normal pressure hydrocephalus (NPH) to those with AD, Iddon and colleagues (1999) found that a pattern of executive dysfunction related to frontal lobe involvement distinguished the former from the latter. In patients with metachromatic leukodystrophy (MLD), a frontal lobe syndrome with impaired executive function has been documented neuropsychologically (Shapiro et al., 1994), and executive dysfunction is the most significantly affected cognitive domain in fragile X tremor ataxia syndrome (FXTAS; Grigsby et al., 2014).

Sustained attention impairment

Attention is a difficult and multifaceted concept in behavioral neurology and neuropsychology. While useful in that it designates a set of important mental operations, the meaning of attention depends on the context in which it is used. In the most general sense, attention refers to the ability to focus on some stimuli while competing distractors are present; this capacity, often called selective attention, operates over a period of seconds, and is usefully tested by the digit span (Mesulam, 2000). When selective attention operates over a period of minutes, sustained attention, also known as concentration or vigilance, is engaged (Filley and Cullum, 1994), and a variety of continuous performance tasks are suitable for assessment of this task (Mesulam, 2000). Sustained attention is also closely related to the notion of working memory, and similar brain regions appear to be involved in each.

In a study testing the idea that sustained attentional disturbances are prominent in white matter disorders, a comparison of MS and AD patients disclosed that sustained attention was markedly affected in the former while relatively normal in the latter (Filley et al., 1989). This study was the first to compare white matter and cortical disease directly from a neurobehavioral perspective, and demonstrated contrasting profiles of attentional and concentration dysfunction in patients with MS versus memory and language impairment in those with AD; from these observations it was proposed that these two diseases represent prototype white matter and cortical dementias (Filley et al., 1989). Attention and concentration deficits were later found to be more common in BD than in AD (Doody et al., 1998), further supporting this distinction. These results are usefully interpreted in light of a neuropsychological comparison of subcortical gray with subcortical white matter disease (Caine et al., 1986); in this study, patients with MS and HD had similar cognitive impairment, but memory dysfunction was more severe in HD, and MS patients showed normal cognitive strategies but lowered mental efficiency. Thus in these respects MS differs from both AD and HD. Sustained attention can also be shown to decline in normal aging (Filley and Cullum, 1994), which not incidentally features a decline in white matter integrity (Bartzokis et al., 2010).

The neuroanatomy of sustained attention is not fully understood, although it is likely that a network of interconnected cerebral structures mediates this capacity. Many lines of evidence implicate the frontal lobes and their connections to more posterior regions (Mesulam, 2000), and some evidence suggests that the right frontal lobe is particularly specialized for sustained attention (Rueckert and Grafman, 1996). It also appears that frontal lobe white matter in particular contributes to this capacity (Filley, 2012).

A study of children with attention-deficit disorder with hyperactivity, for example, found a smaller volume of the right frontal lobe white matter than in normal controls; furthermore, poorer performance on sustained attention tasks was associated with reduced right hemisphere white matter volume (Semrud-Clikeman et al., 2000). More recently, DTI studies in normal children (Karlborg et al., 2013) and adults (Takahashi et al., 2010) have correlated the integrity of right frontal white matter with performance on sustained attention tasks. Evidence also exists for a role of the corpus callosum in sustained attention, as studies of children using tachistoscopic tasks have suggested that interhemispheric transfer of information is important for performance on tests of vigilance (Rueckert, Sorenson, and Levy, 1994; Rueckert et al., 1999).

Consistent with these observations, patients with acquired lesions of the corpus callosum have deficits in sustained attention. In MS, for example, an impairment of vigilance has been correlated with reduced corpus callosum size as assessed by MRI (Rao et al., 1989b). Similar reductions in the size of the corpus callosum have been reported in children with attention-deficit/hyperactivity disorder (Giedd et al., 1994). A considerable body of experimental evidence acquired from normal subjects also supports a prominent role for the corpus callosum in attentional processing (Banich, 1998).

Memory retrieval deficit

Memory, like attention, is a multifaceted and fundamental concept in clinical neuroscience. Many different varieties of memory have been postulated, derived from clinical examples in which specific deficits in memory can follow documented brain lesions (Budson and Price, 2005). For our purposes, two distinctions will prove most helpful. The first is the distinction between declarative and procedural memory. Declarative memory, routinely tested in neurologic encounters, is a mainstay of the mental status examination; two subtypes are episodic (events of personal experience) and semantic (conceptual and factual knowledge). Procedural memory, in contrast, refers to the learning of skills at an unconscious, automatic level, and this form of memory must be evaluated by special neuropsychological tests tapping the capacity for motor learning.

The second distinction involves the related but separable processes of encoding versus retrieval within declarative memory (Cummings, 1990). An encoding deficit, also known as amnesia, is widely thought to indicate hippocampal damage, and among the dementias, AD is by far the most common cause. A retrieval deficit, in contrast, implies that the information is encoded but cannot be readily accessed, and this kind of memory failure implicates extrahippocampal brain regions. The clinician has some capacity to evaluate these aspects of memory by determining if the recall of items that cannot be recalled after a short delay can be improved by one of two methods: (1) cuing the patient with the provision of semantic clues that may trigger a memory, and (2) providing a list of items in which the desired ones are included. If either of these procedures results in improved recall, the patient can be said to have encoded the information but been deficient in its retrieval. The examiner has thus documented preservation of recognition memory, and the patient can be considered to have a retrieval deficit. In the practice of behavioral neurology, this distinction can at times be established during the office or bedside evaluation; but neuropsychological testing can offer a more thorough assessment with standardized measures capturing more of the subtlety of memory impairment. The data on memory retrieval have been primarily derived from this approach, and in this light, it is pertinent to review some neuropsychological studies of memory that have suggested a unique pattern in patients with white matter disorders. The retrieval deficit will first be considered, and then normal procedural memory in a subsequent section.

Early efforts to define the type of declarative memory impairment in white matter disorders were undertaken with MS patients, and a retrieval deficit was found (Rao et al., 1984). As reviewed in Chapter 6, some studies have presented data supporting an alternative idea that the declarative memory deficit of MS patients is more related to difficulty with the acquisition of information than its retrieval (DeLuca, Barbieri-Berger, and Johnson, 1994; DeLuca et al., 1998). It may be that both processes are relevant, given the complex and time-dependent neuropathology of MS (Lafosse et al., 2013). Encoding deficits in MS, for example, may reflect demyelination in the alveus, an intrahippocampal white matter structure (Laule et al., 2008), as well as larger afferent and efferent hippocampal tracts. As gray matter involvement is minimal early in the course of MS (Hauser and Oksenberg, 2006), the initial memory deficits are most likely to be in retrieval.

Similar retrieval deficits have also been documented in ischemic vascular dementia (Lafosse et al., 1997; Libon et al., 1998; Reed et al., 2000); in radiation leukoencephalopathy (Armstrong et al., 2000; Armstrong, Stern, and Corn, 2001); in carbon monoxide intoxication (Chang et al., 2009); in TBI (Timmerman and Brouwer, 1999); in the AIDS dementia complex (ADC; White et al., 1997; Jones and Tranel, 1991); in CADASIL (Chabriat et al., 2009); and in fragile X premutation carriers (Hippolyte et al., 2014), indicating that this pattern of declarative memory loss may be applicable to many other white matter disorders.

Although subtle, these distinctions support the idea that white matter disorders disturb declarative memory in a specific and reproducible fashion. This pattern relates to the selective involvement of white matter tracts that produces disruption of memory retrieval more than encoding. The specific tracts involved have yet to be securely identified, but some information on this issue is available.

On the basis of clinical reports and functional neuroimaging data, Markowitsch (1995) suggested that the uncinate fasciculus is responsible for memory retrieval. Memory retrieval requires the engagement of working memory systems in the frontal lobes to enable the recall of information stored in the temporal lobes, and the tract connecting these regions is the uncinate fasciculus (Markowitsch, 1995). Support for this schema has recently come from functional MRI (fMRI) studies of memory retrieval in normal adults demonstrating a ventral frontotemporal network within which the uncinate fasciculus is situated (Barredo, Oztekin, and Badre, 2015). These data may indicate a specific cognitive role for a white matter tract that has not heretofore been understood to have a firm neurobehavioral affiliation, and invited further study with modern neuroimaging technology applied to a variety of white matter disorders in which memory is affected.

Taking advantage of these technologies, studies of MS (Sepulcre et al., 2008), carbon monoxide intoxication (Chang et al., 2009), and glioma (Papagno et al., 2011) have shown that a variety of frontotemporal tracts, including but not limited to the uncinate fasciculus, participate in memory retrieval. Consistent with this idea, DTI studies of normal elders have demonstrated that decline in the integrity of prefrontal white matter and the genu of the corpus callosum contribute to age-related slowing of memory retrieval (Bucur et al., 2008). As attractive as it may be to assign memory retrieval to one tract, a more complicated system appears to be operative, and a network of white matter structures likely participates in the retrieval of declarative memory (Sepulcre et al., 2008).

As in the case of attentional dysfunction, the retrieval deficit seen in individuals with white matter disorders can be seen as closely related to cognitive slowing. In clinical practice, these patients will often be noted to produce the correct answer to a question if sufficient time is provided, implying that the information is encoded but not easily retrieved. Thus the delay in providing the correct answer may be interpreted as slowed cognition rather than a memory deficit. In other words, the patient is indeed cognitively slow, but the reason for this slowing is a failure of memory retrieval. As intimated earlier, cognitive slowing, while important as a general observation, can be analyzed in more detail and interpreted in terms of cognitive dysfunction. The delineation of specific deficits, most obviously in attention and memory, that contribute to cognitive slowing is an important neuropsychological issue deserving further study.

Visuospatial impairment

Visuospatial function has only lately received attention, but studies that are available suggest an impairment related to white matter dysfunction. Studies on the genetics of normal fiber architecture have shown that the integrity of white matter is associated with full-scale IQ (FSIQ) and performance IQ (PIQ) but not verbal IQ (VIQ) (Chiang et al., 2009). These data indicate a selective relationship of white matter with nonverbal capacities that is in part genetically mediated. Given that diffuse white matter lesions are not strongly associated with language dysfunction, it might be predicted that white matter disorders have more prominent nonverbal manifestations, and this prediction has in fact been upheld.

To begin, focal lesion data clearly support a role of white matter in visuospatial dysfunction. A CT study of 53 patients with visuospatial dysfunction after right hemisphere stroke found that left neglect was highly correlated with damage in the temporoparietal white matter (Samuelsson et al., 1997). Left neglect has also been documented in an MS patient with a right cerebral demyelinative lesion (Graff-Radford and Rizzo, 1987). With respect to the literature on diffuse lesions, cross-sectional and longitudinal studies of diffuse white matter hyperintensities of vascular origin have disclosed that these lesions correlate with perceptual and constructional deficits (Kloppenborg et al., 2014). Similarly, MS patients with diffuse demyelinative lesions score about 10 points lower on the performance subtests of the Wechsler Adult Intelligence Scale than on the verbal subtests (Rao, 1996), and specific visuospatial deficits have been shown on a variety of standard tests of right hemisphere function (Heaton et al., 1985; Rao et al., 1991). Studies of solvent-induced leukoencephalopathy have confirmed that nonverbal abilities are more impaired than verbal skills in patients with toluene dementia (Yamanouchi et al., 1997). This nonverbal-verbal neuropsychological discrepancy has also been observed in children with hydrocephalus (Mataró et al., 2001) and in patients with metachromatic leukodystrophy (MLD; Shapiro et al., 1994). Using DTI, studies in normal young adults have found that visuospatial attention correlates with the integrity of white matter of the right parietal and temporal lobes (Tuch et al., 2005).

With respect to disease states, abstinent alcoholics were then shown to have impaired visuospatial function associated with DTI microstructural white matter involvement in bilateral frontal and temporal regions (Rosenbloom et al., 2009). Most recently, a DTI study of stroke patients correlated microstructural injury in right frontoparietal white matter with chronic left neglect (Lunven et al., 2015).

Psychiatric disturbance

Emotional and personality aspects of WMD have received considerable attention, and psychiatric syndromes have a complex relationship to white matter dysfunction (Filley, 2012). This area of neuropsychiatry is vast and poorly understood, and only a brief account can be offered here; comprehensive reviews have recently addressed intriguing new ideas on the relationship of white matter to psychiatric illness in general (Bartzokis, 2011; Walterfang et al., 2011; Haroutunian et al., 2014). For the purposes of this book, some of the most important observations have been made in patients with known neurologic diseases. Psychosis as an early feature of adult-onset MLD, for example, was noted as a frequent trend (Filley and Gross, 1992; Hyde, Ziegler, and Weinberger, 1992), and the development of this syndrome was interpreted as an early component of a sequential progression to dementia seen in these patients (Filley and Gross, 1992; Shapiro et al., 1994).

Depression in MS has received much attention (Minden and Schiffer, 1990; Feinstein, 2007), and the potential lethality of this problem was better appreciated as a high risk for suicide was documented (Sadovnick et al., 1991). It is likely that depression in MS results at least in part from frontotemporal white matter disease, and exacerbates cognitive dysfunction related to other brain involvement (Feinstein, 2007).

Depression has been reported to be more common in BD patients than in AD patients who are comparably demented (Bennett et al., 1994). In white matter lacunar dementia, the severity of delusions and hallucinations, aggression, irritability, aberrant motor behavior, nighttime behavior, and appetite changes has been correlated with cognitive decline, whereas no such correlations were found in AD (Aharon-Peretz, Kliot, and Tomer, 2000). These data suggest that white matter ischemia and infarcts have a direct impact on psychosis and related syndromes.

A provocative recent contribution to this area has been the proposal that white matter immaturity may predispose to psychiatric disease in adolescence and young adulthood. Adopting a developmental perspective, Bartzokis (2005) suggested that the process of myelination in adolescents and young adults is incomplete, possibly contributing to the high incidence of psychiatric conditions such as schizophrenia, mood disorder, attention-deficit/hyperactivity disorder, and conduct disorder at this time of life. These disorders all tend to reduce the already tenuous inhibitory control of adolescence, thus predisposing to the higher incidence of addiction, the effects of which may further inhibit white matter maturation (Bartzokis, 2005).

Relatively preserved language

One of the most robust observations in the white matter disorders is that language is usually well preserved. In this respect, the classical teachings of clinical neurology are entirely accurate. Genetic studies failing to detect a link between normal white matter and verbal function as measured by VIQ (Chiang et al., 2009) have been mentioned earlier. Among clinical populations, aphasia is uncommon in the setting of white matter disease (Derix, 1994; Filley, 2012), and language impairment, if present, is typically subtle. In the investigation of vascular white matter disease, language has not often been evaluated (Kloppenborg et al., 2014), but cross-sectional studies have not found a correlation between the extent of white matter hyperintensities and language dysfunction (Murray et al., 2010; Price et al., 2012).

In people with MS, aphasia is indeed rare, and a recent large multicenter study found that less than 1% of MS patients experience this syndrome (Lacour et al., 2004). When it does occur, aphasia takes reasonably predictable forms. As expected from the classic model of aphasia localization (Filley, 2011), for example, conduction aphasia can appear in relation to a focal plaque in the left arcuate fasciculus (Arnett et al., 1996). With detailed testing, minor deficits in language can be detected in MS (Kujala, Portin, and Ruutianen, 1996), but these are typically not evident in ordinary discourse or even on routine mental status testing. In comparison to patients with AD, those with MS have little linguistic difficulty (Filley et al., 1989).

Impaired verbal fluency may be seen in some white matter disorders (Derix, 1994, Filley, 2010), reflecting executive dysfunction at least as much as linguistic disturbance. Speech disorders, however, are frequent in white matter disorders. Dysarthria is well known in MS, and can sometimes assume a scanning quality. Articulation deficits are also described in the acquired immunodeficiency syndrome (AIDS; Navia, Jordan, and Price, 1986), toluene leukoencephalopathy (Hormes, Filley, and Rosenberg, 1986), and BD (Babikian and Ropper, 1987). In these disorders, involvement of corticobulbar tracts subserving articulation is plausible.

Despite the fact that language is affected only mildly in WMD, or not at all, it should not be overlooked that white matter still has a prominent role in language. From the stroke literature, for example, it is indeed clear that left perisylvian white matter involvement plays a role in all traditional aphasia syndromes (Alexander, Naeser, and Palumbo, 1987). The resolution of this paradox is that language is highly lateralized and localized, and thus less affected by the diffuse neuropathological distribution of typical white matter disorders. Language is vulnerable to large, focal left perisylvian lesions, most often of vascular origin, but is not typically implicated in WMD, which results from less dramatic but more widely distributed injury to a broad array of tracts elsewhere in the brain. The cortical regions responsible for language processing – Broca's area, Wernicke's area, and adjacent cortices – are interconnected by heavily myelinated tracts that extend relatively short distances (Anderson, Southern, and Powers, 1999) and are therefore less susceptible to most white matter neuropathology. Thus, whereas large left hemisphere infarcts damaging language-related white matter tracts can surely produce aphasia (Alexander, Naeser, and Palumbo, 1987), the diffuse white matter lesions implicated in WMD do not usually lead to aphasia because they mainly affect nonlinguistic tracts, or are of insufficient size to exert a notable effect on language.

Normal extrapyramidal function

Extrapyramidal dysfunction – in the form of tremor, dystonia, chorea, athetosis, tic, myoclonus, and so forth – is traditionally associated with disorders of the subcortical gray matter, and neurologists who detect these signs in the evaluation of dementia patients are usually correct in assuming that white matter disorders are not typically responsible. Despite this useful clinical adage, an initial criticism of the WMD hypothesis questioned the usefulness of the absence of movement disorders based on the observation that these phenomena may be encountered in white matter diseases (Merriam, Hegarty, and Miller, 1990). However, it is well accepted that movement disorders are typically caused by basal ganglia neuropathology, often combined with thalamic and brain stem involvement (Jellinger, 1998), and white matter disorders do so only when myelinated tracts within the deep gray matter are implicated. A large study of older patients seen in memory clinics did in fact detect extrapyramidal signs in 10%, but these were not strongly related to the burden of white matter hyperintensity on MRI (Staekenborg et al., 2010).

Movement disorders reflecting basal ganglia involvement can occasionally occur in white matter disorders that have reached a late stage, as in the case of myoclonus in the AIDS dementia complex (Navia, Jordan, and Price, 1986), or when the leukoencephalopathy is sufficiently widespread to involve the white matter of the basal ganglia, as exemplified by parkinsonism from severe carbon monoxide poisoning (Sohn et al., 2000). In MS, movement disorders are very rare (Ozturk et al., 2002), and some may actually be coincidental to demyelinative disease (Tranchant, Bhatia, and Marsden, 1995).

As few rules in behavioral neurology are absolute, extrapyramidal dysfunction can be seen in white matter disorders, but these cases typically can be explained by some degree of subcortical nuclear involvement, often in the later stages of a white matter disorder, or by an unrelated movement disorder. In the clinic, it remains justified, as a general rule, to associate movement disorders with subcortical gray matter diseases (Ropper, Samuels, and Klein, 2014).

Normal procedural memory

Procedural memory, along with its companion procedural learning, represents an area of cognitive neuroscience that is only peripherally related to clinical neurology and neuropsychology. Patients rarely complain of dysfunction in the performance of previously acquired or newly sought motor skills, and if they do, issues such as joint disease, fatigue, and forgetfulness are often invoked as explanatory. Moreover, procedural memory is challenging to assess and cannot be routinely attempted in a clinical setting. Yet procedural memory is an important cognitive capacity and has relatively secure neuroanatomic correlates.

In WMD, procedural memory has been particularly informative. Studies of MS have found a preservation of procedural memory (Rao et al., 1993), as have investigations of the ADC (White et al., 1997; Jones and Tranel, 1991) and TBI (Timmerman and Brouwer, 1999). Experiments with laboratory mice have demonstrated that recall of a prelearned motor skill does not require active myelination (McKenzie et al., 2014), implying that procedural memory can be preserved as normal in humans with white matter disorders. Procedural memory is also relatively preserved in AD (Grafman et al., 1990). In contrast, HD

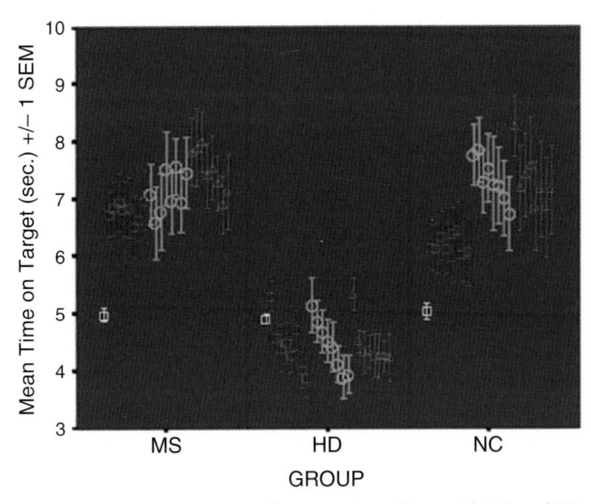

Figure 7.2 Rotary pursuit performance in patients with MS and HD compared to control subjects. HD patients, but not those with MS, show impaired procedural learning (from Lafosse et al., 2007).

patients show impaired procedural memory (Knopman and Nissen, 1991; Gabrieli et al., 1997). These studies suggest that diseases affecting the basal ganglia are most likely to disrupt procedural memory.

To assess the specific role of white matter in procedural memory, Lafosse and colleagues (2007) compared clinically definite MS patients, genetically verified HD patients, and normal controls, and found that, as hypothesized, MS patients and HD patients share a retrieval deficit in declarative memory, but MS patients have normal procedural memory, as tested by rotary pursuit, while HD patients are impaired (Figure 7.2). The findings with respect to spared procedural memory in MS support the notion that procedural memory dysfunction may distinguish white matter disorders from the subcortical gray matter diseases (Lafosse et al., 2007). These neuropsychological results thus generally support a specific pattern of memory loss proposed for WMD, contrasting with both cortical disease, in which there is an encoding deficit in declarative memory and normal procedural memory, and subcortical gray matter diseases, in which there is a retrieval deficit and impairment of procedural memory (Filley, 1998, 2010).

To help conceptualize the essence of WMD, a crucial distinction should be maintained between the core functions of white matter – information transfer – and those of gray matter – information processing (Filley, 2010). White matter is characterized by extensive macroconnectivity, which integrates neuroanatomically distant functionally connected gray matter regions into coherent neural networks, and gray matter is characterized by massive microconnectivity, referring to the extensive synaptic networks by which individual neurons communicate with each other in the processing of information. Both constituents of the brain are necessary for normal behavior. WMD implies that distributed neural networks subserving cognition are less well organized, not as efficient, and ill-suited to integrate the impressive panoply of seamless cognitive operations implied by the concept of information processing (Filley, 2010). Whereas dementia of any type may proceed clinically to the same terminal outcome, the brain–behavior relationships involved in the onset, pathogenesis, and course of WMD are distinctive.

Unresolved issues

Any new proposal such as WMD entails a host of issues that require continued study and resolution. Just as the dichotomy of cortical and subcortical dementia engendered considerable resistance after its promotion in the 1970s and 1980s, so too may WMD seem foreign to those who regard the cortex as the unique repository of cognition. Whereas no one would contend that a patient deprived of all brain white matter by some neuropathological insult would have normal cognition, the precise role of white matter has yet to be fully established. Given the complex structural relationships of white and gray matter, a nuanced approach will be most productive. In other words, there may be relatively few patients in whom pure WMD – or for that matter cortical or subcortical dementia – appears, but these constructs nonetheless organize thinking so that the dynamic interplay of all regions can be considered in furthering the understanding of brain–behavior relationships relevant to dementia.

One important issue derives from the observation that some patients with extensive white matter hyperintensity on MRI may escape any cognitive disturbance (Fein et al., 1990). Examples such as these present a perplexing counterargument that challenges the idea of WMD, but may plausibly be explained by the concept of reserve, or the capacity of an individual to enjoy reduced vulnerability to dementing brain diseases because of premorbid protective factors. Reserve can be of two kinds: brain reserve – in essence a bigger brain with more neurons – or cognitive reserve – a brain with more synapses as a consequence of educational or occupational attainment before disease onset; but the demarcation of these categories is not absolute (Stern, 2009). In cortical dementia such as AD, a protective effect is likely mediated by increased synaptic density within cortical gray matter that counteracts the effects of neuritic plaques and neurofibrillary tangles, and a similar principle may apply to white matter disorders. For example, in neuropsychological studies of both adults with MS (Sumowski et al., 2010) and normal elders (Brickman et al., 2009), all of whom had some MRI white matter lesions, cognitive reserve was found to mitigate the impact of white matter pathology. Thus the highly educated, intellectually active, and socially engaged individual may be able to lessen or even avoid the cognitive impact of white matter lesions because of well-prepared cortical systems in which rich synaptic density can compensate for the specific effects of the newly acquired pathology. In this regard, a recent combined functional MRI and DTI study of normal elders found that performance on executive function and memory tasks was associated with both higher cortical activity and diminished white matter integrity, consistent with the notion of "less wiring, more firing" as a consequence of age-related changes in white matter (Daselaar et al., 2015). Further study of the idea of reserve with respect to the dementias will be of considerable interest.

A major concern with the concept of WMD is the issue of coexistent gray matter neuropathology. One of the most appropriate questions in this work is the degree to which concurrent gray matter involvement may explain the cognitive deficits. Discussion of this issue begins with the accumulated weight of correlational evidence justifying the existence of WMD in many patients with many disorders (Filley, 2012). Toluene leukoencephalopathy remains the most convincing cause of WMD, with confirmatory neuroimaging, neuropsychological, and neuropathological evidence (Yücel et al., 2008; Al-Hajri and Del Bigio, 2010) continuing to support the earlier reports making this claim (Hormes, Filley, and Rosenberg, 1986; Rosenberg et al., 1988b; Filley et al., 1990; Filley et al., 2004). In this disorder, brain myelin appears to be diffusely damaged by the highly lipophilic solvent toluene, leading to dementia that cannot be plausibly attributed to cortical neuronal injury, synaptic loss, or deep gray matter damage.

However, toluene leukoencephalopathy is a unique example of white matter toxicity, and few cognitive disorders can be attributed to exclusive white matter involvement. As discussed in Chapter 5, the relative contributions of white and gray matter changes may both be relevant. It is therefore essential that future studies combine state-of-the-art neuroimaging of both white and gray matter regions with detailed cognitive evaluation to address this issue. An example of such work can be found in an innovative study of Mendez and colleagues (2000) comparing 28 patients with dementia from various causes who had 25% or more of the subcortical white matter affected on conventional MRI with 28 AD patients; the former group had greater difficulty with cognitive speed and sustained attention, but better recognition memory, consistent with the profile of WMD.

Another issue with the concept of WMD has been the lack of a suitable animal model for laboratory study. Experiments with nonhuman animals are indeed hindered by limitations inherent in the use of such animals to investigate human brain–behavior relationships. Nevertheless, some support for the WMD idea is available because some investigators have succeeded in examining selective white matter pathology. The work of Gennarelli and colleagues (1982) on TBI in monkeys, for example, showed that the degree of diffuse axonal injury (DAI) was directly proportional to the length of coma and the quality of outcome. These experimental injuries were very severe, however, and in light of recent human studies suggesting that mild but repetitive TBI may have similar effects on white matter, repetitive mild TBI has been examined in mice; results disclosed ongoing memory impairments and white matter degeneration for up to 12 months after injury (Mouzon et al., 2014). Another useful category of neuropathology that can be studied experimentally is vascular disease. In mouse models of cerebral ischemia (Shibata et al., 2007; Coltman et al., 2011; Miyamoto et al., 2013), bilateral carotid artery stenosis damaging only the brain white matter has been shown to produce selective working memory impairment. Further experiments such as these are likely to add much to our knowledge.

Leaving aside for a moment the intricate details of how much white matter versus gray matter may be implicated in a given neurobehavioral syndrome, it is pertinent to reflect on the corticocentric bias that so dominates current neuroscientific thinking. If a patient has a cognitive deficit syndrome related to a focal cerebral lesion affecting both cortex and white matter, the explanation offered by most neurologists is that the cortical component of the lesion must be the critical area of damage. A left hemisphere stroke causing aphasia, for example, may often involve both cortex and white matter, but the gray matter portion is deemed crucial while the white matter damage is ignored. Such an opinion may be premature, as the contribution of white matter to language has been well demonstrated (Alexander, Naeser, and Palumbo, 1987).

Similarly, the assumption that dementia in patients with ischemic white matter lesions must be related to coexistent AD should be reconsidered in light of data that many such patients have no evidence of cortical amyloid. In one study, for example, 69% of patients with subcortical vascular dementia and severe white matter ischemia had no evidence of cortical amyloid as shown by Pittsburgh compound B (PiB) combined with positron emission tomography (PET) scanning (Lee et al., 2011). Moreover, these individuals performed better on tests of memory than on measures of frontal lobe functions, while those with cortical amyloid on PiB-PET had the opposite pattern (Yoon et al., 2013), again suggesting that white and gray matter lesions exert distinctive effects on cognition. Brain lesions may involve gray matter, white matter, or both, and it would seem that a reasonable and scientific approach is to consider both kinds of lesions in exploring the pathogenesis of neurobehavioral syndromes. While gray matter will not likely be obliged to concede its lofty position as a key neural mediator of human behavior, the white matter is likely to gain respect as a partner in the operations of higher functions, and elucidation of the interplay between the two will greatly expand our understanding.

The timing of neuropathological lesions may offer a helpful perspective as the relative contributions of white and gray matter are considered. As indicated in Chapter 5, the advance of white matter lesions is recognized to be associated with progressive brain compromise in other regions. This principle is most evident in the case of ischemic white matter hyperintensities, which are associated with global brain atrophy over time (Appelman et al., 2009) and produce either ventricular enlargement (Inatomi et al., 2008) or cortical atrophy (Tuladhar et al., 2015). Recent studies have focused on cortical thickness, and longitudinal data are now available to show that the cortex does indeed become thinner over time as white matter hyperintensities accumulate (Smith et al., 2015). The mechanism explaining this progression is likely complex, but the key point may be that early clinical features reflecting white matter disease may blend into those determined by gray matter involvement as time proceeds. This sequence may be typical of many white matter disorders, as will be discussed further later.

Closely related to the issue of coexistent gray matter pathology is the challenge posed by intracortical myelin and its pathology. As reviewed in Chapter 3, small fascicles of myelinated axons coursing through all six layers of the neocortex have been known for more than a century (Nieuwenhuys, 2013). Moreover, some disease states – mainly those involving inflammatory demyelination (Moll et al., 2008) – have been found to feature damage to intracortical myelin. Diseases such as these complicate the distinction between cortical and white matter dysfunction since the white matter of the cortex may be involved along with larger tracts in the subcortical regions. This intracortical myelin damage may secondarily affect the axons, dendrites, and synapses of the cortex so as to produce cortical deficits such as amnesia, aphasia, apraxia, and agnosia. A clinical picture may thus emerge in which neurobehavioral sequelae reflect a commingling of large tract and intracortical white matter involvement.

Currently the importance of intracortical myelin is most evident in MS, where interest in cortical MS has rekindled the supposition that cognitive impairment can be ascribed to gray matter involvement (Lucchinetti et al., 2011). Without doubt, gray matter is affected in MS, and the evidence that this process develops more prominently later in the disease was reviewed in Chapter 6. But even in MS, in which gray matter neuropathology has long been recognized, the WMD model appears justified, at least early in the disease. The resolution of this problem is not yet apparent, but in a thoughtful commentary Feinstein (2007) offered the reasonable statement that whereas white matter disorders may have gray matter involvement that contributes to cognitive impairment and dementia, damage to white matter alone can indeed influence the type of cognitive loss.

Cognitive decline begins early in MS (Amato et al., 2010), and while all patients have white matter lesions, cortical lesions are found with conventional MRI in only 8% of children (Absinta et al., 2011), and, using brain biopsy, only 38% of adults with early disease have cortical lesions (Lucchinetti et al., 2011). Moreover, the cognitive profile of MS resembles other white matter disorders more than AD

(Filley et al., 1989), suggesting that tract demyelination is the major determinant of cognitive decline, at least until later in the course. Studies with high field strength MRI have recently shed further light on this issue. Using 7.0 T MRI to examine both gray and white matter in patients with mean illness duration of 9 years, it has been found that the strongest correlates of cognitive dysfunction are white matter lesion volume and lesions that involve the gray matter–white matter junction ("type 1" plaques), suggesting that cognitive decline early in MS primarily results from tract demyelination that involves both large association tracts and the U fibers connecting adjacent gyri (Nielsen et al., 2013). Such studies promise to more firmly establish the relative contributions of white and gray matter neuropathology to the cognitive profile of MS and other white matter disorders.

In this regard, toluene leukoencephalopathy offers a useful perspective. Here the impact of intracortical myelin can be assessed on the basis of how much leukotoxic damage can be observed within the cortex. When the cortex of these patients has been examined, the intracortical myelin has typically been found normal (Rosenberg et al., 1988b; Filley, Halliday, and Kleinschmidt-DeMasters, 2004) and in just one study was intracortical myelin found to be mildly affected (Kornfeld et al., 1994). While more attention to intracortical myelin in toluene leukoencephalopathy is warranted, it would appear at this point that the primary cause for the WMD pattern in this disorder is involvement of large subcortical tracts.

An issue directly pertaining to the concept of WMD is the notion of a threshold effect. How much white matter damage is required to produce dementia? This question is far from straightforward, and indeed the analysis of many other dementia syndromes faces the same general problem. Whether the damage is sustained in white or gray matter, many variables influence the point at which dementia occurs, including the age of the patient; the degree of brain and cognitive reserve before the disorder begins; the presence or absence of other neurologic, psychiatric, or medical problems; and many incompletely understood genetic factors. Nevertheless, investigators have introduced the idea of a threshold effect whereby a certain amount of white matter must be compromised to reach the point where cognitive impairment becomes evident.

The most comprehensive work on this question has come from the study of demyelinative and ischemic white matter lesions as seen on MRI. In MS, it is generally acknowledged that cognitive decline is correlated with increasing lesion load on MRI (Rao, 1995), and an early effort to establish a cognitive threshold proposed that a cerebral plaque burden of 30 cm^2 was required to impact cognition (Swirsky-Sacchetti et al., 1992). However, it has also become clear that determining a precise threshold at which dementia begins in MS is complicated by the problem of cortical MS (Lucchinetti et al., 2011), which could hasten the onset of dementia, and cognitive reserve (Sumowski et al., 2010), which could have the opposite effect. In other words, two individuals with MS who have exactly the same white matter lesion burden could have a markedly different risk for dementia.

Work has proceeded in parallel on vascular disease, and an early study of individuals with ischemic white matter hyperintensities concluded that a lesion area of greater than 10 cm^2 was associated with disturbances in attentional and frontal lobe skills (Boone et al., 1992). Subsequently, a consensus statement concluded that ischemic involvement of 25% of the cerebral white matter was necessary for the appearance of dementia (Román et al., 1993). Later work with leukoaraiosis (LA) patients also found that 25% could be considered a threshold for the development of cognitive impairment in the domains of executive function, visuospatial ability, and working memory, while declarative memory and language were relatively spared (Price et al., 2005; Libon et al., 2008). Moreover, demented adults with a low burden of LA had impaired episodic memory compared with working memory, whereas those with moderate LA had equal impairment on episodic and working memory, and severe LA was associated with selective impairment of working memory (Price et al., 2005; Libon et al., 2008).

Yet these studies have focused only on macrostructural white matter lesions, and, as will be discussed in the following chapter, microstructural lesions can also be usefully investigated. The question of a threshold effect is clearly influenced by the sensitivity of neuroimaging techniques used to identify white matter pathology, and abnormalities found in the normal-appearing white matter (NAWM) promise to restructure the study of what happens first in white matter disorders, and how these changes may impact cognition. As has been true throughout the MRI era, improvements in technology will permit a more elegant approach to the study of white matter–cognition relationships, and study of the earliest visible manifestations of white matter pathology will be of great interest.

Another issue arises with respect to clinical outcomes of patients with white matter disorders. If it is indeed true that white matter involvement exerts a specific effect on cognition, improvement of white matter lesion burden should produce a salutary clinical effect. One of the ways to assess the strength of the construct of WMD is to consider data on whether the resolution of white matter lesions leads to reversal of the neurobehavioral syndrome produced. That is, if spontaneous recovery from, or treatment of, white matter lesions produces improvement of the clinical deficit, much more credence can be gained as to the neurobehavioral importance of the lesion(s). Spontaneous recovery, however gratifying it may be, is difficult to use for investigating the role of white matter lesions, but outcome studies following treatment are indeed helpful. As will be discussed in Chapter 11, a number of categories of white matter disorder offer examples of specific conditions in which clinical improvement after treatment can be seen in parallel with resolution of or reduction in white matter lesion burden. With further refinement of neuroimaging that can securely identify specific lesions before and after treatment, the impact of these lesions, particularly those that affect one tract and alter one cognitive domain, can be carefully evaluated.

A final issue looming large over all of these unresolved questions is uncertainty revolving around the secure determination of what can be considered normal white matter. As discussed in Chapter 2, the ever-expanding capacity of advanced neuroimaging to reveal subtle aspects of white matter structure calls into question what can be characterized as normal. Whereas the studies reviewed earlier do suggest that white matter disease of any sort can accumulate to produce specific cognitive deficits, it should be recalled that MRI detects only macrostructural white matter lesions, and that the NAWM often harbors microstructural changes that may be of uncertain significance. The work on the NAWM illustrates how the understanding of how white matter contributes to cognitive function is far from complete, and more study using the most sensitive available techniques combined with careful clinical correlation will be needed to clarify these important issues.

References

Aharon-Peretz J, Kliot D, Tomer R. Behavioral differences between white matter lacunar dementia and Alzheimer's Disease: a comparison on the Neuropsychiatric Inventory. Dement Geriatr Gogn Disord 2000; 11: 294–298.

Albert ML. Subcortical dementia: historical review and personal view. Neurocase 2005; 11: 243–245.

Albert ML, Feldman RG, Willis AL. The "subcortical dementia" of progressive supranuclear palsy. J Neurol Neurosurg Psychiatry 1974; 37: 121–130.

Alexander MP, Naeser MA, Palumbo CL. Correlations of subcortical CT lesion sites and aphasia profiles. Brain 1987; 110: 961–991.

Al-Hajri Z, Del Bigio MR. Brain damage in a large cohort of solvent abusers. Acta Neuropathol 2010; 119: 435–445.

Al-Hasani OH, Smith C. Traumatic white matter injury and toxic leukoencephalopathies. Expert Rev Neurother 2011; 11: 1315–1324.

American Psychiatric Association. *Diagnostic and statistical manual of mental disorders*. 5th ed. *DSM-V*. Arlington, VA: American Psychiatric Association, 2013.

Anderson B, Southern BD, Powers RE. Anatomic asymmetries of the posterior superior temporal lobes: a postmortem study. Neuropsychiatry Neuropsychol Behav Neurol 1999; 12: 247–254.

Appelman AP, Exalto LG, van der Graaf Y, et al. White matter lesions and brain atrophy: more than shared risk factors? A systematic review. Cerebrovasc Dis 2009; 28: 227–242.

Armstrong CL, Corn BW, Ruffer JE, et al. Radiotherapeutic effects on brain function: double dissociation of memory systems. Neuropsychiatry Neuropsychol Behav Neurol 2000; 13: 101–111.

Armstrong CL, Stern CH, Corn BW. Memory performance used to detect radiation effects on cognitive function. Appl Neuropsychol 2001; 8: 129–139.

Arnett PA, Rao SM, Bernardin L, et al. Relationship between frontal lobe lesions and Wisconsin Card Sorting Test performance in patients with multiple sclerosis. Neurology 1994; 44: 420–425.

Arnett PA, Rao SM, Hussain M, et al. Conduction aphasia in multiple sclerosis: a case report with MRI findings. Neurology 1996; 47: 576–578.

Babikian V, Ropper AH. Binswanger's disease: a review. Stroke 1987; 18: 2–12.

Banich MT. The missing link: the role of interhemispheric interaction in attentional processing. Brain Cogn 1998; 36: 128–157.

Barredo J, Öztekin I, Badre D. Ventral fronto-temporal pathway supporting cognitive control of episodic memory retrieval. Cereb Cortex 2015; 25: 1004–1019.

Bartzokis G. Brain myelination in prevalent neuropsychiatric developmental disorders: primary and comorbid addiction. Adolesc Psychiatry 2005; 29: 55–96.

Bartzokis G. Neuroglialpharmacology: white matter pathophysiologies and psychiatric treatments. Front Biosci 2011; 16: 2695–2733.

Bartzokis G, Lu PH, Tingus K, Mendez MF, et al. Lifespan trajectory of myelin integrity and maximum motor speed. Neurobiol Aging 2010; 31: 1554–1562.

Bendlin BB, Fitzgerald ME, Ries ML, et al. White matter in aging and cognition: a cross-sectional study of microstructure in adults aged eighteen to eighty-three. Dev Neuropsychol 2010; 35: 257–277.

Bennett DA, Gilley DW, Lee S, Cochran EJ. White matter changes: neurobehavioral manifestations of Binswanger's Disease and clinical correlates in Alzheimer's Disease. Dementia 1994; 5: 148–152.

Bleuler E. *Textbook of psychiatry*. (trans. Brill AA). New York: Macmillan, 1924.

Bonelli RM, Cummings JL. Frontal-subcortical dementias. Neurologist 2008; 14: 100–107.

Boone KB, Miller BL, Lesser IM, et al. Neuropsychological correlates of white-matter lesions in healthy elderly subjects: a threshold effect. Arch Neurol 1992; 49: 549–554.

Brown RG, Marsden CD. "Subcortical dementia": the neuropsychological evidence. Neuroscience 1988; 25: 363–387.

Bucur B, Madden DJ, Spaniol J, et al. Age-related slowing of memory retrieval: contributions of perceptual speed and cerebral white matter integrity. Neurobiol Aging 2008; 29: 1070–1079.

Budson AE, Price BH. Memory dysfunction. N Engl J Med 2005; 352: 692–699.

Caine ED, Bamford KA, Schiffer RB, et al. A controlled neuropsychological comparison of Huntington's disease and multiple sclerosis. Arch Neurol 1986; 43: 249–254.

Chabriat H, Joutel A, Dichgans M, et al. Cadasil. Lancet Neurol 2009; 8: 643–653.

Chang CC, Lee YC, Chang WN, et al. Damage of white matter tract correlated with neuropsychological deficits in carbon monoxide intoxication after hyperbaric oxygen therapy. J Neurotrauma 2009; 26: 1263–1270.

Charcot JM. *Lectures on the diseases of the nervous system delivered at La Salpêtrière*. London: New Sydenham Society, 1877.

Chiang MC, Barysheva M, Shattuck DW, et al. Genetics of brain fiber architecture and intellectual performance. J Neurosci 2009; 29: 2212–2224.

Coltman R, Spain A, Tsenkina Y, et al. Selective white matter pathology induces a specific impairment in spatial working memory. Neurobiol Aging 2011; 32: 2324. e7–e12.

Cummings JL, ed. *Subcortical dementia*. New York: Oxford University Press, 1990.

Cummings JL, Benson DF. Subcortical dementia: review of an emerging concept. Arch Neurol 1984; 41: 874–879.

Darvesh S, Freedman M. Subcortical dementia: a neurobehavioral approach. Brain Cogn 1996; 31: 230–249.

Daselaar SM, Iyengar V, Davis SW, et al. Less wiring, more firing: low-performing older adults compensate for impaired white matter with greater neural activity. Cereb Cortex 2015; 25: 983–990.

DeLuca J, Barbieri-Berger S, Johnson SK. The nature of memory acquisition in multiple sclerosis: acquisition versus retrieval. J Clin Exp Neuropsychol 1994; 16: 183–189.

DeLuca J, Gaudino EA, Diamond BJ, et al. Acquisition and storage deficits in multiple sclerosis. J Clin Exp Neuropsychol 1998; 20: 376–390.

Demaree HA, DeLuca J, Gaudino EA, Diamond BJ. Speed of information processing as a key deficit in multiple sclerosis: implications for rehabilitation. J Neurol Neurosurg Psychiatry 1999; 67: 661–663.

Derix MMA. *Neuropsychological differentiation of dementia syndromes*. Lisse: Swets and Zeitlinger, 1994.

Doody RS, Massman PJ, Mawad M, Nance M. Cognitive consequences of subcortical magnetic resonance imaging changes in Alzheimer's Disease: comparison to small vessel ischemic vascular dementia. Neuropsychiatry Neuropsychol Behav Neurol 1998; 11: 191–199.

Drebing CE, Moore LH, Cummings JL, et al. Patterns of neuropsychological performance among forms of subcortical dementia. Neuropsychiatry Neuropsychol Behav Neurol 1994; 7: 57–66.

Fein G, Van Dyke C, Davenport L, et al. Preservation of normal cognitive functioning in elderly subjects with extensive white-matter lesions of long duration. Arch Gen Psychiatry 1990; 47: 220–223.

Feinstein A. *The clinical neuropsychiatry of multiple sclerosis*. 2nd ed. Cambridge: Cambridge University Press, 2007.

Filley CM. The behavioral neurology of cerebral white matter. Neurology 1998; 50: 1535–1540.

Filley CM. White matter: organization and functional relevance. Neuropsychol Rev 2010; 20: 158–173.

Filley CM. *Neurobehavioral anatomy*. 3rd ed. Boulder: University Press of Colorado, 2011.

Filley CM. *The behavioral neurology of white matter*. 2nd ed. New York: Oxford University Press, 2012.

Filley CM, Franklin GM, Heaton RK, Rosenberg NL. White matter dementia: clinical disorders and implications. Neuropsychiatry Neuropsychol Behav Neurol 1988; 1: 239–254.

Filley CM, Heaton RK, Nelson LM, Burks JS, Franklin GM. A comparison of dementia in Alzheimer's Disease and multiple sclerosis. Arch Neurol 1989; 46: 157–161.

Filley CM, Heaton RK, Rosenberg NL. White matter dementia in chronic toluene abuse. Neurology 1990; 40: 532–534.

Filley CM, Gross KF. Psychosis with cerebral white matter disease. Neuropsychiatry Neuropsychol Behav Neurol 1992; 5: 119–125.

Filley CM, Cullum CM. Attention and vigilance function in normal aging. Appl Neuropsychol 1994; 1: 29–32.

Filley CM, Thompson LL, Sze C-I, et al. White matter dementia in CADASIL. J Neurol Sci 1999; 163: 163–167.

Filley CM, Kleinschmidt-DeMasters BK. Toxic leukoencephalopathy. N Engl J Med 2001; 345: 425–432.

Filley CM, Halliday W, Kleinschmidt-DeMasters BK. The effects of toluene on the central nervous system. J Neuropathol Exp Neurol 2004; 63: 1–12.

Filley CM, Kozora E, Brown MS, et al. White matter microstructure and cognition in non-neuropsychiatric systemic lupus erythematosus. Cogn Behav Neurol 2009; 22: 38–44.

Fornazzari L, Pollanen MS, Myers V, Wolf A. Solvent abuse–related toluene leukoencephalopathy. J Clin Forensic Med 2003; 10: 93–95.

Franklin GM, Nelson LM, Filley CM, Heaton RK. Cognitive loss in multiple sclerosis: case reports and review of the literature. Arch Neurol 1989; 46: 162–167.

Gabrieli JD, Stebbins GT, Singh J, et al. Intact mirror-tracing and impaired rotary-pursuit skill learning in patients with Huntington's disease: evidence for dissociable memory systems in skill learning. Neuropsychology 1997; 11: 272–281.

Gallassi R, Morreale A, Montagna P, et al. Binswanger's disease and normal-pressure hydrocephalus: clinical and neuropsychological comparison. Arch Neurol 1991; 48: 1156–1159.

Gennarelli TA, Thibault LA, Adams JH, et al. Diffuse axonal injury and traumatic coma in the primate. Ann Neurol 1982; 12: 564–574.

Geschwind N. Disconnexion syndromes in animals and man. Brain 1965; 88: 237–294, 585–644.

Giedd JN, Castellanos FX, Casey BJ, et al. Quantitative morphology of the corpus callosum in attention deficit hyperactivity disorder. Am J Psychiatry 1994; 151: 665–669.

Graff-Radford NR, Rizzo M. Neglect in a patient with multiple sclerosis. Eur Neurol 1987; 26: 100–103.

Grafman J, Weingartner H, Newhouse PA, et al. Implicit learning in patients with Alzheimer's disease. Pharmacopsychiatry 1990; 23: 94–101.

Grigsby J, Cornish K, Hocking D, et al. The cognitive neuropsychological phenotype of carriers of the FMR1 premutation. J Neurodev Disord 2014; 6: 28.

Haász J, Westlye ET, Fjær S, et al. General fluid-type intelligence is related to indices of white matter structure in middle-aged and old adults. Neuroimage 2013; 83: 372–383.

Haroutunian V, Katsel P, Roussos P, et al. Myelination, oligodendrocytes, and serious mental illness. Glia 2014; 62: 1856–1877.

Harris JG, Filley CM. CADASIL: neuropsychological findings in three generations of an affected family. J Int Neuropsychol Soc 2001; 7: 768–774.

Hauser SL, Oksenberg JR. The neurobiology of multiple sclerosis: genes, inflammation, and neurodegeneration. Neuron 2006; 52: 61–76.

Heaton RK, Nelson LM, Thompson DS, et al. Neuropsychological findings in relapsing-remitting and chronic-progressive multiple sclerosis. J Consul Clin Psychol 1985; 53: 103–110.

Hippolyte L, Battistella G, Perrin AG, et al. Investigation of memory, executive functions, and anatomic correlates in asymptomatic FMR1 premutation carriers. Neurobiol Aging 2014; 35: 1939–1946.

Hormes JT, Filley CM, Rosenberg NL. Neurologic sequelae of chronic solvent vapor abuse. Neurology 1986; 36: 698–702.

Howard MO, Bowen SE, Garland EL, et al. Inhalant use and inhalant use disorders in the United States. Addict Sci Clin Pract 2011; 6: 18–31.

Huber SJ, Shuttleworth EC, Paulson GW, et al. Cortical vs subcortical dementia: neuropsychological differences. Arch Neurol 1986; 43: 392–394.

Hyde TM, Ziegler JC, Weinberger DR. Psychiatric disturbances in metachromatic leukodystrophy: insights into the neurobiology of psychosis. Arch Neurol 1992; 49: 401–406.

Iddon JL, Pickard JD, Cross JJL, et al. Specific patterns of cognitive impairment in patients with idiopathic normal pressure hydrocephalus and Alzheimer's disease: a pilot study. J Neurol Neurosurg Psychiatry 1999; 67: 723–732.

Inatomi Y, Yonehara T, Hashimoto Y, Hirano T, Uchino M. Correlation between ventricular enlargement and white matter changes. J Neurol Sci 2008; 269: 12–17.

Jellinger KA. Neuropathology of movement disorders. Neurosurg Clin N Am 1998; 9: 237–362.

Jones RD, Tranel D. Preservation of procedural memory in HIV-positive patients with subcortical dementia. J Clin Exp Neuropsychol 1991; 13: 74.

Karlborg B, Skak Madsen K, Vestergaard M, et al. Sustained attention is associated with right superior longitudinal fasciculus and superior parietal white matter microstructure in children. Hum Brain Mapp 2013; 34: 3216–3232.

Kloppenborg RP, Nederkoorn PJ, Geerlings MI, van den Berg E. Presence and progression of white matter hyperintensities and cognition: a meta-analysis. Neurology 2014; 82: 2127–2138.

Knopman D, Nissen MJ. Procedural learning is impaired in Huntington's disease: evidence from the serial reaction time task. Neuropsychologia 1991; 29: 245–254.

Kochunov P, Coyle T, Lancaster J, et al. Processing speed is correlated with cerebral health markers in the frontal lobes as quantified by neuroimaging. Neuroimage 2010; 49: 1190–1199.

Kornfeld M, Moser AB, Moser HW, et al. Solvent vapor abuse leukoencephalopathy: comparison to adrenoleukodystrophy. J Neuropathol Exp Neurol 1994; 53: 389–398.

Krupp L, Elkins LE. Fatigue and declines in cognitive functioning in multiple sclerosis. Neurology 2000; 55: 934–939.

Kujala P, Portin R, Ruutianen J. Language functions in incipient cognitive decline in multiple sclerosis. J Neurol Sci 1996; 141: 79–86.

Lacour A, De Seze J, Revenco E, et al. Acute aphasia in multiple sclerosis: a multicenter study of 22 patients. Neurology 2004; 62: 974–977.

Lafosse J, Reed BR, Mungas D, et al. Fluency and memory differences between ischemic vascular dementia and Alzheimer's disease. Neuropsychology 1997; 11: 514–522.

Lafosse JM, Corboy JR, Leehey MA, et al. MS vs. HD: can white matter and subcortical gray matter pathology be distinguished neuropsychologically? J Clin Exp Neuropsychol 2007; 29: 142–154.

Lafosse JM, Mitchell SM, Corboy JR, Filley CM. The nature of verbal memory impairment in multiple sclerosis: a list-learning and meta-analytic study. J Int Neuropsychol Soc 2013; 19: 995–1008.

Laule C, Kozlowski P, Leung E, et al. Myelin water imaging of multiple sclerosis at 7 T: correlations with histopathology. Neuroimage 2008; 40: 1575–1580.

Lee JH, Kim SH, Kim GH, et al. Identification of pure subcortical vascular dementia using 11C-Pittsburgh compound B. Neurology 2011; 77: 18–25.

Libon DJ, Bogdanoff B, Cloud BS, et al. Declarative and procedural learning, quantitative measures of the hippocampus, and subcortical white alterations in Alzheimer's disease and ischaemic vascular dementia. J Clin Exp Neuropsychol 1998; 20: 30–41.

Libon DJ, Price CC, Giovannetti T, et al. Linking MRI hyperintensities with patterns of neuropsychological impairment: evidence for a threshold effect. Stroke 2008; 39: 806–813.

Litvan I, Grafman J, Vendrell P, Martinez JM. Slowed information processing in multiple sclerosis. Arch Neurol 1988; 45: 281–285.

Lucchinetti CF, Popescu BF, Bunyan RF, et al. Inflammatory cortical demyelination in early multiple sclerosis. N Engl J Med 2011; 365: 2188–2197.

Lunven M, Thiebaut de Schotten M, Bourlon C, et al. White matter lesional predictors of chronic visual neglect: a longitudinal study. Brain 2015; 138: 746–760.

Markowitsch HJ. Which brain regions are critically involved in the retrieval of old episodic memory? Brain Res Rev 1995; 21: 117–127.

Mataró M, Junqué C, Poca MA, Sahuquillo J. Neuropsychological findings in congenital and acquired childhood hydrocephalus. Neuropsychol Rev 2001; 11: 169–178.

Mayeux R, Stern Y, Rosen J, Benson F. Is "subcortical dementia" a recognizable clinical entity? Ann Neurol 1983; 14: 278–283.

McHugh PR, Folstein MF. Psychiatric syndromes of Huntington's chorea: a clinical and phenomenologic study. In: Benson DF, Blumer D, eds. *Psychiatric aspects of neurologic disease*. Vol. 1. New York: Grune and Stratton, 1975: 267–285.

McKenzie IA, Ohayon D, Li H, et al. Motor skill learning requires active central myelination. Science 2014; 346: 318–322.

McKhann G, Drachman D, Folstein M, et al. Clinical diagnosis of Alzheimer's disease: report of the NINCDS-ADRDA Work Group under the auspices of Department of Health and Human Services Task Force on Alzheimer's Disease. Neurology 1984; 34: 939–944.

McKinney AM, Kieffer SA, Paylor RT, et al. Acute toxic leukoencephalopathy: potential for reversibility clinically and on MRI with diffusion-weighted and FLAIR imaging. AJR 2009; 193: 192–206.

Mendez MF, Perryman KM, Bronstein YL. White matter dementias: neurobehavioral aspects and etiology. J Neuropsychiatry Clin Neurosci 2000; 12: 133.

Mendez MF, Cummings JL. *Dementia, a clinical approach*. 3rd ed. Philadelphia: Butterworth Heinemann, 2003.

Merriam AE, Hegarty A, Miller A. A proposed etiology for psychotic symptoms in white matter dementia. Neuropsychiatry Neuropsychol Behav Neurol 1989; 2: 225–228.

Merriam AE, Hegarty AM, Miller A. The mental disabilities of metachromatic leukodystrophy: implications concerning the differentiation of cortical, subcortical, and white matter dementias. Neuropsychiatry Neuropsychol Behav Neurol 1990; 3: 217–225.

Mesulam M-M. Attentional networks, confusional states, and neglect syndromes. In: Mesulam M-M, ed. *Principles of behavioral and cognitive neurology*. 2nd ed. New York: Oxford University Press, 2000: 174–256.

Minden SL, Schiffer RB. Affective disorders in multiple sclerosis: review and recommendations for clinical research. Arch Neurol 1990; 47: 98–104.

Miyamoto N, Maki T, Pham LD, et al. Oxidative stress interferes with white matter renewal after prolonged cerebral hypoperfusion in mice. Stroke 2013; 44: 3516–3521.

Moll NM, Rietsch AM, Ransohoff AJ, et al. Cortical demyelination in PML and MS: similarities and differences. Neurology 2008; 70: 336–343.

Mouzon BC, Bachmeier C, Ferro A, et al. Chronic neuropathological and neurobehavioral changes in a repetitive mild traumatic brain injury model. Ann Neurol 2014; 75: 241–254.

Murray ME, Senjem ML, Petersen RC, et al. Functional impact of white matter hyperintensities in cognitively normal elderly subjects. Arch Neurol 2010; 67: 1379–1385.

Navia BA, Jordan BD, Price RW. The AIDS dementia complex: I. Clinical features. Ann Neurol 1986; 19: 517–524.

Nielsen AS, Kinkel RP, Madigan N, et al. Contribution of cortical lesion subtypes at 7T MRI to physical and cognitive performance in MS. Neurology 2013; 81: 641–649.

Nieuwenhuys R. The myeloarchitectonic studies on the human cerebral cortex of the Vogt-Vogt school, and their significance for the interpretation of functional neuroimaging data. Brain Struct Funct 2013; 218: 303–352.

Ozturk V, Idiman E, Sengun IS, Yuksel Z. Multiple sclerosis and parkinsonism: a case report. Funct Neurol 2002; 17: 145–147.

Papagno C, Miracapillo C, Casarotti A, et al. What is the role of the uncinate fasciculus? Surgical removal and proper name retrieval. Brain 2011; 134: 405–414.

Parvizi J. Corticocentric myopia: old bias in new cognitive sciences. Trends Cogn Sci 2009; 13: 354–359.

Penke L, Muñoz Maniega S, Murray C, et al. A general factor of brain white matter integrity predicts information processing speed in healthy older people. J Neurosci 2010; 30: 7569–7574.

Price CC, Jefferson AL, Merino JG, Heilman KM, Libon DJ. Subcortical vascular dementia: integrating neuropsychological and neuroradiologic data. Neurology 2005; 65: 376–382.

Price CC, Mitchell SM, Brumback B, et al. MRI-leukoaraiosis thresholds and the phenotypic expression of dementia. Neurology 2012; 79: 734–740.

Prins ND, Scheltens P. White matter hyperintensities, cognitive impairment and dementia: an update. Nat Rev Neurol 2015; 11: 157–165.

Rao SM. White matter dementias. In: Parks RW, Zec RF, Wilson RS, eds. *Neuropsychology of Alzheimer's disease and other dementias*. New York: Oxford University Press, 1993: 438–456.

Rao SM. White matter disease and dementia. Brain Cogn 1996; 31: 250–268.

Rao SM, Hammeke TA, McQuillen MP, et al. Memory disturbance in chronic-progressive multiple sclerosis. Arch Neurol 1984; 41: 625–631.

Rao SM, Bernardin L, Leo GJ, et al. Cerebral disconnection in multiple sclerosis: relationship to atrophy of the corpus callosum. Arch Neurol 1989b; 46: 918–920.

Rao SM, Leo GJ, Bernardin L, Unverzagt F. Cognitive dysfunction in multiple sclerosis: I. Frequency, patterns, and prediction. Neurology 1991; 41: 685–691.

Rao SM, Grafman J, DiGiulio D, et al. Memory dysfunction in multiple sclerosis: its relation to working memory, semantic encoding, and implicit learning. Neuropsychology 1993; 7: 364–374.

Reed BR, Eberling JL, Mungas D, et al. Memory failure has different mechanisms in subcortical stroke and Alzheimer's Disease. Ann Neurol 2000; 48: 275–284.

Riva D, Bova SM, Bruzzone MG. Neuropsychological testing may predict early progression of asymptomatic adrenoleukodystrophy. Neurology 2000; 54: 1651–1655.

Román GC, Tatemichi TK, Erkinjuntti T, et al. Vascular dementia: diagnostic criteria for research studies; report of the NINDS-AIREN International Workshop. Neurology 1993; 43: 250–260.

Ropper AH, Samuels MA, Klein JP. *Adams and Victor's principles of neurology*. 10th ed. New York: McGraw-Hill, 2014.

Rosenberg NL, Spitz MC, Filley CM, et al. Central nervous system effects of chronic toluene abuse – clinical, brainstem evoked response and magnetic resonance imaging studies. Neurotoxicol Teratol 1988a; 10: 489–495.

Rosenberg NK, Kleinschmidt-DeMasters BK, Davis KA, et al. Toluene abuse causes diffuse central nervous system white matter changes. Ann Neurol 1988b; 23: 611–614.

Rosenbloom MJ, Sassoon SA, Pfefferbaum A, Sullivan EV. Contribution of regional white matter integrity to visuospatial construction accuracy, organizational strategy, and memory for a complex figure in abstinent alcoholics. Brain Imaging Behav 2009; 3: 379–390.

Rueckert LM, Sorenson L, Levy J. Callosal efficiency is related to sustained attention. Neuropsychologia 1994; 32: 159–173.

Rueckert L, Grafman J. Sustained attention deficits in patients with right frontal lesions. Neuropsychologia 1996; 34: 953–963.

Rueckert L, Baboorian D, Stavropoulos K, Yasutake C. Individual differences in callosal efficiency: correlation with attention. Brain Cogn 1999; 41: 390–410.

Sadovnick AD, Eisen K, Ebers GC, Paty DW. Cause of death in patients attending multiple sclerosis clinics. Neurology 1991; 41: 1193–1196.

Samuelsson H, Jensen C, Ekholm S, et al. Anatomical and neurological correlates of acute and chronic visuospatial neglect following right hemisphere stroke. Cortex 1997; 33: 271–285.

Saunders JBDM, O'Malley CD. *The illustrations from the works of Andreas Vesalius of Brussels.* New York: Dover, 1973.

Schmahmann JD, Pandya DN. *Fiber pathways of the brain.* New York: Oxford University Press, 2006.

Schmahmann JD, Smith EE, Eichler FS, Filley CM. Cerebral white matter: neuroanatomy, clinical neurology, and neurobehavioral correlates. Ann N Y Acad Sci 2008; 1142: 266–309.

Schwid R, Tyler CM, Scheid EA, et al. Cognitive fatigue during a test requiring sustained attention: a pilot study. Mult Scler 2003; 9: 503–508.

Semrud-Clikeman M, Steingard RJ, Filipek P, et al. Using MRI to examine brain–behavior relationships in males with attention deficit disorder with hyperactivity. J Am Acad Child Adolesc Psychiatry 2000; 39: 477–484.

Sepulcre J, Masdeu JC, Sastre-Garriga J, et al. Mapping the brain pathways of declarative verbal memory: evidence from white matter lesions in the living human brain. Neuroimage 2008; 42: 1237–1243.

Shapiro EG, Lockman LA, Knopman D, Krivit W. Characteristics of the dementia in late-onset metachromatic leukodystrophy. Neurology 1994; 44: 662–665.

Shibata M, Yamasaki N, Miyakawa T, et al. Selective impairment of working memory in a mouse model of chronic cerebral hypoperfusion. Stroke 2007; 38: 2826–2832.

Smith EE, O'Donnell M, Dagenais G, et al. Early cerebral small vessel disease and brain volume, cognition, and gait. Ann Neurol 2015; 77: 251–261.

Sohn YH, Jeong Y, Kim HS, et al. The brain lesion responsible for parkinsonism after carbon monoxide poisoning. Arch Neurol 2000; 57: 1214–1218.

Spikman JM, van Zomeren AH, Deelman BG. Deficits of attention after closed-head injury: slowness only? J Clin Exp Neuropsychol 1996; 18: 755–767.

Staekenborg SS, de Waal H, Admiraal-Behloul F, et al. Neurological signs in relation to white matter hyperintensity volumes in memory clinic patients. Dement Geriatr Cogn Disord 2010; 29: 301–308.

Stern Y. Cognitive reserve. Neuropsychologia 2009; 47: 2015–2028.

Sumowski JF, Wylie GR, Chiaravalloti N, DeLuca J. Intellectual enrichment lessens the effect of brain atrophy on learning and memory in multiple sclerosis. Neurology 2010; 74: 1942–1945.

Swirsky-Sacchetti T, Field HL, Mitchell DR, et al. The sensitivity of the Mini-Mental State Exam in the white matter dementia of multiple sclerosis. J Clin Psychol 1992; 48: 779–786.

Takahashi M, Iwamoto K, Fukatsu H, et al. White matter microstructure of the cingulum and cerebellar peduncle is related to sustained attention and working memory: a diffusion tensor imaging study. Neurosci Lett 2010; 477: 72–76.

Tanridag O, Kirshner HS. Magnetic resonance imaging and CT scanning in neurobehavioral syndromes. Psychosomatics 1987; 28: 517–528.

Tierney MC, Snow WG, Reid DW, et al. Psychometric differentiation of dementia: replication and extension of the findings of Storandt and coworkers. Arch Neurol 1987; 44: 720–722.

Timmerman ME, Brouwer WH. Slow information processing after very severe closed head injury: impaired access to declarative knowledge and intact application and acquisition of procedural knowledge. Neuropsychologia 1999; 37: 467–478.

Tranchant C, Bhatia KP, Marsden CD. Movement disorders in multiple sclerosis. Mov Disord 1995; 10: 418–423.

Tuladhar AM, Reid AT, Shumskaya E, et al. Relationship between white matter hyperintensities, cortical thickness, and cognition. Stroke 2015; 46: 425–432.

Tuch DS, Salat DH, Wisco JJ, et al. Choice reaction time performance correlates with diffusion anisotropy in white matter pathways supporting visuospatial attention. Proc Natl Acad Sci 2005; 102: 12212–12217.

Turken A, Whitfield-Gabrieli S, Bammer R, et al. Cognitive processing speed and the structure of white matter pathways: convergent evidence from normal variation and lesion studies. Neuroimage 2008; 42: 1032–1044.

von Stockert FG. Subcorficale demenz. Arch Psychiatry 1932; 97: 77–100.

Walterfang M, Velakoulis D, Whitford TJ, Pantelis C. Understanding aberrant white matter development in schizophrenia: an avenue for therapy? Expert Rev Neurother 2011; 11: 971–987.

Weinstein M, Silverstein ML, Nader T, Turnbull A. Sustained attention and related perceptuomotor functions. Percept Mot Skills 1999; 89: 387–388.

White DA, Taylor MJ, Butters N, et al. Memory for verbal information in individuals with HIV-associated dementia complex; HNRC Group. J Clin Exp Neuropsychol 1997; 19: 357–366.

Whitehouse PJ. The concept of subcortical and cortical dementia: another look. Ann Neurol 1986; 19: 1–6.

Yamanouchi N, Okada S, Kodama K, et al. Effects of MRI abnormalities on WAIS-R performance in solvent abusers. Acta Neurol Scand 1997; 96: 34–39.

Yoon CW, Shin JS, Kim HJ, et al. Cognitive deficits of pure subcortical vascular dementia vs. Alzheimer disease: PiB-PET-based study. Neurology 2013; 80: 569–573.

Yücel M, Takagi M, Walterfang M, Lubman DI. Toluene misuse and long-term harms: a systematic review of the neuropsychological and neuroimaging literature. Neurosci Biobehav Rev 2008; 32: 910–926.

Chapter 8

Mild cognitive dysfunction: a precursor syndrome

In the past, when the understanding of cognitive disorders was more limited than it is today, dementia was often considered as a unitary and invariant syndrome of acquired intellectual decline. An immediate corollary of this view was that the cerebral cortex was necessarily damaged. Yet it is now widely accepted that the syndrome of dementia is a highly variable clinical problem with many nuances and subtleties. No two dementia patients are alike in all respects, and the neuropathology underlying the dementia syndrome is unique in every case. Thus, while the term is a useful descriptive construct, it is increasingly clear that every dementia has its own neurobehavioral profile, specific neuropathological basis, and singular natural history.

As experience grew with white matter dementia (WMD), the variable features of its phenomenology became apparent even as the deficits and strengths reviewed in the previous chapter were recognized. One of the most obvious aspects of the clinical presentation of affected patients was a wide range of severity. Similar to any other dementia syndrome, WMD therefore came to be seen as a spectrum including the categories of mild, moderate, or severe, depending to a large extent on how much aggregate neuropathology exists. From this observation, a further insight naturally suggested itself: a precursor syndrome may exist that is manifested by cognitive dysfunction that does not reach the level of dementia but is nevertheless clinically important. This hypothetical syndrome, later termed mild cognitive dysfunction (MCD), was also postulated to depend on the total burden of white matter neuropathology. The idea thus began to take shape that a continuum of cognitive loss – beginning before dementia sets in and proceeding through its most severe stages – can be associated with advancing degrees of white matter involvement. Indeed, the majority of patients with the disorders discussed in this book are likely to present with a syndrome of cognitive impairment that does not reach the level of dementia but nevertheless has significant clinical implications. In this chapter, MCD will be considered in detail as the putative precursor of WMD. As this account is developed, an instructive comparison to the well-known mild cognitive impairment (MCI), the proposed precursor of Alzheimer's Disease (AD), will become apparent.

Background

As the problem of dementia becomes ever more ominous in the absence of curative treatment for most cases, a great deal of effort has come to be focused on identifying the earliest sign of the disorder. Widespread agreement exists that finding neuropathology of any kind while it produces mild or even no symptoms offers the best opportunity for effective intervention. A major component of this process is the making of an accurate diagnosis at the earliest possible time, surely a high priority in any medical setting. Another approach to the problem is the current focus on biomarkers, which are being sought in the blood, the cerebrospinal fluid, and the living brain with neuroimaging techniques (Ahmed et al., 2014). An accurate biomarker has the appeal of potentially allowing for diagnosis even before any clinical evidence of dementia appears, and the possibilities for prevention and treatment that could follow are of course attractive. The majority of work on biomarkers has been devoted to AD, but other neurodegenerative diseases are also being studied with this objective in mind (Ahmed et al., 2014).

Turning to the topic of white matter, WMD is a syndrome based on the correlation of cerebral white matter lesions with a specific cognitive profile. The early years of the magnetic resonance imaging (MRI) era made possible the research leading to this understanding, and this development unquestionably permitted the in vivo study of white matter that neurologists of the past could not have attempted. Yet the visualization of

Table 8.1 Three stages of severity in toxic leukoencephalopathy

	Clinical features	MRI appearance	Neuropathology
Mild	Confusion, inattention, forgetfulness	Periventricular white matter hyperintensity	Intramyelinic edema
Moderate	Apathy, abulia, dementia	Diffuse white matter hyperintensity	Myelin loss with preserved axons
Severe	Akinetic mutism, stupor, coma, death	Confluent white matter disease with necrotic areas	Axonal loss, white matter necrosis

BOX 8.1 Some conditions in which the normal-appearing white matter may be abnormal

- Metachromatic leukodystrophy
- Phenylketonuria
- Neurofibromatosis
- Tuberous sclerosis
- Myotonic dystrophy
- Fragile X tremor ataxia syndrome
- Multiple sclerosis
- Human immunodeficiency virus infection
- Systemic lupus erythematosus
- Alcoholism
- Hypoxia
- Critical illness
- Delirium
- Leukoaraiosis
- Traumatic brain injury
- Glioma
- Normal pressure hydrocephalus
- Aging
- Autism
- Attention-deficit/hyperactivity disorder
- Aggression
- Bipolar disorder
- Schizophrenia
- Alzheimer's Disease

macrostructural white matter lesions has proven to be only the first step in the interrogation of myelinated systems in the brain. Neuropathology of myelin, axons, and glial cells can also be studied at the microscopic level, and changes in the microstructure of white matter have also been recognized with the use of ever-improving MRI techniques. Recent advances in neuroimaging have in fact revealed a most interesting new finding, which is that the seemingly unaffected white matter on conventional MRI, now known as the normal-appearing white matter (NAWM), may not in fact be normal when examined with more sensitive techniques. These techniques, among them magnetic resonance spectroscopy (MRS), magnetization transfer imaging (MTI), and diffusion tensor imaging (DTI), permit the investigation of NAWM and regularly uncover microstructural abnormalities. A rapidly expanding, and remarkably diverse, list of conditions can now be assembled in which the NAWM is not normal when queried by one or more of these methods (Box 8.1). Given the neurobehavioral importance of macrostructural white matter lesions, an appropriate next question concerns the potential effects of more subtle changes in the NAWM.

Studies of WMD as well as clinical experience suggest the existence of a less severe cognitive syndrome associated with less obvious white matter neuropathology. A good example of the potentially wide range of white matter involvement can be seen in toxic leukoencephalopathy, in which a spectrum of MRI and neuropathological changes occurs, with the resultant neurobehavioral dysfunction being concomitantly mild, moderate, or severe (Table 8.1) (Filley and Kleinschmidt-DeMasters, 2001; Filley et al., 2004). A dose-response effect is strongly implicated in this conceptualization, such that milder cases can often be completely reversed if recognized, and this aspect highlights the clinical imperative to prevent the problem, especially its more severe forms, if at all possible. The main point is that diffuse toxicity of white matter produces a relatively predictable sequence of adverse events, and that parallel neurobehavioral sequelae can be predicted to follow. Whereas the details of this sequence may vary to some extent among other white matter disorders, which are of course associated with many different etiologies, the idea of progressive involvement producing more serious illness is crucial. The concept of a spectrum of white matter alterations can be extended to suggest that NAWM abnormalities from potentially any etiology may be associated with subtle cognitive loss even before macrostructural lesions appear on routine MRI.

In this context, the category of inflammatory white matter disease became relevant as a clinical model for studying the effects of NAWM changes on cognition. Inflammatory disease begins at the microstructural level, and subtle neuropathology is likely well before changes become evident on conventional MRI. Systemic lupus erythematosus (SLE) presented itself as an ideal disease for studying of this phenomenon because it is an illness that frequently affects cognition at an early stage, typically affects young adults who generally harbor little or no other neuropathology, and features white matter hyperintensities as its most common conventional MRI finding (Kozora and Filley, 2011). MRS studies of frontal NAWM in fact disclosed that increased choline, a metabolic marker of inflammation and demyelination, correlated with impaired processing speed, attention, and executive function in SLE patients whose gray and white matter volumes did not differ from controls (Filley et al., 2009). From a pathophysiological perspective, the elevation of choline suggested immune-related myelinopathy in SLE since the axonal marker N-acetyl aspartate (NAA) was normal (Filley et al., 2009). In terms of brain–behavior relationships, however, the observation of microstructural white matter change correlating with subtle cognitive impairment had implications extending far beyond SLE.

Definition and characterization

Based on the MRS findings generated from the study of cognitive dysfunction in SLE, and in light of parallel observations made in the context of other white matter disorders, the term MCD was introduced (Kozora and Filley, 2011). MCD can be defined as a syndrome of cognitive slowing, inattention, and executive dysfunction resulting from insidious cerebral white matter pathology (Kozora et al., 2013). As specifically defined in SLE patients, MCD is a syndrome of nondisabling cognitive impairment appearing early in the disease, and the correlation of cognitive dysfunction with increased choline suggests that, al least in some SLE patients, MCD results from subtle white matter neuropathology. Whereas the origin of the elevated choline is not clear, a plausible explanation is an inflammatory myelinopathy related to the autoimmune pathogenesis of SLE (Filley et al., 2009).

Although first described in SLE, MCD may also apply to other disorders in which white matter is involved, and many possibilities in improving early diagnosis and treatment are apparent. To invoke one example of the potential widespread generalizability of the MCD concept, a striking similarity between the working memory deficits of SLE and multiple sclerosis (MS) has been observed (Benedict, Shucard, and Zivadinov, 2008; Covey et al., 2012). The presence of demyelination in both diseases, and in other autoimmune disorders (Theodoridou and Settas, 2006), is relevant in this context, and implies a neuropathological commonality underlying the similar cognitive profiles. The early cognitive deficits of many other white matter disorders also resemble those noted in SLE and MS (Filley, 2012), suggesting that white matter involvement may produce a relatively uniform profile of impairment that can be identified early in the course and used to monitor disease progression and treatment. The profile appears to differ from that produced by cortical disease, and may thus have wide applicability to the white matter disorders. More study is needed to confirm the emerging relationship of microstructural white matter neuropathology and cognition, but this model may inform the understanding of how subtle white matter changes disrupt cognition well before the onset of dementia. From a theoretical perspective, the deficits of MCD are remarkably similar to, but less severe than, those of WMD (Filley et al., 1989; Lafosse et al., 2007), further supporting the legitimacy of WMD as a dementia syndrome.

MCD is quite similar to the category of mild neurocognitive disorder that has been introduced in the recently revised *Diagnostic and Statistical Manual of Mental Disorders* (*DSM-5*; American Psychiatric Association, 2013). Under this heading are included individuals who experience a modest decline from their previous level of performance as a result of their disorder, but who can still maintain independence in everyday activities (American Psychiatric Association, 2013). Because one of the cognitive domains in which mild neurocognitive disorder can manifest is executive function, the deficits in working memory commonly found as a result of subtle white matter dysfunction (Filley, 2012; Kozora et al., 2013) would justify the tentative generalization that MCD is one form of mild neurocognitive disorder. But this situation may only reflect the uncertainty of a field struggling to objectify a highly subjective mental state. As the underlying structural basis of mild forms of cognitive loss becomes better understood, it is surely to be hoped that some consistency of terminology develops, and that clinical syndromes can be securely based on the neuropathology involved.

It should be pointed out, however, that the idea of an early syndrome of cognitive loss in neurologic disease is not new. In addition to mild neurocognitive disorder (American Psychiatric Association, 2013), many similar proposals of new syndromes of this type have appeared for more than 50 years. Some of the more notable of these proposals are benign senescent forgetfulness (Kral, 1962); age-associated memory impairment (Crook et al., 1986); cognitive impairment, no dementia (CIND; Graham et al., 1997); and mild cognitive impairment (MCI; Petersen et al., 1999). MCI has been by far the best recognized, and will be discussed later in this chapter.

Given the plethora of proposed intermediate syndromes of cognitive impairment, the introduction of yet another may prove to be of uncertain value. The problem of how to capture the essence of a mild cognitive disturbance for clinical and research purposes is not trivial. However, the firm grounding of MCD in the setting of measurable white matter neuropathology observed in vivo distinguishes this approach from all others, and offers the opportunity to specifically identify the impact of damage to myelinated systems in isolation.

The broad spectrum of white matter pathology

As one thinks about MCD, the relevance of the concept can be seen to extend far beyond patients with SLE who have cognitive dysfunction not reaching the level of dementia. Disturbance of tissue function must begin at some point, and because the definition of dementia requires that the syndrome is acquired, it can be assumed that pathology sets in to disrupt the function of a given tissue that has previously been normal. Thus a variety of white matter disorders may progress through an early stage during which pathology is less severe than later in the course, and concomitant cognitive changes at the pre-dementia stage can be expected.

The work discussed previously on SLE clearly suggests an inflammatory process affecting brain white matter and leading to MCD. This principle is immediately apparent with regard to other inflammatory diseases such as MS and the systemic autoimmune diseases that can involve the white matter (Chapter 6). Another implication of the SLE data, however, is that inflammation as a general pathological mechanism may exert similar effects even in the absence of a known and clinically diagnosed chronic inflammatory disorder. Perhaps the brain, and particularly the white matter, is vulnerable to lesser degrees of inflammatory insult than that which characterizes SLE and related diseases.

Recent years have witnessed a surge of interest in the potentially deleterious effects of systemic inflammation on the brain, largely stimulated by the recognition that activated microglia can be found in the brains of people with AD, and the possibility that inflammation may play a role in AD etiopathogenesis (Akiyama et al., 2000; Bettcher and Kramer, 2014). The potential adverse brain effects of inflammation related to systemic infection have been emphasized not only in AD, but in MS, stroke, and even normal aging (Teeling and Perry, 2009). In such conditions, the activated microglial cells have been hypothesized to produce pro-inflammatory cytokines, which then contribute to a range of pathologies via inflammatory cascades that go on to produce tissue damage (Teeling and Perry, 2009). By analogy to SLE, this notion implies that systemic inflammation may produce brain myelinopathy as one step on the path to more severe involvement. Indeed, recent DTI studies have shown that, among nondemented adults in both middle life (Miralbell et al., 2012) and late life (Arfanakis et al., 2013), measures of systemic inflammation such as the circulating marker C-reactive protein correlate with both reduced microstructural integrity of NAWM and measurable cognitive impairment. The idea of systemic inflammation exerting subtle effects on the white matter deserves further study as another means by which MCD might be substantiated. The topic of inflammation as a research agenda will be further considered in Chapter 12.

A related disorder featuring early white matter involvement producing a syndrome akin to MCD is MS, a disease well known to affect cognitive function in some 40% to 70% of patients (Amato, Zipoli, and Portaccio, 2006), and in which estimates of dementia prevalence reach as high as 25% (Benedict and Bobholz, 2007). Experience from the neurology clinic suggests that many people with MS suffer with insidious cognitive decline before dementia occurs, and even before notable sensorimotor features of MS appear (Filley, 2000), inviting the speculation that this early cognitive loss may in fact be a form of MCD. The NAWM is an important concept in MS, as it was in this disease that the notion first became apparent that white matter may be damaged beyond the obvious demyelinative lesions on conventional MRI (Filippi, Tortorella, and Bozzali, 1999). Evidence for the suspicion that NAWM harbors tissue damage relevant to neurobehavioral status comes from DTI studies of MS showing that lower fractional anisotropy in the NAWM predicts cognitive impairment (Akbar et al., 2010).

A similar situation has become evident among individuals with human immunodeficiency virus (HIV) infection, in whom an early cognitive syndrome known as mild neurocognitive disorder (MND) may develop (Antinori et al., 2007). With the advent of increasingly effective antiretroviral therapy, the dementia of HIV infection – HIV-associated dementia – has actually become less common, while MND has become more so (Sacktor and Robertson, 2014). Subtle white matter involvement may thus be even more important because individuals with HIV are living longer. In nondemented HIV patients, the integrity of NAWM has been found to be compromised (Stebbins et al., 2007), and in view of MRS correlations between frontal white matter changes and cognitive impairment in demented HIV patients (Mohamed et al., 2010; Leite et al., 2013), MND has much in common with MCD. Indeed, DTI studies have shown that slow processing speed and executive dysfunction correlate with diffusely diminished fractional anisotropy in the NAMW of nondemented HIV patients (Tate et al., 2010).

Another example, from the literature on vascular dementia, derives from the concept of vascular cognitive impairment (VCI), intended to capture the entire spectrum of cognitive deficits related to vascular damage in the brain (O'Brien et al., 2003; Selnes and Vinters, 2006). In VCI that has not reached the level of dementia, the term "VCI–no dementia" has been used to highlight the early phase of the illness that could be more readily reversible than vascular dementia if promptly recognized (Román et al., 2004). It has been known for some time, for example, that even a single white matter lacune – an obvious lesion on conventional MRI – may exert measurable cognitive effects that diminish mental effort and compromise everyday performance (Van Zandvoort et al., 1998). The incomplete infarction of leukoaraiosis (LA) may have similar effects, and in many cases this syndrome of VCI–no dementia may result from a mild degree of ischemic white matter hyperintensity (Sun et al., 2014). The concept of MCD becomes relevant in light of diffusion-weighted imaging studies that have shown attentional dysfunction to correlate with microstructural injury in the frontal lobe NAWM in patients who also have LA (Viana-Baptista et al., 2008).

More recently, the problem of cognitive dysfunction related to cancer chemotherapy – popularly known as "chemobrain" – has garnered considerable notice, and a deficit profile quite similar to that of MCD has been correlated with DTI measures of white matter integrity in both cross-sectional and longitudinal studies (Deprez et al., 2013). Radiation therapy for brain malignancy may produce a similar effect, as DTI studies have recently disclosed damage to NAWM in glioma patients who had received cranial irradiation (Hope et al., 2015). Moreover, working memory dysfunction has been associated with reduced NAWM volume in brain tumor patients who underwent radiation therapy (Jacola et al., 2014). In practice, brain tumor patients are commonly treated with both chemotherapy and radiation, and damage to the NAWM again appears plausible in the pathogenesis of cognitive dysfunction. Consistent with the profile of deficits characteristic of MCD, attentional dysfunction has been associated with NAWM injury in such patients (Mulhern et al., 2004).

Primary brain neoplasms may themselves produce a quite similar impact by virtue of their predilection for white matter (Chapter 6). Very few studies exist regarding the early cognitive dysfunction produced by brain tumors, as almost all of the research on cognition and brain neoplasia has concentrated on the effects of treatment and prediction of tumor recurrence. Yet clinical experience suggests that early cognitive loss can be a common feature of brain malignancy, even before more obvious manifestations such as headache and seizures. Available studies of patients with brain tumors examined before treatment have found cognitive dysfunction (Tucha et al., 2000; Reijneveld et al., 2001), but, unfortunately, neuroimaging data were not provided. A particularly illustrative example of the early effects of neoplastic white matter disease, however, is the infiltrative malignancy gliomatosis cerebri, as reviewed in Chapter 6. This neoplasm has a clear predilection for cerebral white matter, and neurobehavioral changes have been reported as the most common and persistent clinical features (Artigas et al., 1985; Filley et al., 2003). Another brain neoplasm exhibiting the relationship between infiltrative white matter neoplasia and cognitive decline is lymphomatosis cerebri (Bakshi et al., 1999; Rollins et al., 2005; Deutsch and Mendez, 2015). Further study of the initial cognitive features of brain neoplasia is clearly warranted, as the early diagnosis of these tumors is critical and may be enhanced by defining the early stage as MCD.

In the category of hydrocephalus, little is known about the initial cognitive loss in patients with normal pressure hydrocephalus (NPH), but it is generally agreed that the onset of symptoms is insidious (Williams and Relkin, 2013). A similarity between the cognitive features of NPH and those of normal aging has been emphasized, as has the early prominence of forgetfulness, apathy, and executive dysfunction (Devito et al., 2005). In view of postmortem findings suggesting the gradual but progressive involvement of periventricular white matter (Leinonen et al., 2012), a premonitory clinical state of subtle cognitive decline is likely in NPH. As the frontal white matter bears the heaviest burden (Akai et al., 1987), a profile of cognitive deficits similar to those of MCD may thus be an early clinical manifestation of NPH, possibly even before more obvious signs of gait disorder and incontinence appear.

Finally, the genetic diseases of white matter may also feature an early phase of cognitive impairment that could be considered MCD. The inherited neurogenerative disease fragile X tremor ataxia syndrome (FXTAS) serves as an example. Recent studies with MRS and DTI in individuals with the fragile X mental retardation 1 (*fMR1*) premutation, but who do not yet have FXTAS, have disclosed microstructural white matter disease in the middle cerebellar peduncle and anterior corpus callosum that correlates with executive dysfunction and slowed processing speed (Filley et al., 2015). In this study, both MRS and DTI were able to identify clinically significant white matter disease before dementia was apparent.

These concepts are not as tightly defined by a singular neuropathology as in the original description of MCD, but the principle of early white matter disease producing subtle cognitive dysfunction obtains nevertheless. The idea of MCD represents an approach complementary to that of WMD by emphasizing the earliest neurobiological features of cognitive impairment. By requiring the correlation of early cognitive dysfunction with insidious neuropathology in a well-defined component of the brain, MCD offers a unique neurobiological advantage that may not only clarify the larger syndrome of WMD but also help illuminate the role of white matter in normal cognition.

This discussion naturally recalls one of the foundational principles of behavioral neurology, which is that the location of neuropathology determines the clinical manifestation to a greater extent than the type of damage present. This adage is nowhere more relevant than in the white matter disorders of the brain. In addition to location, however, increasing evidence also points to the severity of damage as another powerful determinant of the clinical sequelae. The relationship of MCD to WMD can be seen as based in white matter dysfunction that includes both macrostructural and microstructural involvement. Figure 8.1 depicts in schematic form the proposed general relationship between cognitive decline and white matter involvement of varying severity. The categories of MCD and WMD require further study using a range of disease models, as distinctions between these syndromes need clarification and correlation with neuropathological changes, but the notion of increasing white matter change producing advancing degrees of cognitive loss serves as a paradigm for exploring the entire range of white matter involvement.

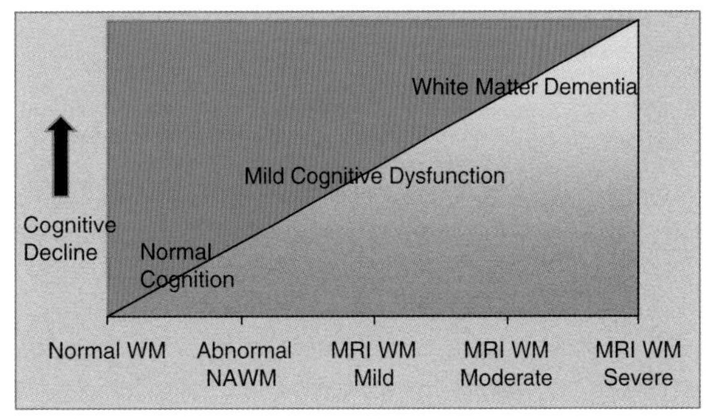

Figure 8.1 Proposed schematic relationship between white matter and cognition (WM – white matter, NAWM – normal-appearing white matter, MRI – magnetic resonance imaging).

Distinction from mild cognitive impairment

A syndrome obviously related to MCD in behavioral neurology is MCI (Petersen, 2011), which is being intensively studied as a putative precursor to AD. Introduced in the late 1990s (Petersen et al., 1999), the concept of MCI has proven to be highly influential in terms of both research on AD and clinical practice. As a concept signifying neuropathological changes in the brain, MCI is most commonly associated with cortical dysfunction, in particular hippocampal volume loss. Although not all cases of MCI in fact feature hippocampal atrophy, perhaps the major value of MCI has been in targeting what has been assumed to be the early stage of AD so that diagnosis and, at some point when more effective medications

Table 8.2 Mild cognitive dysfunction compared to mild cognitive impairment

Mild cognitive dysfunction	Mild cognitive impairment
White matter involvement	Gray matter involvement
One type	Multiple types
Clinically and radiologically defined	Clinically defined
Frontal white matter localization	Hippocampus is putative site for amnestic MCI
Neuroimaging biomarkers available	Biomarkers not firmly established
Myelin loss with or without axonal loss	Neuronal cell body and synapse loss
Applicable to any age	Applicable only to aging
Relevant to all white matter disorders	Relevant to neurodegenerative disease
Treatment of disorder may be effective	No treatment known to be effective

are available, treatment can be improved. Whereas many controversies continue as MCI is studied in greater detail, a focus on understanding the earliest manifestations of dementia, in this case AD, is surely a major step forward.

MCD is a parallel construct in the white matter disorders, and is conceptualized as the putative precursor to WMD. As might be expected, MCD does not readily correspond to one of the currently recognized subtypes of MCI (Petersen, 2011). Because MCD is founded on pathology in white matter, its profile naturally differs from that MCI, the most familiar form of which – amnestic MCI – is postulated to result from gray matter atrophy, most notably in the medial temporal regions, including the hippocampus. Thus the specific profile of deficits in MCD merits a separate category. Many differences in fact exist between MCD and MCI (Table 8.2), and, while the understanding of MCD is still preliminary, a syndrome that is relevant to the cognitive effects of white matter dysfunction of any etiology may prove useful in contrast to MCI as a syndrome of gray matter degeneration. Additional advantages of the use of MCD include its reliance on readily available in vivo neuroimaging technology, its applicability to any age, and its potential reversibility.

As discussed earlier, however, it can be questioned whether yet another attempt to capture the premonitory features of a dementia syndrome is warranted. Perhaps MCI should simply be applied to the white matter disorders causing dementia without the need for MCD. This view has merit, and medicine does risk subdividing its many disorders into so many categories that every patient may at times seem to deserve his or her own unique diagnostic label. But the distinct neurobiology of white matter tracts does pertain to a large portion of brain tissue that has undeniable importance for cognition, and impels a more specific descriptor of the pre-dementia stage of potentially all white matter disorders. Evidence supporting the concept has been adduced, and in the spirit of investigating the entire range of dementing disorders, MCD appears to have a legitimate role. At the very least, MCD can stimulate thinking about the relatively neglected area of white matter and cognition, just as the notion of MCI has done for cortical disease since its introduction.

References

Ahmed RM, Paterson RW, Warren JD, et al. Biomarkers in dementia: clinical utility and new directions. J Neurol Neurosurg Psychiatry 2014; 85: 1426–1434.

Akai K, Uchigasaki S, Tanaka U, Komatsu A. Normal pressure hydrocephalus: neuropathological study. Acta Pathol Jpn 1987; 37: 97–110.

Akbar N, Lobaugh NJ, O'Connor P, et al. Diffusion tensor imaging abnormalities in cognitively impaired multiple sclerosis patients. Can J Neurol Sci 2010; 37: 608–614.

Akiyama H, Barger S, Barnum S, et al. Inflammation and Alzheimer's disease. Neurobiol Aging 2000; 21: 383–421.

Amato MP, Zipoli V, Portaccio E. Multiple sclerosis-related cognitive changes: a review of cross-sectional and longitudinal studies. J Neurol Sci 2006; 245: 41–46.

American Psychiatric Association. *Diagnostic and statistical manual of mental disorders*. 5th ed. *DSM-V*. Washington, DC: American Psychiatric Association, 2013.

Antinori A, Arendt G, Becker JT, et al. Updated research nosology for HIV-associated neurocognitive disorders. Neurology 2007; 69: 1789–1799.

Arfanakis K, Fleischman DA, Grisot G, et al. Systemic inflammation in non-demented elderly human subjects: brain microstructure and cognition. PLoS One 2013; 8: e73107.

Artigas J, Cervos-Navarro J, Iglesias JR, Ebhardt G. Gliomatosis cerebri: clinical and histological findings. Clin Neuropathol 1985; 4: 135–148.

Bakshi R, Mazziotta JC, Mischel PS, et al. Lymphomatosis cerebri presenting as a rapidly progressive dementia: clinical, neuroimaging and pathologic findings. Dement Geriatr Cogn Disord 1999; 10: 152–157.

Benedict RH, Bobholz JH. Multiple sclerosis. Semin Neurol 2007; 27: 78–85.

Benedict RH, Shucard JL, Zivadinov R, Shucard DW. Neuropsychological impairment in systemic lupus erythematosus: a comparison with multiple sclerosis. Neuropsychol Rev 2008; 18: 149–166.

Bettcher BM, Kramer JH. Longitudinal inflammation, cognitive decline, and Alzheimer's disease: a mini-review. Clin Pharmacol Ther 2014; 96: 464–469.

Covey TJ, Shucard JL, Shucard DW, Stegen S, Benedict RH. Comparison of neuropsychological impairment and vocational outcomes in systemic lupus erythematosus and multiple sclerosis patients. J Int Neuropsychol Soc 2012; 18: 530–540.

Crook T, Bartus RT, Ferris SH, et al. Age-associated memory impairment: proposed diagnostic criteria and measures of clinical change; report of a National Institute of Mental Health work group. Dev Neuropyschol 1986; 2: 261–276.

Deprez S, Billiet T, Sunaert S, Leemans A. Diffusion tensor MRI of chemotherapy-induced cognitive impairment in non-CNS cancer patients: a review. Brain Imaging Behav 2013; 7: 409–435.

Deutsch MB, Mendez MF. Neurocognitive features distinguishing primary central nervous system lymphoma from other possible causes of rapidly progressive dementia. Cogn Behav Neurol 2015; 28: 1–10.

Devito EE, Pickard JD, Salmond CH, et al. The neuropsychology of normal pressure hydrocephalus (NPH). Br J Neurosurg 2005; 19: 217–224.

Filippi M, Tortorella C, Bozzali M. Normal-appearing white matter changes in multiple sclerosis: the contribution of magnetic resonance techniques. Mult Scler 1999; 5: 273–282.

Filley CM. Clinical neurology and executive dysfunction. Semin Speech Lang 2000; 21: 95–108.

Filley CM. White matter dementia. Ther Adv Neurol Disord 2012; 5: 267–277.

Filley CM, Franklin GM, Heaton RK, Rosenberg NL. White matter dementia: clinical disorders and implications. Neuropsychiatry Neuropsychol Behav Neurol 1988; 1: 239–254.

Filley CM, Heaton RK, Nelson LM, et al. A comparison of dementia in Alzheimer's disease and multiple sclerosis. Arch Neurol 1989; 46: 157–161.

Filley CM, Kleinschmidt-DeMasters BK. Toxic leukoencephalopathy. N Engl J Med 2001; 345: 425–432.

Filley CM, Kleinschmidt-DeMasters BK, Lillehei KO, et al. Gliomatosis cerebri: neurobehavioral and neuropathological observations. Cogn Behav Neurol 2003; 16: 149–159.

Filley CM, Halliday W, Kleinschmidt-DeMasters BK. The effects of toluene on the central nervous system. J Neuropathol Exp Neurol 2004; 63: 1–12.

Filley CM, Kozora E, Brown MS, et al. White matter microstructure and cognition in non-neuropsychiatric systemic lupus erythematosus. Cogn Behav Neurol 2009; 22: 38–44.

Filley CM, Brown MS, Onderko K, et al. White matter disease and cognitive impairment in FMR1 premutation carriers. Neurology 2015; 84: 2146–2152.

Graham JE, Rockwood K, Beattie BL, et al. Prevalence and severity of cognitive impairment with and without dementia in an elderly population. Lancet 1997; 349: 1793–1796.

Hope TR, Vardal J, Bjørnerud A, et al. Serial diffusion tensor imaging for early detection of radiation-induced injuries to normal-appearing white matter in high-grade glioma patients. J Magn Reson Imaging 2015; 41: 414–423.

Jacola LM, Ashford JM, Reddick WE, et al. The relationship between working memory and cerebral white matter volume in survivors of childhood brain tumors treated with conformal radiation therapy. J Neurooncol 2014; 119: 197–205.

Kozora E, Filley CM. Cognitive dysfunction and white matter abnormalities in systemic lupus erythematosus. J Int Neuropsychol Soc 2011; 17: 1–8.

Kozora E, Arciniegas DB, Duggan E, et al. White matter abnormalities and working memory impairment in systemic lupus erythematosus. Cogn Behav Neurol 2013; 26: 63–72.

Kral VA. Senescent forgetfulness: benign and malignant. Can Med Assoc J 1962; 86: 257–260.

Lafosse JM, Corboy JR, Leehey MA, et al. MS vs. HD: can white matter and subcortical gray matter pathology be distinguished neuropsychologically? J Clin Exp Neuropsychol 2007; 29: 142–154.

Leinonen V, Koivisto AM, Savolainen S, et al. Post-mortem findings in 10 patients with presumed normal-pressure hydrocephalus and review of the literature. Neuropathol Appl Neurobiol 2012; 38: 72–86.

Leite SC, Corrêa DG, Doring TM, et al. Diffusion tensor MRI evaluation of the corona radiata, cingulate gyri, and corpus callosum in HIV patients. J Magn Reson Imaging 2013; 38: 1488–1493.

Miralbell J, Soriano JJ, Spulber G, et al. Structural brain changes and cognition in relation to markers of vascular dysfunction. Neurobiol Aging 2012; 33: 1003. e9–e17.

Mohamed MA, Barker PB, Skolasky RL, et al. Brain metabolism and cognitive impairment in HIV infection: a 3-T magnetic resonance spectroscopy study. Magn Reson Imaging 2010; 28: 1251–1257.

Mulhern RK, White HA, Glass JO, et al. Attentional functioning and white matter integrity among survivors of malignant brain tumors of childhood. J Int Neuropsychol Soc 2004; 10: 180–199.

O'Brien JT, Erkinjuntti T, Reisberg B, et al. Vascular cognitive impairment. Lancet Neurol 2003; 2: 89–98.

Petersen RC. Clinical practice: mild cognitive impairment. N Engl J Med 2011; 364: 2227–2234.

Petersen RC, Smith GE, Waring SC, et al. Mild cognitive impairment: clinical characterization and outcome. Arch Neurol 1999; 56: 303–308.

Reijneveld JC, Sitskoorn MM, Klein M, et al. Cognitive status and quality of life in patients with suspected versus proven low-grade gliomas. Neurology 2001; 56: 618–623.

Rollins KE, Kleinschmidt-DeMasters BK, Corboy JR, et al. Lymphomatosis cerebri as a cause of white matter dementia. Hum Pathol 2005; 36: 282–290.

Román GC, Sachdev P, Royall DR, et al. Vascular cognitive disorder: a new diagnostic category updating vascular cognitive impairment and vascular dementia. J Neurol Sci 2004; 226: 81–87.

Sacktor N, Robertson K. Evolving clinical phenotypes in HIV-associated neurocognitive disorders. Curr Opin HIV AIDS 2014; 9: 517–520.

Selnes OA, Vinters HV. Vascular cognitive impairment. Nat Clin Pract Neurol 2006; 2: 538–547.

Stebbins GT, Smith CA, Bartt RE, et al. HIV-associated alterations in normal-appearing white matter: a voxel-wise diffusion tensor imaging study. J Acquir Immune Defic Syndr 2007; 46: 564–573.

Sun X, Liang Y, Wang J, Chen K, et al. Early frontal structural and functional changes in mild white matter lesions relevant to cognitive decline. J Alzheimers Dis 2014; 40: 123–134.

Tate DF, Conley J, Paul RH, et al. Quantitative diffusion tensor imaging tractography metrics are associated with cognitive performance among HIV-infected patients. Brain Imaging Behav 2010; 4: 68–79.

Teeling JL, Perry VH. Systemic infection and inflammation in acute CNS injury and chronic neurodegeneration: underlying mechanisms. Neuroscience 2009; 158: 1062–1073.

Theodoridou A, Settas L. Demyelination in rheumatic diseases. J Neurol Neurosurg Psychiatry 2006; 77: 290–295.

Tucha O, Smely C, Preier M, Lange KW. Cognitive deficits before treatment among patients with brain tumors. Neurosurgery 2000; 47: 324–333.

Van Zandvoort MJ, Kappelle LJ, Algra A, De Haan EH. Decreased capacity for mental effort after single supratentorial lacunar infarct may affect performance in everyday life. J Neurol Neurosurg Psychiatry 1998; 65: 697–702.

Viana-Baptista M, Bugalho P, Jordão C, et al. Cognitive function correlates with frontal white matter apparent diffusion coefficients in patients with leukoaraiosis. J Neurol 2008; 255: 360–636.

Williams MA, Relkin NR. Diagnosis and management of idiopathic normal-pressure hydrocephalus. Neurol Clin Pract 2013; 3: 375–385.

Chapter 9

Diagnosis

The clinical impact of white matter dementia (WMD) and mild cognitive dysfunction (MCD) can be realized in terms of improving diagnosis, prognostication, and treatment options. The first step in the evaluation of patients with cognitive complaints is of course an accurate diagnosis (Taber, Hurley, and Yudofsky, 2010). The process of diagnostic evaluation is not markedly different from that of any possible cognitive disorder (Box 9.1), but certain aspects of the evaluation are especially relevant to the disorders of white matter. As in every clinical setting, maintaining suspicion for the problem will improve the likelihood of its detection, and thus enhance all further aspects of care.

It need hardly be stated that WMD and MCD are not diagnoses that will be found on standard diagnostic lists, and third-party payers are not likely to accept these terms as reimbursable entities. While it is true that conventional diagnoses such as multiple sclerosis (MS), Binswanger's Disease (BD), cerebral autosomal-dominant arteriopathy with subcortical infarcts and leukoencephalopathy (CADASIL), and metachromatic leukodystrophy (MLD) may be usefully classified within one these categories, WMD and MCD are at this point clinical research constructs meant to focus attention on a specific neural correlate of dementia. The intent of highlighting WMD and MCD is to expand thinking about white matter and cognition so that clinical care can be more securely focused on the specific neuropathology involved, and research can better establish the contributions of white matter and its dysfunction to human behavior. This chapter is thus not intended to replace any existing diagnostic methods or strategies, but to elaborate on the manner in which established diagnostic approaches can help disclose white matter disorders with more accuracy and lead to better understanding of their neurobehavioral impact. As the cortical-subcortical dementia distinction informed behavioral neurology a generation ago, an emphasis on white matter can widen the spectrum of disorders that manifest with cognitive dysfunction, and in general stimulate a more nuanced approach to brain–behavior relationships in the dementias.

Clinical evaluation

Individuals with cognitive impairment related to white matter involvement come to clinical evaluation via one of three primary routes: (1) a white matter disorder is known, in most cases supported by a brain neuroimaging study, usually magnetic resonance imaging (MRI); (2) white matter abnormalities of potential significance have been disclosed by MRI or another neuroimaging study; or (3) the medical history suggests the possibility of brain white matter neuropathology. In all of these scenarios, the time-honored methods of careful history taking and thorough physical examination are crucial, with special emphasis on mental status testing.

A diagnosed white matter disorder may pose little or no challenge if the cognitive impairment is obvious and no other disorder is likely to explain the problem. A young adult chronic toluene abuser with no other notable medical history who has dementia associated with severe, diffuse MRI white matter hyperintensity serves an illustrative example. Similarly, a genetically proven case of MLD in an adult who first developed psychosis and then dementia as confluent MRI white matter hyperintensity advanced over several years poses no diagnostic difficulty. Far more often, however, the patient has a complex clinical picture that may include a disease that also affects gray matter, such as MS, or one that prominently affects other organs outside the nervous system, such as systemic lupus erythematosus (SLE). In these cases, clinical judgment must be applied to ascertain the extent to which white matter involvement explains cognitive impairment.

More difficult is the situation in which white matter abnormalities have been identified by neuroimaging

BOX 9.1 Diagnosis of white matter dementia and mild cognitive dysfunction

- Clinical evaluation
- Laboratory testing
- Neuroimaging
- Neuropsychology
- Brain biopsy

and cognitive impairment is an issue, but no clear diagnosis has been made. Many patients seen in MS clinics, for example, have minor degrees of nonspecific white matter hyperintense lesions that are not clearly related to demyelination. In these cases, clinical assessment should first be applied to determine the primary diagnosis so that any cognitive disturbances can be properly interpreted. If a white matter disorder is diagnosed, the appropriateness of diagnosing WMD or MCD can be determined, and if no such disorder is found, the origin of cognitive symptoms can be sought elsewhere.

The clinical history may be highly suggestive or even diagnostic. A patient with a known leukodystrophy, MS, human immunodeficiency virus (HIV) infection, inhalant abuse, or cerebrovascular disease who develops progressive cognitive decline in the absence of other etiologies of dementia may well qualify for the descriptor WMD or MCD. In a patient with unexplained MRI white matter abnormalities and cognitive decline, the medical, psychiatric, family, and social history may all be relevant and can help guide the diagnostic evaluation. White matter involvement may produce a picture of rapidly progressive dementia, prompting an urgent evaluation, as in some cases of infectious disease (Jones et al., 1988), inflammatory disease (Kirk, Kertesz, and Polk, 1991), demyelination (Hardy and Chataway, 2013), and neoplasia (Filley et al., 2003; Rollins et al., 2005; Deutsch and Mendez, 2015).

Also challenging is the patient with symptoms that could suggest the presence of a white matter disorder affecting cognition. These symptoms include a host of complaints, ranging from fatigue, lassitude, somnolence, and apathy to inattention, multitasking difficulty, impaired word finding, and memory loss. As MRI is a rather costly procedure, and these many diverse symptoms can be due to a great variety of medical, neurologic, and psychiatric disorders that do not implicate brain white matter, clinical evaluation is important as the initial step to find alternative explanations. But MRI is at times an appropriate diagnostic test to consider.

Before turning to neuroimaging, other information from the history and elemental neurologic examination may prove helpful. Seizures and movement disorders are relatively uncommon in white matter disorders affecting cognition because these phenomena reflect pathology in cortical and deep gray matter, respectively (Filley, 2012). In contrast, other signs can be quite helpful. Corticospinal dysfunction often indicates tract damage and can be useful for distinguishing a problem such as BD, MS, HIV-associated dementia, cobalamin deficiency, and normal pressure hydrocephalus (NPH) from cortical disorders such as Alzheimer's Disease (AD), in which cognitive impairment is not accompanied by motor dysfunction until late in the course. Gait disorder is common in white matter disorders, and urinary incontinence may also occur; both reflect disruption of frontal lobe tracts. Gait disorder in older people has been repeatedly correlated with frontal lobe white matter dysfunction as measured by MRI and diffusion tensor imaging (DTI) (Srikanth et al., 2010; de Laat et al., 2011; Annweiler and Montero-Odasso, 2012; Callisaya et al., 2013; Smith et al., 2015), and whereas this problem is sometimes referred to as "lower body parkinsonism," a more appropriate term may be "cerebrovascular gait disorder" (Rektor, Rektorová, and Kubová, 2006). Urinary incontinence can also occur with frontal white matter dysfunction of various etiologies (Vigliani et al., 1999; Graff-Radford, 2007; Sakakibara et al., 2012). Incontinence is of course a defining clinical feature of NPH, and can also be a result of cerebrovascular white matter lesions interfering with the normal inhibitory function of medial frontal lobe structures controlling micturition (Andrew and Nathan, 1964; Sakakibara et al., 2012). Recent neuro-urological studies have in fact shown that overactivity of the bladder detrusor muscle in older people, popularly known as overactive bladder, is more related to white matter lesions than to the pathology of AD (Sakakibara et al., 2014).

The mental status examination is a key component of the evaluation in patients suspected of WMD or MCD. This examination, always a time-intensive process requiring considerable sensitivity to clinical subtleties, can be particularly challenging in the diagnosis of cognitive decline related to white matter involvement, because language is normal or nearly so in these patients, and deficits are more apparent in cognitive speed, executive function, and attention. Whereas the relative subtlety of these deficits means that the cognitive deficits of many impaired patients may remain undetected as other sensorimotor features of the illness often dominate the clinical encounter, a detailed mental status examination can provide the critical information (Arciniegas, 2013), and neuropsychological testing can be equally helpful (Cullum, 2013). Detailed neurobehavioral or neuropsychological evaluation may not always be feasible, however, so brief clinical measures may be called upon. The popular Mini-Mental State Examination (MMSE; Folstein, Folstein, and McHugh, 1975) is heavily weighted toward language, and relatively insensitive to the executive dysfunction of patients with white matter disorders (Franklin et al., 1988; Swirsky-Sacchetti et al., 1992; Román and Royall, 1999; Xu et al., 2014). Other, more useful tests include the Montreal Cognitive Assessment (MoCA; Nasreddine et al., 2005), the Frontal Assessment Battery (FAB; Dubois et al., 2000), and the Clock Drawing Test (CDT; Cosentino et al., 2004). The MoCA (Griebe et al., 2011; Xu et al., 2014), the FAB (Kanno et al., 2011), and the CDT (Kim et al., 2009) have all been found sensitive to white matter dysfunction in various disorders. The MoCA may be the most convenient of these measures as it incorporates executive function and clock drawing tasks into a 30-point format; another advantage is that it enables the testing of memory retrieval, another clinical feature central to the assessment of WMD and MCD.

Laboratory testing

As in any dementia evaluation, the search for reversible causes includes laboratory testing of blood and sometimes other tissues (Miller and Boeve, 2009). A comprehensive metabolic panel, complete blood count, thyroid-stimulating hormone (TSH), and vitamin B_{12} level are routinely obtained, and in selected cases, rapid protein reagin (RPR), HIV, Lyme disease serology, erythrocyte sedimentation rate (ESR), C-reactive protein (CRP), antinuclear antibody (ANA), urinary toxicology screening, and genetic testing for CADASIL and leukodystrophies can be considered. All of these tests can detect various white matter disorders, including the TSH, elevation of which is diagnostic of hypothyroidism; although not widely appreciated, thyroid hormones contribute to normal brain myelination, and recent DTI studies of hypothyroid patients have found a correlation between impaired memory and microstructural white matter damage (Singh et al., 2014). Lumbar puncture is indicated for dementia that is rapidly progressive (Paterson, Takada, and Geschwind, 2012), and white matter involvement is sometimes found to be responsible, as many infectious, inflammatory, demyelinative, and neoplastic diseases can be detected that feature an abrupt onset and fulminant clinical course. In many cases, problems such as hypothyroidism, B_{12} deficiency, and HIV infection will have been detected by primary care evaluation, but any potentially reversible cause of white matter dysfunction should always be kept in mind. In contrast, a test helpful for excluding white matter involvement is electroencephalography (EEG), which can support the diagnosis of a seizure disorder or nonconvulsive status epilepticus; in selected cases, the use of continuous EEG in dedicated epilepsy monitoring units can be required (Maganti and Rutecki, 2013). Finally, in recognition of the increasingly apparent role of sleep disorders in producing cognitive complaints, evaluation with polysomnography may be beneficial (Colrain, 2011).

Neuroimaging

MRI is clearly the procedure of choice in this context, and, for white matter disorders, computed tomography (CT) is inadequate. As discussed in Chapter 2, the advent of MRI both revolutionized general neurology and inaugurated the detailed study of the behavioral neurology of white matter without the necessity of neuropathological correlation. The utility of MRI in the diagnosis of dementing disorders has been well documented, and many of the disorders identified feature prominent white matter abnormalities (Pantano, Caramia, and Pierallini, 1999). Although gray matter of the cortex and subcortical regions is often affected, complicating the relationship between clinical phenomenology and neuropathology, MRI allows detailed views of white matter lesions that can be generally correlated with cognitive deficits. As in any cognitive evaluation that includes neuroimaging, careful inspection of the MRI by the behavioral neurologist can be most informative, often adding helpful interpretation to the reading provided by the radiologist (Miller and Boeve, 2009). The primary data used to develop the constructs of WMD and MCD are in fact derived from clinical research showing that brain MRI white matter lesions correlate with cognitive deficits.

Whereas MRI has been essential to progress in the dementias, it is clear that the sensitivity of the technique to brain pathology may not be matched by its specificity. That is, MRI can detect a multitude of lesions, especially in white matter, but it is often unclear exactly what those lesions may be. A white matter lesion in the periventricular region of an adult, for example, may be determined by genetic, demyelinative, infectious, inflammatory, toxic, metabolic, ischemic, traumatic, neoplastic, or hydrocephalic pathology, and the clinician may be hard-pressed to settle on a single etiology. A related point is that whereas MRI can be diagnostic of a white matter disorder such as MS, and can even establish the basis of cognitive impairment in many cases, it can also disclose nonspecific white matter abnormalities that have no impact on the patient's cognition. Thus MRI can be considered very sensitive to white matter lesions, but the specificity of these findings is a topic better left to the clinician who has a more complete understanding of the clinical picture. This discrepancy between the sensitivity and specificity of MRI is a theme that appears once again in the next section, albeit in a different context.

The newer techniques of DTI, magnetization transfer imaging (MTI), and magnetic resonance spectroscopy (MRS) remain research tools at this point. All require extra time for patients in the scanner, and often significant postacquisition time for data analysis, and the cost of these requirements cannot be justified without clear evidence of patient benefit. It is to be hoped, however, that some clinical utility of these techniques, which after all are all noninvasive and without important risk, will be realized as technology advances and the need for assessing the integrity of white matter tracts for patient care is appreciated. Not only are there likely to be advances in the identification and characterization of tracts seen to be damaged on conventional MRI, but the presumably vast terra incognita of lesions within the normal-appearing white matter (NAWM) will become accessible to the eagerly curious eyes of behavioral neurologists.

Neuropsychology

The field of neuropsychology, a close companion of behavioral neurology, has been essential to the establishment of white matter–cognition relationships (Heaton et al., 1985; Filley and Cullum, 1994; Harris and Filley, 2001; Lafosse et al., 2007; Kozora and Filley, 2011; Kozora et al., 2013; Grigsby, 2014). Combined with MRI and other evolving technologies, neuropsychological assessment has been invaluable in documenting consistent patterns of cognitive impairment in many disorders that inform the concepts of WMD and MCD (Filley, 2012; Cullum, 2013).

In the clinic, individuals with white matter disorders who have had neuropsychological testing can often be readily understood to have WMD or MCD because brain MRI is available. However, more difficulty arises when neuropsychological evaluation suggests a white matter disorder but no such diagnosis has been made and brain MRI has not been obtained. In these cases, it should be remembered that, like MRI, neuropsychological testing is in general more sensitive than it is specific, and that cognitive deficits consistent with white matter neuropathology can be equally indicative of subcortical gray matter involvement or a wide range of psychiatric disorders such as depression and anxiety. A careful clinical approach using the available data will be most useful in interpreting the findings of neuropsychological assessment.

The profile of deficits in WMD has been discussed in Chapter 7, and remains the basis for suspecting the development of this syndrome from a neuropsychological perspective. Accordingly, MCD would manifest as a similar profile but with less severe impairments, prominently featuring deficits in processing speed and working memory, and the important clinical datum that usual social and occupational function is not compromised. This assessment is crucial in many cases, and can help distinguish a white matter disorder from others impacting cognition.

Neuropsychological testing can take many forms depending on the professional orientation of the examiner and the specific measures selected, and the intent here is not to propose an invariant assessment method or battery of tests. One perspective that is particularly useful in white matter disorders, however, is the Boston Process Approach, a strong academic tradition in neuropsychology championed by Edith Kaplan during her many years at the Boston Veterans Administration Medical Center in the latter half of the twentieth century (Libon et al., 2013). This approach emphasizes the process by which a patient carries out a given task rather than considering only the test score obtained. Test scores in comparison to normative data are considered, but close attention is also paid to the analysis of errors that emerge as a patient undertakes a given task (Libon et al., 2013). The philosophy motivating this approach is one that considers the reason for test failure as much as the failure itself. Given the subtlety of cognitive impairment that can occur in WMD, which is still more evident in MCD, the Boston Process Approach readily lends itself to the assessment of these problems.

An illustrative example of the advantage of the Boston Process Approach can be found in the California Verbal Learning Test (CVLT), a widely used neuropsychological assessment instrument introduced by Kaplan and her colleagues (Delis et al., 1987). The CVLT provides a detailed analysis of memory performance by using various measures that permit the disambiguation of various factors that underlie memory failure. By focusing on the process by which a patient takes on a memory task, the reason for an impaired performance becomes clearer. Of particular importance for the evaluation of patients with suspected WMD and MCD, the CVLT specifically tests for recognition memory, which, if preserved, supports the criterion of retrieval deficit that is included in the clinical profile of white matter disorders affecting cognition (Chapter 7). The Boston Process Approach can also be applied to other domains implicated in WMD and MCD, such as processing speed, working memory, and executive function.

The centrality of slowed processing speed in the disorders of white matter deserves special emphasis. Many neurobehavioral disorders can manifest cognitive slowing, but a specific relationship of this deficit with white matter damage is being increasingly well established (Chapter 7). One of the most useful measures for quantitating this problem is the Paced Auditory Serial Addition Test (PASAT), first developed for use in traumatic brain injury (Gronwall and Wrightson, 1981) and now widely applicable to white matter disorders (Benedict et al., 2008; Kozora et al., 2013). The PASAT can be quite frustrating for patients at times, suggesting the need for alternative means of quantitating slowed cognition, but assessment of this aspect of white matter dysfunction is critical.

One of the areas in which neuropsychological testing for WMD and MCD could be expanded is in the evaluation of procedural learning and memory. As reviewed in Chapter 7, this domain is one of the key areas in which the distinction between WMD and subcortical gray matter dementia can be clarified. Acquisition of motor skills is typically only mildly impaired or even unaffected in patients with white matter disorders (Lafosse et al., 2007), in contrast to those with lesions of the basal ganglia (Martone et al., 1984) and the cerebellum (Sanes, Dimitrov, and Hallett, 1990). Thus the preservation of procedural learning and memory would be useful to document, since this testing can help differentiate patients with white matter disorders from other patients expected to manifest deficits, such as those with Parkinson's Disease and cerebellar disorders (Yamadori et al., 1996). Yet the acquisition of motor skills is not typically tested in clinical evaluations, and this aspect of the cognitive profile is usually not available. Procedural learning and memory are more readily tested in experimental settings with measures such as rotary pursuit and mirror drawing (Gabrieli et al., 1997; Lafosse et al., 2007), but these methods, however useful, are difficult to apply in the clinic and may yield equivocal results. The development of other, more convenient measures for the assessment of procedural learning and memory would be welcome.

Brain biopsy

The use of brain biopsy permits direct examination of brain tissue during life, and is thus highly informative. This procedure is rarely implemented, however, as it is of course invasive and fraught with potential complications. Brain biopsy involves obvious hazard to the patient in terms of operative and anesthetic risk, postoperative complications, and later effects that may develop such as intracranial and wound infections, intracranial hemorrhage, and seizures. Moreover, neurosurgeons are understandably reluctant to consider brain biopsy in many cases of dementia because of the specter of possible prion disease that almost inevitably arises. The reasoning behind this reluctance is that obscure dementias for which a noninvasive diagnosis has not been found, particularly those with rapid progression, may often mean the presence of prion involvement that introduces considerable risk of contamination of neurosurgical instruments as well as some hazard to the operative personnel. In the vast majority of cases, the need for brain biopsy is indeed obviated by the noninvasive methods discussed earlier.

Brain biopsy, however, can be very useful in selected cases (Warren et al., 2005). The procedure deserves mention here as a reminder that clinical problems can arise in which the white matter lesion or lesions remain perplexing to all involved despite the use of every nonsurgical diagnostic effort, and the clinical treatment may be altered as a result of the surgery. An example of such a problem is the patient with extensive cerebral white matter lesions that could represent a leukodystrophy, demyelination, an infection, inflammation, a vascular disorder, leukotoxicity, or a neoplasm (Warren et al., 2005). In such cases, particularly those that are rapidly progressive and have defied diagnosis, brain biopsy may be not only indicated but lifesaving. The recently described tumefactive MS (Hu and Lucchinetti, 2009), for example, often proves perplexing because it can closely resemble other brain lesions such a stroke or a neoplasm, and biopsy can be definitive for confirming demyelination as the etiology of this unusual mass (Hardy and Chataway, 2013). Brain biopsy may also prove crucial in diagnosing puzzling cases that were found to be the rare neoplasm gliomatosis cerebri (Filley et al., 2003) and the similarly uncommon lymphomatosis cerebri (Rollins et al., 2005; Deutsch and Mendez, 2015). Other cases will often prove to have no potential for reversibility, but benefit can still be achieved by accurate diagnosis. One such example is adult-onset leukoencephalopathy with axonal spheroids, a rare disorder that can present as a rapidly progressive dementia and mimic cortical frontotemporal syndromes (Wong, Chow, and Hazrati, 2011). In all cases of suspected brain white matter involvement, it need hardly be stated that acquisition of a sufficient biopsy specimen including white matter is critical; the biopsy should therefore include a portion of deep white matter as well as overlying gray matter and meninges.

It is well to remember, however, that even brain biopsy may prove insufficient to provide a firm diagnosis; findings may be equivocal because the specimen does not include enough tissue to yield a clear diagnosis, steroid or other therapy has altered the findings to impair diagnostic specificity, or the disorder is unique and requires further genetic or other investigation to establish its identity. Thus even the gold standard of neuropathology may sometimes prove inadequate for declaring a clear diagnosis, and clinicians are reminded once again of the humbling complexity that can accompany the neurologic disorders to which humans are susceptible.

References

Andrew J, Nathan PW. Lesions on the anterior frontal lobes and disturbances of micturition and defaecation. Brain 1964; 87: 233–262.

Annweiler C, Montero-Odasso M. Vascular burden as a substrate for higher-level gait disorders in older adults: a review of brain mapping literature. Panminerva Med 2012; 54: 189–204.

Arciniegas DB. Mental status examination. In: Arciniegas DB, Anderson CA, Filley CM, eds. *Behavioral neurology & neuropsychiatry*. Cambridge: Cambridge University Press, 2013: 344–393.

Benedict RH, Shucard JL, Zivadinov R, Shucard DW. Neuropsychological impairment in systemic lupus erythematosus: a comparison with multiple sclerosis. Neuropsychol Rev 2008; 18: 149–166.

Callisaya ML, Beare R, Phan TG, et al. Brain structural change and gait decline: a longitudinal population-based study. J Am Geriatr Soc 2013; 61: 1074–1079.

Colrain IM. Sleep and the brain. Neuropsychol Rev 2011; 21: 1–4.

Cosentino S, Jefferson A, Chute DL, et al. Clock drawing errors in dementia: neuropsychological and neuroanatomical considerations. Cogn Behav Neurol 2004; 17: 74–84.

Cullum CM. Neuropsychological assessment. In: Arciniegas DB, Anderson CA, Filley CM, eds. *Behavioral neurology & neuropsychiatry*. Cambridge: Cambridge Univerisity Press, 2013: 394–405.

de Laat KF, van Norden AG, Gons RA, et al. Diffusion tensor imaging and gait in elderly persons with cerebral small vessel disease. Stroke 2011; 42: 373–379.

Delis DC, Kramer JH, Kaplan E, Ober BA. *The California Verbal Learning Test*. San Antonio, TX: Psychological Corporation, 1987.

Deutsch MB, Mendez MF. Neurocognitive features distinguishing primary central nervous system lymphoma from other possible causes of rapidly progressive dementia. Cogn Behav Neurol 2015; 28: 1–10.

Dubois B, Slachevsky A, Litvan I, Pillon B. The FAB: a Frontal Assessment Battery at bedside. Neurology 2000; 55: 1621–1626.

Filley CM. *The behavioral neurology of white matter*. 2nd ed. New York: Oxford University Press, 2012.

Filley CM, Cullum CM. Attention and vigilance functions in normal aging. Appl Neuropsychol 1994; 1: 29–32.

Filley CM, Kleinschmidt-DeMasters BK, Lillehei KO, et al. Gliomatosis cerebri: neurobehavioral and neuropathological observations. Cogn Behav Neurol 2003; 16: 149–159.

Folstein MF, Folstein SE, McHugh PR. “Mini-Mental State”: a practical method for grading the cognitive state of patients for the clinician. J Psychiatr Res 1975; 12: 189–198.

Franklin GM, Heaton RK, Nelson LM, et al. Correlation of neuropsychological and MRI findings in chronic/progressive multiple sclerosis. Neurology 1988; 38: 1826–1829.

Gabrieli JD, Stebbins GT, Singh J, et al. Intact mirror-tracing and impaired rotary-pursuit skill learning in patients with Huntington's disease: evidence for dissociable memory systems in skill learning. Neuropsychology 1997; 11: 272–281.

Graff-Radford NR. Normal pressure hydrocephalus. Neurol Clin 2007; 25: 809–832.

Griebe M, Förste, A, Wessa M, et al. Loss of callosal fibre integrity in healthy elderly with age-related white matter changes. J Neurol 2011; 258: 1451–1459.

Grigsby J, Cornish K, Hocking D, et al. The cognitive neuropsychological phenotype of carriers of the FMR1 premutation. J Neurodev Disord 2014; 6: 28.

Gronwall D, Wrightson P. Memory and information processing capacity after closed head injury. J Neurol Neurosurg Psychiatry 1981; 44: 889–895.

Hardy TA, Chataway J. Tumefactive demyelination: an approach to diagnosis and management. J Neurol Neurosurg Psychiatry 2013; 84: 1047–1053.

Harris JG, Filley CM. CADASIL: neuropsychological findings in three generations of an affected family. J Int Neuropsychol Soc 2001; 7: 768–774.

Heaton RK, Nelson LM, Thompson DS, et al. Neuropsychological findings in relapsing-remitting and chronic-progressive multiple sclerosis. J Consul Clin Psychol 1985; 53: 103–110.

Hu W, Lucchinetti CF. The pathological spectrum of CNS inflammatory demyelinating diseases. Semin Immunopathol 2009; 31: 439–453.

Jones HR Jr, Ho DD, Forgacs P, et al. Acute fulminating fatal leukoencephalopathy as the only manifestation of human immunodeficiency virus infection. Ann Neurol 1988; 23: 519–522.

Kanno S, Abe N, Saito M, et al. White matter involvement in idiopathic normal pressure hydrocephalus: a voxel-based diffusion tensor imaging study. J Neurol 2011; 258: 1949–1957.

Kim YS, Lee KM, Choi BH, et al. Relation between the clock drawing test (CDT) and structural changes of brain in dementia. Arch Gerontol Geriatr 2009; 48: 218–221.

Kirk A, Kertesz A, Polk MJ. Dementia with leukoencephalopathy in systemic lupus erythematosus. Can J Neurol Sci 1991; 18: 344–348.

Kozora E, Filley CM. Cognitive dysfunction and white matter abnormalities in systemic lupus erythematosus. J Int Neuropsychol Soc 2011; 17: 1–8.

Kozora E, Arciniegas DB, Duggan E, et al. White matter abnormalities and working memory impairment in systemic lupus erythematosus. Cogn Behav Neurol 2013; 26: 63–72.

Lafosse JM, Corboy JR, Leehey MA, et al. MS vs. HD: can white matter and subcortical gray matter pathology be distinguished neuropsychologically? J Clin Exp Neuropsychol 2007; 29: 142–154.

Libon DJ, Swenson R, Ashendorf L, et al. Edith Kaplan and the Boston Process Approach. Clin Neuropsychol 2013; 27: 1223–1233.

Maganti RK, Rutecki P. EEG and epilepsy monitoring. Continuum (Minneap Minn) 2013; 19 (3 Epilepsy): 598–622.

Martone M, Butters N, Payne M, et al. Dissociations between skill learning and verbal recognition in amnesia and dementia. Arch Neurol 1984; 41: 965–970.

Miller BL, Boeve BF, eds. *The behavioral neurology of dementia*. Cambridge: Cambridge University Press, 2009.

Nasreddine ZS, Phillips NA, Bédirian V, et al. The Montreal Cognitive Assessment, MoCA: a brief screening tool for mild cognitive impairment. J Am Geriatr Soc 2005; 53: 695–699.

Pantano P, Caramia F, Pierallini A. The role of MRI in dementia. Ital J Neurol Sci 1999; 20 (5 Suppl): S250–S253.

Paterson RW, Takada LT, Geschwind MD. Diagnosis and treatment of rapidly progressive dementias. Neurol Clin Pract 2012; 2: 187–200.

Rektor I, Rektorová I, Kubová D. Vascular parkinsonism – an update. J Neurol Sci 2006; 248: 185–191.

Rollins KE, Kleinschmidt-DeMasters BK, Corboy JR, et al. Lymphomatosis cerebri as a cause of white matter dementia. Hum Pathol 2005; 36: 282–290.

Román GC, Royall DR. Executive control function: a rational basis for the diagnosis of vascular dementia. Alzheimer Dis Assoc Disord 1999; 13 Suppl 3: S69–S80.

Sakakibara R, Panicker J, Fowler CJ, et al. Vascular incontinence: incontinence in the elderly due to ischemic white matter changes. Neurol Int 2012; 4: e13.

Sakakibara R, Panicker J, Fowler CJ, et al. Is overactive bladder a brain disease? The pathophysiological role of cerebral white matter in the elderly. Int J Urol 2014; 21: 33–38.

Sanes JN, Dimitrov B, Hallett M. Motor learning in patients with cerebellar dysfunction. Brain 1990; 113: 103–120.

Singh S, Trivedi R, Singh K, et al. Diffusion tensor tractography in hypothyroidism and its correlation with memory function. J Neuroendocrinol 2014; 26: 825–833.

Smith EE, O'Donnell M, Dagenais G, et al. Early cerebral small vessel disease and brain volume, cognition, and gait. Ann Neurol 2015; 77: 251–261.

Srikanth V, Phan TG, Chen J, et al. The location of white matter lesions and gait – a voxel-based study. Ann Neurol 2010; 67: 265–269.

Swirsky-Sacchetti T, Field HL, Mitchell DR, et al. The sensitivity of the Mini-Mental State Exam in the white matter dementia of multiple sclerosis. J Clin Psychol 1992; 48: 779–786.

Taber KH, Hurley RA, Yudofsky SC. Diagnosis and treatment of neuropsychiatric disorders. Annu Rev Med 2010; 61: 121–133.

Vigliani MC, Duyckaerts C, Hauw JJ, et al. Dementia following treatment of brain tumors with radiotherapy administered alone or in combination with nitrosourea-based chemotherapy: a clinical and pathological study. J Neurooncol 1999; 41: 137–149.

Warren JD, Schott JM, Fox NC, et al. Brain biopsy in dementia. Brain 2005; 128: 2016–2025.

Wong JC, Chow TW, Hazrati LN. Adult-onset leukoencephalopathy with axonal spheroids and pigmented glia can present as frontotemporal dementia syndrome. Dement Geriatr Cogn Disord 2011; 32: 150–158.

Xu Q, Cao WW, Mi JH, et al. Brief screening for mild cognitive impairment in subcortical ischemic vascular disease: a comparison study of the Montreal Cognitive Assessment with the Mini-Mental State Examination. Eur Neurol 2014; 71: 106–114.

Yamadori A, Yoshida T, Mori E, Yamashita H. Neurological basis of skill learning. Brain Res Cogn Brain Res 1996; 5: 49–54.

Chapter 10

Prognosis

The prognosis of white matter disorders that may lead to white matter dementia (WMD) or its precursor mild cognitive dysfunction (MCD) is a complex topic because of the diversity of neuropathological insults that may prove responsible. Determining the outcome of WMD and MCD will be improved by greater understanding of alterations in white matter neurobiology, which is steadily advancing within each of the neuropathological categories that can exert effects on white matter. In this chapter, the prognosis of cognitive impairment in white matter disorders will be considered without regard to the treatments that can be offered in order to explore the inherent properties of myelinated systems that stand out as unique. Treatment will be taken up in Chapter 11, but at this point the important determinants of outcome in the absence of treatment deserve attention. Table 10.1 lists major factors influencing the prognosis of WMD and MCD.

Natural history

The wide range of white matter disorders of course means that prognosis of WMD and MCD is highly variable depending on the specific disease, intoxication, or injury present as the underlying cause. As in medicine generally, every disorder has its own natural history, and one of the most important tasks of a physician is to understand these patterns and thus acquire at least some capacity to predict outcome and timing. Comparatively little is known about the prognosis of cognitive impairment in white matter disorders, and the clinician is often obliged to offer informed speculation when considering these questions. By way of background, the details of specific white matter disorders are discussed elsewhere (Filley, 2012), and selected key points about prognosis will be considered here.

The diverse nature of neuropathology affecting white matter means that prognosis for cognitive improvement ranges from very favorable, as in the case of self-limited acute confusional state from cranial irradiation (Rimkus et al., 2014), to very poor, as in leukodystrophies (Orchard and Tolar, 2010) and gliomatosis cerebri (Chen et al., 2013). Many intermediate prognostic levels can be seen, such as the slowly progressive dementia of Binswanger's Disease (BD; Caplan, 1995), the static dementia of severe toluene leukoencephalopathy (Dingwall et al., 2011), cognitive impairment after moderate traumatic brain injury (TBI) (Dikmen et al., 2003), and the relapsing-remitting pattern of many patients with multiple sclerosis (MS) (Amato, Zipoli, and Portaccio, 2006).

The severity of the primary neuropathology is a critical determinant of outcome, as white matter damage may be as mild as transient intramyelinic edema or as severe as relentless necrosis involving myelin, axons, and oligodendrocytes (Filley and Kleinschmidt-DeMasters, 2001; Filley, 2012). The age of the patient also impacts outcome in many cases, as both the very young and the very old have less well developed white matter and may be more susceptible to damage (Bartzokis et al., 2010). Coexistent medical, surgical, or psychiatric problems may of course exert a negative impact as well, just as they might in any disorder. In this regard, it is noteworthy that the presence of more than one white matter disorder may also be a predictor of poor

Table 10.1 Factors influencing the prognosis of white matter dementia and mild cognitive dysfunction

Natural history
Disease severity
Age
Comorbid disorders
Presence of axonal loss
Brain and cognitive reserve
Premorbid white matter structure
Premorbid white matter function
Plasticity
Cognitive engagement
Physical activity

prognosis; for example, TBI patients fare worse in the long term if they also have severe leukoaraiosis (LA) (Henninger et al., 2014).

An important generalization about cognitive prognosis in all white matter disorders can be made on the basis of the microscopic study of white matter lesions. Whereas myelin injury may impose its own degree of dysfunction, it is now known that axonal loss clearly implies a worse prognosis in many white matter disorders (Trapp et al., 1998; Medana and Esiri, 2003). This principle has been most emphasized in MS, in which the clinical impact of demyelinative plaques is far more deleterious if the neuropathology also includes axonal loss (Trapp et al., 1998). The loss of axons has also been associated with a worse prognosis in TBI, vascular white matter disease, human immunodeficiency virus (HIV) infection, leukodystrophies, and the metabolic disorder central pontine myelinolysis (Medana and Esiri, 2003). As discussed earlier, diffuse axonal injury (DAI) is a key neuropathology in TBI, and the degree of DAI is likely the most important lesion in determining the severity of neurobehavioral deficits (Smith, Meaney, and Shull, 2003).

In vascular disease, the degree of axonal loss present within areas of LA is variable (Gouw et al., 2011), but when dementia develops from the accumulation of LA, axonal loss appears to be important (Nitkunan et al., 2008). Recent neuroimaging evidence has suggested that white matter axons are damaged in BD, but relatively intact in normal pressure hydrocephalus (NPH), consistent with the worse prognosis of BD in comparison with the potential reversibility of NPH (Tullberg et al., 2009). In toluene leukoencephalopathy, axonal loss is uncommon, suggesting that reversibility may be possible in many exposed individuals (Filley, Halliday, and Kleinschmidt-DeMasters, 2004). Reversibility is in fact well recognized in the metabolic disorder of cobalamin deficiency, and may plausibly be related to the observation that loss of axons is less pronounced than myelin damage (Adams and Kubik, 1944).

Finally, systemic lupus erythematosus (SLE) may involve only myelin injury (Filley et al., 2009), but axonal loss can be seen in some cases with reduced N-acetyl aspartate (NAA) on magnetic resonance spectroscopy (MRS) (Kozora et al., 2008), and at autopsy (Sibbitt et al., 2010), suggesting that SLE can damage central axons in addition to myelin. The MRS data in SLE are particularly intriguing because they directly apply to the MCD construct. By enabling the assessment of axonal integrity at an early stage of a white matter disorder, MRS may provide the opportunity to use a noninvasive modality to detect early cognitive dysfunction at a stage when the prognosis is more favorable (Filley et al., 2009; Kozora and Filley, 2011).

At present, however, conventional MRI remains the procedure of choice for assessing the advance of white matter pathology. One advantage enjoyed by clinicians in the MRI era is that a readily available neuroimaging modality can be employed to assess the structure of white matter in the course of disease. Longitudinal follow-up is substantially informed by the use of MRI to assess the state of white matter over time, enabling monitoring of the natural history of the disorder by direct visualization of the affected neuroanatomy. In MS, for example, MRI has become essential for ongoing clinical management as well as diagnosis (Simon, 2014). Figure 10.1 illustrates the utility of MRI in documenting progression of specific white matter involvement in this disease, showing the advance of corpus callosum atrophy over 2 years. Many other white matter lesions can be seen, including focal areas of demyelination, ischemia, and other neuropathology, and atrophy of the brain as a whole can be readily assessed. Whereas clinical assessment is of course the mainstay of long-term follow-up, and resource considerations require careful consideration of the relative costs and benefits of MRI in each case, the opportunity to see the tissue in question using a noninvasive procedure with no apparent risk should not be overlooked. Particularly as treatments for white matter disorders advance, MRI will serve an

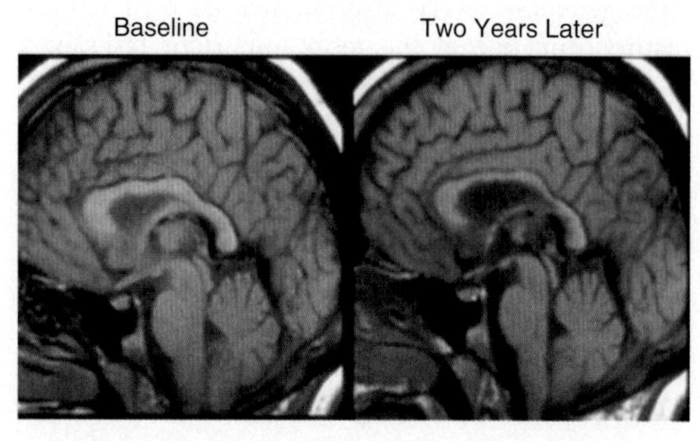

Figure 10.1 Sagittal T1-weighted MRI scans demonstrating progressive atrophy of the corpus callosum in an individual with MS (courtesy of John R. Corboy, MD).

increasingly important role in the assessment of interventions to treat a wide array of white matter lesions.

Brain and cognitive reserve

In 1937, the noted British neurologist Sir Charles Symonds proposed the notion that the effects of brain lesions were determined not only by the insult sustained but also by the preexisting condition of the brain. "In other words," Symonds wrote in a discussion of the mental sequelae of head injury, "it is not only the kind of injury that matters, but the kind of head" (Symonds, 1937). This idea reflects a general understanding among clinicians that any brain affliction can be seen as producing its effects on cognition not only by virtue of the specific location and severity of neuropathology, but also because of the state of the brain at the time the disorder begins. In an effort to develop this concept in more detail, recent studies in clinical neuroscience have proposed the idea of a reserve capacity that functions to modify, delay, or even prevent the onset of neurobehavioral disorders (Stern, 2002, 2009). Following Symonds's lead, the concept has since been applied not only to TBI but to vascular injury, MS, HIV infection, Parkinson's Disease, schizophrenia and other neuropsychiatric disorders, aging, and the degenerative dementias (Satz, 1993; Allen, Bruss, and Damasio, 2005; Stern, 2012).

The reserve concept posits that the brain may be protected against the ravages of cognitive disorders by either genetic endowment or environmental influences that can mitigate the effect of neuropathology. A distinction has been drawn between *brain reserve*, the physical attributes of an individual's brain – mainly its size and number of neurons – that may reduce the individual's susceptibility to the effects of brain disease (Satz, 1993, 2012), and *cognitive reserve*, the previously acquired neural resources of an individual brain that allow effective task performance even in the presence of brain disease (Stern, 2009). Brain reserve is determined by the innate, congenital, and developmental aspects of brain organization, and thus invokes many genetic factors as well as a range of environmental variables such as prenatal care, nutrition, and the characteristics of child rearing. Cognitive reserve is a function of the extent of engagement in cognitive stimulation, which largely involves educational attainment, occupational accomplishment, and socialization across the life span. Brain reserve can therefore be considered a passive phenomenon, based essentially on the general health of the brain being affected by acquired insult, whereas cognitive reserve implicates an active process that increases brain capabilities by the individual's frequent engagement in cognitive activities (Stern, 2002, 2009). Another implication of this distinction is that brain reserve involves the advantages conferred by the premorbid *structure* of the brain, while cognitive reserve implies that premorbid brain *function* has been enhanced by a cognitively stimulating lifestyle (Stern, 2009, 2012).

In the dementias, brain and cognitive reserve have been most investigated in the cortical dementias, notably Alzheimer's Disease (AD), in which it has become clear that these advantages do indeed offer some degree of protection. Brain reserve, indexed by brain size, appears by itself to be protective, as the appearance of dementia related to AD neuropathology is decreased in people with larger brains (Katzman et al., 1988; Schofield et al., 1997). While an overly large brain can of course be associated with cognitive impairment or dementia because of neuropathology related to excessive and thus dysfunctional brain mass (Miles et al., 2009), a larger brain in normal adults, within the standard range of brain size, appears to be mildly protective against AD.

Cognitive reserve also seems to be of benefit, as educational and occupational attainment can also provide some degree of protection from AD (Stern, 2012). This phenomenon first became clear in epidemiological studies from China examining the effect of education on the prevalence of AD (Zhang et al., 1990). The disease cannot be completely prevented by such factors, as the application of demanding mental tasks does not reverse the neuropathology, and indeed the tempo of cognitive decline may be similar in all cases once the reserve capacity of the brain is exhausted (Filley and Cullum, 1997). However, it is generally thought that intellectually stimulating activities offer a salutary means of increasing the integrity of the cortex as it copes with the onset of AD neuropathology. Given that patients with AD have reduced synaptic density that correlates with cognitive impairment (DeKosky and Scheff, 1990), the demonstration of increased synaptic density in laboratory animals exposed to enriched environments (Greenough and Bailey, 1988) assumes special relevance. Experimental animal evidence continues to support the notion that increased synaptic density plays an important role in the mediation of cognitive reserve (Petrosini et al., 2009), and the contribution of neurogenesis is increasingly seen as likely to be important as well (Brown et al., 2003). Thus the number of both synapses and neurons in the cerebral cortices may be important as protective advantages in AD that are enhanced by environmental stimulation.

An intriguing study of normal aging recently appeared that supports the role of brain and cognitive reserve in mitigating the cognitive effects of age-related white matter loss (Daselaar et al., 2015). In older adults whose cognitive function was examined together with functional MRI (fMRI) and diffusion tensor imaging (DTI) data, cortical activity was found to be inversely related to lower white matter integrity in closely related cerebral areas (Daselaar et al., 2015). This finding was interpreted as evidence of the concept of "less wiring, more firing," implying that compensatory activity of cortical regions is recruited to accomplish a relevant cognitive task in the setting of less efficient white matter (Daselaar et al., 2015). The mechanism of such a phenomenon is almost certainly increased synaptic activity.

Among the white matter disorders, MS has been best studied, and neuropsychological data suggest that brain and cognitive reserve can indeed protect against cognitive dysfunction in this disease (Sumowski, Chiaravalloti, and DeLuca, 2009; Langdon, 2011; Sumowski et al., 2014). The mechanism may be similar to that postulated in AD; that is, cortical synaptic density and perhaps neuronal numbers are increased in MS patients who have experienced greater intellectual stimulation, and this advantage may help compensate for the white matter (and to some extent gray matter) neuropathology of the disease. Studies with fMRI have shown that cognitive reserve in MS may rely on the activity of the default mode network, which includes the anterior and posterior cingulate cortices, medial frontal regions, precuneus, and medial and lateral temporal lobes (Sumowski et al., 2010). Patients with MS display considerable variability in their cognitive impairment, and in part this observation may be due to the individuals' premorbid intellectual ability, which in turn relates to both maximal lifetime brain growth and educational and occupational enrichment that mitigates the impact of the neuropathology (Sumowski et al., 2014). Studies in other white matter disorders, including TBI (Kesler et al., 2003), ischemic white matter disease (Dufouil, Alperovitch, and Tzourio, 2003), and HIV infection (Farinpour et al., 2003), also support the notion that reserve can be beneficial in modifying the impact of neuropathology. Thus evidence is accumulating that the cognitive burden imposed by white matter neuropathology may be modified by the capacity of the cerebral cortex to compensate because of an increase in the number of its synapses and neurons.

While these data are of considerable interest in the process of assessing the prognosis of potentially any dementing disease, they apply largely to the notion of plasticity in the cerebral cortex. More intriguing still is the recent idea that experience-dependent neural changes may also occur in the white matter, and have important effects on the cognitive prognosis of white matter disorders.

Plasticity

A fascinating idea pertinent to the recovery of damaged white matter is the notion of plasticity, more generally known as neural plasticity. Operationally defined as the ability of the central nervous system to adapt to environmental changes or acquired lesions (Sharma, Classen, and Cohen, 2013), neural plasticity has recently drawn considerable neuroscientific attention in light of emerging evidence that the brain may possess more adaptive capacity than formerly thought. Long known to be a property of gray matter related to synaptic function, particularly in the cerebral cortex (Majewska and Sur, 2006), plasticity in this conventional sense likely plays a critical role in recovery after many neurologic and neuropsychiatric disorders (Ward and Frackowiak, 2004). However, plasticity has also recently been observed to occur in the cerebral white matter (Fields, 2010; Zatorre, Fields, and Johansen-Berg, 2012; Boulanger and Messier, 2014). This rather arresting notion immediately seems counterintuitive to most neurologists and neuroscientists, accustomed as they have become to a corticocentric perspective. The white matter is often regarded as providing little more than structural connectivity between gray matter regions, acting only to transfer information, and the remarkable capacity of the brain to exhibit plastic changes in response to experience has been seen by most as an exclusive property of gray matter. But this view requires reconsideration.

White matter plasticity is a measurable phenomenon that has been shown both in normal individuals, such as piano players whose pyramidal tract integrity correlated with number of hours practiced (Bengtsson et al., 2005), and in neurologic patients, such as those with Broca's aphasia in whom the right arcuate fasciculus volume increased as melodic intonation therapy improved language performance (Schlaug, Marchina, and Norton, 2009). A recent review of the DTI literature on the effects of musical training in normal people concluded that, among many white matter tracts that may be potentially altered by musical training, the corpus callosum is the one where a beneficial effect of music on white matter connectivity is most compelling (Moore et al., 2014). Equally intriguing are findings indicating that bilingualism is associated with the maintenance of white matter integrity (Luk et al., 2011; Li, Legault, and Litcofsky, 2014), implying that the regular use of more than one language may recruit mechanisms of plasticity within myelinated tracts. Furthermore, DTI data gathered from the fornix of both rats and humans have suggested that structural changes indicative of plasticity may occur after as little as 2 hours of engagement in a learning task (Hofstetter et al., 2013).

These observations suggest that individuals with WMD and MCD may benefit from engagement in cognitive activity that helps restore white matter integrity. But there is also reason to think that physical activity may have similar effects. Emerging neuroimaging evidence, for example, has shown that lifelong physical exercise not only can reduce the number of MRI white matter hyperintensities, but can also increase white matter microstructural integrity (Tseng et al., 2013; Herting et al., 2014).

Laboratory observations have helped elucidate the means by which such changes occur, and the discovery of white matter synapses has been pivotal in this work. White matter plasticity may be mediated by novel glutamatergic axo-oligodendroglial synapses lying within the white matter, which appear to be capable of inducing oligodendrocytes to myelinate distal axonal segments upon stimulation of the proximal axon (Alix and Domingues, 2011; Wake, Lee, and Fields, 2011; Boulanger and Messier, 2014). Thus an increase in the electrical activity coursing through an axon leads to greater distal myelination. In a white matter tract relevant to the task involved, the result of this phenomenon is an expansion of tract volume, and a concomitant increase in white matter integrity.

The specific impact of cognitive engagement and physical activity on white matter is thus becoming clear, and the clinical benefits of this form of plasticity are likely to be substantial. While changes in gray matter would also be expected with such regular habits, the effects on white matter may be equally or perhaps even more apparent. The prognosis of WMD and MCD may thus be meaningfully improved by such activities as playing a musical instrument, learning another language, and staying fit.

More study is needed to understand the application of white matter plasticity to clinical populations, and an obvious setting where this work could be readily accomplished is in the area of stroke rehabilitation (Johansson, 2011; Cumming, Marshall, and Lazar, 2013; Chen et al., 2014). Patients with a single ischemic stroke, featuring both a quantifiable cognitive deficit and a discrete white matter lesion, present a valuable opportunity to assess the impact of various rehabilitation strategies on the role of white matter plasticity in cognitive recovery. But the implications for recovery after any white matter lesion may be profound, and many opportunities for investigation can be imagined. These ideas naturally blend in with the treatment of white matter disorders affecting cognition, and will be further considered in the chapter to follow.

On a larger scale, data on white matter plasticity such as these may inform decision making in the arena of public policy. Whereas these concerns extend beyond the scope of routine medical practice, the promotion of healthy lifestyles that support and maintain white matter integrity under the assault of accumulating insults such as ischemic, traumatic, and leukotoxic injury may warrant focused attention as a public health objective. Societal policies aimed at improving the capacity of the brain to endure the effects of acquired insults, and then to respond more effectively when they occur, have the potential to offer significant benefits to the population as a whole.

References

Adams RD, Kubik CS. Subacute degeneration of the brain in pernicious anemia. N Engl J Med 1944; 231: 1–9.

Alix JJ, Domingues AM. White matter synapses: form, function, and dysfunction. Neurology 2011; 76: 397–404.

Allen JS, Bruss J, Damasio H. The aging brain: the cognitive reserve hypothesis and hominid evolution. Am J Hum Biol 2005; 17: 673–689.

Amato MP, Zipoli V, Portaccio E. Multiple sclerosis–related cognitive changes: a review of cross-sectional and longitudinal studies. J Neurol Sci 2006; 245: 41–46.

Bartzokis G, Lu PH, Tingus K, et al. Lifespan trajectory of myelin integrity and maximum motor speed. Neurobiol Aging 2010; 31: 1554–1562.

Bengtsson SL, Nagy Z, Skare S, et al. Extensive piano practicing has regionally specific effects on white matter development. Nat Neurosci 2005; 8: 1148–1150.

Boulanger JJ, Messier C. From precursors to myelinating oligodendrocytes: contribution of intrinsic and extrinsic factors to white matter plasticity in the adult brain. Neuroscience 2014; 269: 343–366.

Brown J, Cooper-Kuhn CM, Kemperman G, et al. Enriched environment and physical activity stimulate hippocampal but not olfactory bulb neurogenesis. Eur J Neurosci 2003; 17: 2042–2046.

Caplan LR. Binswanger's disease – revisited. Neurology 1995; 45: 626–633.

Chen J, Venkat P, Zacharek A, Chopp M. Neurorestorative therapy for stroke. Front Hum Neurosci 2014; 8: 382.

Chen S, Tanaka S, Giannini C, et al. Gliomatosis cerebri: clinical characteristics, management, and outcomes. J Neurooncol 2013; 112: 267–275.

Cumming TB, Marshall RS, Lazar RM. Stroke, cognitive deficits, and rehabilitation: still an incomplete picture. Int J Stroke 2013; 8: 38–45.

Daselaar SM, Iyengar V, Davis SW, et al. Less wiring, more firing: low-performing older adults compensate for impaired white matter with greater neural activity. Cereb Cortex 2015; 25: 983–990.

DeKosky ST, Scheff SW. Synapse loss in frontal cortex biopsies in Alzheimer's disease: correlation with cognitive severity. Ann Neurol 1990; 27: 457–464.

Dikmen SS, Machamer JE, Powell JM, Temkin NR. Outcome 3 to 5 years after moderate to severe traumatic brain injury. Arch Phys Med Rehabil 2003; 84: 1449–1457.

Dingwall KM, Maruff P, Fredrickson A, Cairney S. Cognitive recovery during and after treatment for volatile solvent abuse. Drug Alcohol Depend 2011; 118: 180–185.

Dufouil C, Alperovitch A, Tzourio C. Influence of education on the relationship between white matter lesions and cognition. Neurology 2003; 60: 831–836.

Farinpour R, Miller EN, Satz P, et al. Psychosocial risk factors of HIV morbidity and mortality: findings from the Multicenter AIDS Cohort Study (MACS). J Clin Exp Neuropsychol 2003; 25: 654–670.

Fields RD. Neuroscience. Change in the brain's white matter. Science 2010; 330: 768–769.

Filley CM. *The behavioral neurology of white matter*. 2nd ed. New York: Oxford University Press, 2012.

Filley CM, Cullum CM. Education and cognitive function in Alzheimer's disease. Neuropsychiatry Neuropsychol Behav Neurol 1997; 10: 48–51.

Filley CM, Kleinschmidt-DeMasters BK. Toxic leukoencephalopathy. N Engl J Med. 2001; 345: 425–432.

Filley CM, Halliday W, Kleinschmidt-DeMasters BK. The effects of toluene on the central nervous system. J Neuropathol Exp Neurol 2004; 63: 1–12.

Filley CM, Kozora E, Brown MS, et al. White matter microstructure and cognition in non-neuropsychiatric systemic lupus erythematosus. Cogn Behav Neurol 2009; 22: 38–44.

Gouw AA, Seewann A, van der Flier WM, et al. Heterogeneity of small vessel disease: a systematic review of MRI and histopathology correlations. J Neurol Neurosurg Psychiatry 2011; 82: 126–135.

Greenough WT, Bailey CH. The anatomy of a memory: convergence of results across a diversity of tests. Trends Neurosci 1988; 11: 142–147.

Henninger N, Izzy S, Carandang R, et al. Severe leukoaraiosis portends a poor outcome after traumatic brain injury. Neurocrit Care 2014; 21: 483–495.

Herting MM, Colby JB, Sowell ER, Nagel BJ. White matter connectivity and aerobic fitness in male adolescents. Dev Cogn Neurosci 2014; 7: 65–75.

Hofstetter S, Tavor I, Tzur Moryosef S, Assaf Y. Short-term learning induces white matter plasticity in the fornix. J Neurosci 2013; 33: 12844–12850.

Johansson BB. Current trends in stroke rehabilitation: a review with focus on brain plasticity. Acta Neurol Scand 2011; 123: 147–159.

Katzman R, Terry R, DeTeresa R, et al. Clinical, pathological, and neurochemical changes in dementia: a subgroup with preserved mental status and numerous neocortical plaques. Ann Neurol 1988; 23: 138–144.

Kesler SR, Adams HF, Blasey CM, et al. Premorbid intellectual functioning, education, and brain size in traumatic brain injury: an investigation of the cognitive reserve hypothesis. Appl Neuropsychol 2003; 10: 153–162.

Kozora E, Hanly JG, Lapteva L, Filley CM. Cognitive dysfunction in systemic lupus erythematosus: past, present, and future. Arthritis Rheum 2008; 58: 3286–3298.

Kozora E, Filley CM. Cognitive dysfunction and white matter abnormalities in systemic lupus erythematosus. J Int Neuropsychol Soc 2011; 17: 1–8.

Langdon DW. Cognition in multiple sclerosis. Curr Opin Neurol 2011; 24: 244–249.

Li P, Legault J, Litcofsky KA. Neuroplasticity as a function of second language learning: anatomical changes in the human brain. Cortex 2014; 58: 301–324.

Luk G, Bialystok E, Craik FI, Grady CL. Lifelong bilingualism maintains white matter integrity in older adults. J Neurosci 2011; 31: 16808–16813.

Majewska AK, Sur M. Plasticity and specificity of cortical processing networks. Trends Neurosci 2006; 29: 323–329.

Medana IM, Esiri MM. Axonal damage: a key predictor of outcome in human CNS diseases. Brain 2003; 26: 515–530.

Miles L, DeGrauw TJ, Dinopoulos A, et al. Megalencephalic leukoencephalopathy with subcortical cysts: a third confirmed case with literature review. Pediatr Dev Pathol 2009; 12: 180–186.

Moore E, Schaefer RS, Bastin ME, et al. Can musical training influence brain connectivity? Evidence from diffusion tensor MRI. Brain Sci 2014; 4: 405–427.

Nitkunan A, Charlton RA, McIntyre DJ, et al. Diffusion tensor imaging and MR spectroscopy in hypertension and presumed cerebral small vessel disease. Magn Reson Med 2008; 59: 528–534.

Orchard PJ, Tolar J. Transplant outcomes in leukodystrophies. Semin Hematol 2010; 47: 70–78.

Petrosini L, De Bartolo P, Foti F, et al. On whether the environmental enrichment may provide cognitive and brain reserves. Brain Res Rev 2009; 61: 221–239.

Rimkus C de M, Andrade CS, Leite C da C, et al. Toxic leukoencephalopathies, including drug, medication, environmental, and radiation-induced encephalopathic syndromes. Semin Ultrasound CT MR 2014; 35: 97–117.

Satz P. Brain reserve capacity on symptom onset after brain injury: a formulation and review of evidence for threshold theory. Neuropsychology 1993; 7: 273–295.

Schlaug G, Marchina S, Norton A. Evidence for plasticity in white-matter tracts of patients with chronic Broca's aphasia undergoing intense intonation-based speech therapy. Ann N Y Acad Sci 2009; 1169: 385–394.

Schofield PW, Logroscino G, Andrews HF, et al. An association between head circumference and Alzheimer's disease in a population-based study of aging and dementia. Neurology 1997; 49: 30–37.

Sharma N, Classen J, Cohen LG. Neural plasticity and its contribution to functional recovery. Handb Clin Neurol 2013; 110: 3–12.

Sibbitt WL Jr, Brooks WM, Kornfeld M, et al. Magnetic resonance imaging and brain histopathology in neuropsychiatric systemic lupus erythematosus. Semin Arthritis Rheum 2010; 40: 32–52.

Simon JH. MRI outcomes in the diagnosis and disease course of multiple sclerosis. Handb Clin Neurol 2014; 122: 405–425.

Smith DH, Meaney DF, Shull WH. Diffuse axonal injury in head trauma. J Head Trauma Rehabil 2003; 18: 307–316.

Stern Y. What is cognitive reserve? Theory and research application of the reserve concept. J Int Neuropsychol Soc 2002; 8: 448–460.

Stern Y. Cognitive reserve. Neuropsychologia 2009; 47: 2015–2028.

Stern Y. Cognitive reserve in ageing and Alzheimer's disease. Lancet Neurol 2012; 11: 1006–1012.

Sumowski JF, Chiaravalloti N, DeLuca J. Cognitive reserve protects against cognitive dysfunction in multiple sclerosis. J Clin Exp Neuropsychol 2009; 31: 913–926.

Sumowski JF, Wylie GR, Deluca J, Chiaravalloti N. Intellectual enrichment is linked to cerebral efficiency in multiple sclerosis: functional magnetic resonance imaging evidence for cognitive reserve. Brain 2010; 133: 362–374.

Sumowski JF, Rocca MA, Leavitt VM, et al. Brain reserve and cognitive reserve protect against cognitive decline over 4.5 years in MS. Neurology 2014; 82: 1776–1783.

Symonds CP. Mental disorder following head injury (Section of Psychiatry). Proc R Soc Med 1937; 30: 1081–1094.

Trapp BD, Peterson J, Ransohoff RM, et al. Axonal transection in the lesions of multiple sclerosis. N Engl J Med 1998; 338: 278–285.

Tseng BY, Gundapuneedi T, Khan MA, et al. White matter integrity in physically fit older adults. Neuroimage 2013; 82: 510–516.

Tullberg M, Ziegelitz D, Ribbelin S, Ekholm S. White matter diffusion is higher in Binswanger Disease than in idiopathic normal pressure hydrocephalus. Acta Neurol Scand 2009; 120: 226–234.

Wake H, Lee PR, Fields RD. Control of local protein synthesis and initial events in myelination by action potentials. Science 2011; 333: 1647–1651.

Ward NS, Frackowiak RS. Towards a new mapping of brain cortex function. Cerebrovasc Dis 2004; 17 Suppl 3: 35–38.

Zatorre RJ, Fields RD, Johansen-Berg H. Plasticity in gray and white: neuroimaging changes in brain structure during learning. Nat Neurosci 2012; 15: 528–536.

Zhang M, Katzman R, Salmon D, et al. The prevalence of dementia and Alzheimer's disease in Shanghai, China: impact of age, gender and education. Ann Neurol 1990; 27: 428–437.

Chapter 11

Treatment

The treatment of white matter dementia (WMD) and mild cognitive dysfunction (MCD) centers on the treatment of the underlying disorder deemed responsible for the syndrome. As such, this topic is well covered in general textbooks of neurology and internal medicine, and specific regimens will not be considered here. In clinical practice, each patient will of course require his or her individual attention, and medical, surgical, rehabilitative, and psychiatric interventions may all be considered. The goal of this chapter will be to pursue selected aspects of treatment that are relevant to WMD and MCD by virtue of their capacity to effect specific improvements in cognitive function. That is, whereas textbooks and reviews detailing standard treatment of white matter disorders are intended to address the clinical features broadly considered, the following account will take up what is known of how these treatments actually impact cognition.

A more intriguing question for the purposes of this book, and one much more difficult to answer, concerns the determination of whether these treatments exert their beneficial effects via an influence on the macroscopic or microscopic structure of white matter tracts. This critical question has been studied only infrequently, as it necessarily entails the acquisition of neuroimaging data as a component of treatment outcome, but some information is available. Table 11.1 lists the disorders in which some evidence for a beneficial therapeutic effect on white matter has been found.

Table 11.1 White matter disorders with preliminary evidence that treatment improves cognitive dysfunction by an effect on white matter

Disorder	Treatment
Multiple sclerosis	Immunomodulatory agents
Systemic lupus erythematosus	Immunosuppressive drugs
Human immunodeficiency virus infection	Antiretroviral therapy
Cobalamin deficiency	Vitamin B_{12} replacement
Normal pressure hydrocephalus	Shunt insertion
Metachromatic leukodystrophy	Stem cell transplantation

Medical

Medical treatment of white matter disorders is the area of therapy most commonly employed with patients with WMD or MCD. At least until other modalities become available, some of which will be considered in Chapter 13, most of the available treatments for these patients will involve pharmacotherapy as well as other noninvasive modalities.

In the vascular category, the primary approach remains preventive, and a considerable portion of the neurologist's daily work is dedicated to primary and secondary stroke prevention (Grossman and Broderick, 2013). While these efforts often prove effective, less can be expected once the damage is done and dementia has set in. However, medical therapy with the cholinesterase inhibitors and memantine has been studied to a considerable extent in vascular dementia and vascular cognitive impairment (Demaerschalk and Wingerchuk, 2007). Among these agents, the most evidence exists for the cholinesterase inhibitors, providing some basis for the treatment of patients with ischemic white matter disease. Autopsy studies of patients with Binswanger's Disease (BD) have shown damage to ascending cholinergic neurons similar to that seen in Alzheimer's Disease (AD) (Tomimoto et al., 2005), helping justify efforts to treat dementia in BD with drugs such as donepezil and galantamine. No study of this kind of treatment in BD as a well-defined entity has appeared, and while the use of donepezil in vascular dementia (Román et al., 2010) and galantamine in vascular cognitive impairment (Birks and Craig, 2006) has some experimental support, whether white matter dysfunction is specifically addressed by these medications remains conjectural.

Toxic leukoencephalopathy is by definition a disorder caused by exogenous white matter toxins, and an increasing number of leukotoxic agents have been identified by clinical observation combined with magnetic resonance imaging (MRI) (Filley and Kleinschmidt-DeMasters, 2001; Rimkus et al., 2014). Removal of the toxin and appropriate supportive care can often lead to partial or complete recovery (Rimkus et al., 2014), implying that many of these disorders involve myelin injury but preservation of axons. The clinical recovery is often evident in parallel with steady resolution of neuroimaging changes (Rimkus et al., 2014). With the increasing recognition of toxic leukoencephalopathy as MRI is more widely used, attention has been called to the syndrome of acute toxic leukoencephalopathy, and the treatment of this disorder is generally thought to be more successful than that of more chronic forms of intoxication (Rimkus et al., 2014). Dementia from long-standing toluene abuse, for example, may be irreversible, as will be considered further later.

Medical therapy has also been investigated for individuals with traumatic brain injury (TBI), in whom white matter is damaged by diffuse axonal injury (DAI). As discussed later, the first line treatment for cognitive impairment after TBI is considered to be rehabilitative, and, in general, the use of medications is regarded as adjunctive (Arciniegas, Wortzel, and Frey, 2013). However, several medications may find utility in selected cases (Wortzel and Arciniegas, 2012). The best-studied agents that can be considered in TBI are amantadine, methylphenidate, bromocriptine, donepezil, and rivastigmine (Wortzel and Arciniegas, 2012). Amantadine has been found to improve cognitive recovery in patients with severe TBI (Meythaler et al., 2002), and was recently found effective in hastening functional recovery in patients with TBI of sufficient severity to produce the vegetative or minimally conscious state (Giacino et al., 2012). Methylphenidate was observed in several studies of adult and childhood TBI patients to be helpful for memory and attentional problems, although larger studies are needed (Siddall, 2005). Bromocriptine has been found efficacious for executive dysfunction following mild to severe TBI (McDowell, Whyte, and D'Esposito, 1998). The cholinesterase inhibitors donepezil (Zhang et al., 2004) and rivastigmine (Tenovuo, Alin, and Helenius, 2009) have been observed in some studies to improve attention and memory after TBI. All of these treatments are based on augmentation of neurotransmitter systems – principally dopaminergic or cholinergic – and it is of interest that DAI is associated with a reduction in dopamine turnover in the brain (Meythaler et al., 2002) and has also been implicated in the pathogenesis of cholinergic dysfunction after TBI (Arciniegas et al., 1999). Further study is warranted on whether the cognitive benefit of these medications observed after TBI signifies a specific effect on damaged white matter and, if so, what fiber systems are involved.

Perhaps the most thoroughly studied white matter disorder – with the necessary caveat that gray matter is also involved to a variable extent – is multiple sclerosis (MS). Among many questions in MS is whether immunosuppressive and immunomodulatory treatment in MS can effect cognitive improvement (Tumani and Uttner, 2007). Treatment of cognitive dysfunction in MS has been explored in recent years, as it has been recognized that cognitive dysfunction is a major source of disability, and some treatment trials have included cognitive measures among the study outcomes. For acute exacerbations, corticosteroids remain the mainstay of conventional treatment, and it is plausible, although not established, that cognitive decline in the context of an acute exacerbation responds to this intervention.

More pertinent for this account is the use of immunomodulatory drugs, four of which – interferon β-1-a, interferon β-1-b, glatiramer, and natalizumab – have assumed a prominent position in MS therapeutics. The rationale for these drugs in relapsing-remitting MS is persuasive: This form of the disease, if untreated, can be associated with progressive brain atrophy (Simon, 1999), and treatment can reduce relapse rate as well as lessen MRI white matter disease burden (Rudick et al., 1997). An early study of interferon β-1-b in MS did find improvement in a visual reproduction test after 4 years of therapy (Pliskin et al., 1996), while the use of glatiramer in MS patients did not affect cognitive function compared to those treated with a placebo (Weinstein et al., 1999). A comprehensive study of this kind was a prospective placebo-controlled trial of interferon β-1-a in MS that showed significant benefit in information processing, memory, visuospatial ability, and executive function (Fischer et al., 2000). More recently, an open-label study of natalizumab in MS showed promise for improving both cognition and mood (Lang, Reiss, and Mäurer, 2012). One important implication of these studies is that they may justify the use of immunomodulatory drugs in MS for cognitive dysfunction alone. Therapy with these agents could thus plausibly improve or stabilize cognitive function because of a disease-modifying effect.

Post-marketing studies of four standard immunomodulatory drugs have revealed evidence of a positive effect on MS cognition (Comi, 2010). Despite the need for more study, these agents are generally thought to show promise for improving cognition by reducing the accumulation of white matter lesions and brain atrophy (Comi, 2010). Inclusion of cognitive measures in future clinical trials has been advocated (Comi, 2010), and an underappreciated benefit of immunomodulatory drugs in MS may be a positive effect on cognitive dysfunction.

Another intriguing possibility for the pharmacological treatment of cognitive loss in MS is 4-aminopyridine, a potent inhibitor of voltage-gated potassium channels that improves impulse conduction through demyelinative lesions and is now used to treat gait disorder (Jensen et al., 2014). Whereas evidence for an improvement in cognition has thus far not appeared, there is ample rationale for presuming a benefit might be found (Jensen et al., 2014).

In the inflammatory disorders, preliminary evidence for the cognitive benefit of treating white matter dysfunction can be found in the literature. The treatment of cognitive impairment in these diseases remains empirical, with corticosteroids the mainstay of therapy, and provocative clues can be found regarding the idea that treatment directed against white matter disease could be effective. In systemic lupus erythematosus (SLE), evidence that inflammatory microstructural involvement is related to MCD (Filley et al., 2009; Kozora et al., 2013) raises the possibility that anti-inflammatory therapy may address this form of neuropathology early in the disease. Consistent with this idea, a volumetric MRI study of early SLE patients showed that those who received immunosuppressive medications had greater white matter volume in several brain regions (Xu et al., 2010). While cognitive evaluation showed no association of white matter volumes with cognition, the only measure used was the Mini-Mental State Examination (MMSE; Folstein, Folstein, and McHugh, 1975), and more sensitive cognitive assessment might be more revealing. The data from this study (Xu et al., 2010) thus imply that the putative inflammatory myelinopathy of early SLE (Filley et al., 2009) may be a target of immunosuppressive treatment, and that MCD or WMD could be addressed with this approach. In this regard, a recent case report found that a young woman with neuropsychiatric SLE who was treated with corticosteroids and azathioprine improved her MMSE (Folstein, Folstein, and McHugh, 1975) score from 16 to 30 while diffusion tensor imaging (DTI) demonstrated higher fractional anisotropy (FA) of the corpus callosum (Lee et al., 2014).

In the infectious category, investigation of white matter changes associated with human immunodeficiency virus (HIV) infection has been pursued since the first reports of dementia related to the acquired immunodeficiency syndrome (AIDS) in the 1980s (Navia, Jordan, and Price, 1986; Navia et al., 1986). White matter changes were noted to be prominent both on neuroimaging and at postmortem in the AIDS dementia complex (ADC), now known as HIV-associated dementia (HAD), and whereas other regions such as the basal ganglia also sustain damage from HIV infection, initial reports supported the idea that improvement in cognition with antiretroviral therapy may relate to restoration of normal white matter. One of the first studies to show this effect was that of Tozzi and colleagues (1993), which found improvement of MRI white matter burden and on cognition as measured by the Wisconsin Card Sorting Test in some ADC patients treated with zidovudine. Soon therafter, protease inhibitors were found to have a similar effect on cognition in HIV patients (Filippi et al., 1998). Highly active antiretroviral therapy also proved helpful for both cognition and white matter lesions in ADC (Thurnher et al., 2000).

However, a cure for dementia in AIDS has not been found, and white matter injury has been shown to continue even among HIV patients receiving antiretroviral treatment (Cardenas et al., 2009). Indeed, while gains have undeniably been made in enhancing longevity and quality of life, the main impact of antiretroviral therapy seems to have been prevention of HIV complications such as opportunistic infections and neoplasms, and both white and gray matter injury continues to impair cognition even as patients rarely progress to dementia (Gongvatana et al., 2013). Data now suggest that HIV exerts damage to many brain regions through a complex pathogenesis, but the role of white matter injury continues to merit attention. An instructive recent case report documented that, in an HIV patient with HAD who was on antiretroviral therapy and had extensive MRI white matter hyperintensity, the dementia was completely reversed within 2 months of the addition of zidovudine to the treatment regimen, in concert with dramatic improvement of the MRI white matter changes (Hoogland and Portegies, 2014).

A disorder of white matter for which evidence of reversible leukoencephalopathy has often been presented is cobalamin deficiency. Several case studies using MRI have supported this claim, noting that clinical and neuroradiological improvement of leukoencephalopathy may occur in parallel with cobalamin replacement (Chatterjee et al., 1996; Stojsavljević et al., 1997; Su et al., 2000; Graber et al., 2010). Most cases of cobalamin deficiency are related to insufficient dietary vitamin B_{12}, but genetic causes are also recognized, and these too have been observed to respond to cobalamin replacement (Biotti et al., 2014). Recent findings from community-based studies that vitamin B_{12} supplementation can decrease the conversion from mild cognitive impairment to dementia while simultaneously reducing MRI white matter lesion burden (Blasko et al., 2012) offer solid support for the classification of cobalamin deficiency as a WMD. Although questions remain about the pathophysiological relationship between leukoencephalopathy and deficiency of this vitamin (Stabler, 2013), very low levels of cobalamin are associated with WMD, reversibility of cognitive and neuroimaging abnormalities can be seen with B_{12} treatment, and routine use of cobalamin appears to help prevent both dementia and white matter lesions.

Brain neoplasia has been little studied with respect to whether treatment can bring about cognitive improvement because of an effect on white matter involvement, but a report of patients with lymphomatosis cerebri is instructive (Deutsch and Mendez, 2015). In this series, among 6 of the 12 patients who had cognitive assessment, treatment with regimens including corticosteroids, radiation, and chemotherapy produced cognitive improvement (Deutsch and Mendez, 2015). In a study of patients with recurrent glioblastoma multiforme, the anti-angiogenic drug bevacizumab was found to reduce the volume of abnormal fluid-attenuated inversion recovery (FLAIR) signal and the volume of contrast enhancement (Ellingson et al., 2011), implying that chemotherapy may reduce white matter disease burden. These reports suggest that investigation is warranted in the assessment of the extent to which treatment of brain neoplasia may improve cognition in conjunction with regression of white matter disease.

Hydrocephalus is traditionally considered a surgical condition (see next section), but pharmacotherapy may have a role in certain cases. In a small study of patients with normal pressure hydrocephalus (NPH), the carbonic anhydrase inhibitor acetazolamide was recently shown to significantly reduce the volume of periventricular white matter hyperintensities and, in some patients, improve gait (Alperin et al., 2014). Given that acetazolamide acts by reducing the formation of cerebrospinal fluid (CSF) from the choroid plexi, it may be that the periventricular lesions of NPH can be reversed by a reduction in CSF volume. NPH remains a vexing disease with many unanswered dilemmas to be resolved, but evidence is mounting that the cognitive dysfunction that develops and sometimes can be improved may originate in damage to periventricular white matter (Akai et al., 1987; Del Bigio, 1993; Del Bigio et al., 1994; Leinonen et al., 2012). Acetazolamide has also been used successfully to control progressive hydrocephalus in a preterm infant with intraventricular hemorrhage (Miner, 1986).

The genetic white matter disorders have proven very difficult to treat, and early demise is still the unfortunate expectation in many individuals, most of whom are infants or children. The leukodystrophies have attracted the most interest in terms of treatment, as the possibility of hematopoietic stem cell transplantation (HSCT) became available in recent decades (Krivit, Peters, and Shapiro, 1999). This procedure remains the most promising therapeutic approach to these diseases. Currently, the use of HSCT is thought to be appropriate for individuals early in the course of metachromatic leukodystrophy (MLD), adrenoleukodystrophy, and Krabbe's Disease, and referral to a specialized clinical research center is recommended (Vanderver et al., 2014). Results of this procedure have often been disappointing because the treated patients had disease that was too far advanced for the restored enzyme activity to be effective (Biffi et al., 2008; Orchard and Tolar, 2010). The efficacy of prompt treatment, however, was recently shown in a 5-year-old girl with MLD in whom early treatment with HSCT led to stable cognitive function and normal school performance at age 15 (Krägeloh-Mann et al., 2013). Of special interest in this case, MRI white matter lesions regressed over 10 years, while on magnetic resonance spectroscopy (MRS), choline declined and N-acetyl aspartate (NAA) increased (Krägeloh-Mann et al., 2013). Thus both macrostructural and microstructural markers of leukodystrophy improved as cognition stabilized, implying that the direct treatment of the white matter disease enhanced cognitive function.

Most recently, a small controlled study of young adults with MLD showed that HSCT led to sustained neuropsychological and MRI stability, suggesting that adults with this disease may also benefit from this treatment modality (Solders et al., 2014). While the small numbers of patients in these reports highlight the need for more investigation, these studies offer support both for the early treatment of MLD and related disorders and for the restoration of white matter as important for normal cognition.

Surgical

In everyday neurologic practice, the surgical treatment of WMD and MCD is currently limited to patients with hydrocephalus, and the problem of NPH in older people brings up this issue in all its complexity. The selection of patients who may have NPH and could benefit from surgical insertion of a diversionary shunt is fraught with uncertainties (Graff-Radford, 2007; Wilson and Williams, 2010). Many patients, for example, are referred for neurologic evaluation on the basis of MRI scans that have been read as suggestive of possible NPH, when in fact the clinical picture is not consistent with this diagnosis. Moreover, whereas favorable shunting response rates exceeding 50% have been reported (Gustafson and Hagberg, 1978), further study has suggested that the gait disorder responds better to shunting than does the dementia, and that improvement in many patients may not be sustained (Klassen and Ahlskog, 2011). However, clinicians recognize that meaningful clinical improvement can occur in this disease with surgical treatment, and NPH remains an important concern in clinical neurology. As reviewed in Chapter 6, the neuropathology of hydrocephalus is characterized by a predominance of injury in the periventricular white matter (Akai et al., 1987; Del Bigio, 1993; Del Bigio et al., 1994; Leinonen et al., 2012). In NPH, this injury may be accompanied by cortical changes of AD, the white matter lesions of BD, or both, complicating not only patient selection but the assessment of shunt response. However, some studies have demonstrated that NPH patients who respond to shunting have reduced white matter disease burden that correlates with improved cognition (Tullberg et al., 2002; Akiguchi et al., 2008). In the study of Akiguchi and colleagues, shunted NPH patients who had reductions of white matter lesion ratings also had improved scores on cognitive measures, including the MMSE (Folstein, Folstein, and McHugh, 1975), the Frontal Assessment Battery (Dubois et al., 2000), and Form A of the Trail Making Test (Ehrenstein, Heister, and Cohen, 1982).

Other potential surgical avenues include applications of gene therapy (Leone et al., 2000) and stem cell therapeutics (Goldman, 2007; Tran, Ho, and Jandial, 2010). While these appear to have some promise, much more fundamental research is needed before modalities involving this kind of intervention can be routinely applied to brain white matter disorders. This topic will be further explored in Chapter 13.

Any enthusiasm for the surgical treatment of WMD, however, should be viewed in light of experience gained from the era of surgery for psychiatric illness in the mid-twentieth century (Anderson and Arciniegas, 2004). Before the introduction of major tranquilizers beginning with chlorpromazine in the 1950s, severe forms of schizophrenia and other psychiatric diseases were often treated with psychosurgical procedures that mainly targeted the frontal lobe white matter. In general, the idea motivating these procedures was that psychosis originated in the frontal lobes, and disconnecting these regions from other brain areas by lobotomy or leucotomy could reduce the severity of psychotic ideation. Whereas some patients may have had amelioration of severe psychosis by these procedures, many were not helped or were clearly worsened, and the operations were typically performed in a shockingly inappropriate – even barbaric – manner (Anderson and Arciniegas, 2004). Moreover, a paucity of useful information was gathered on long-term outcome because of little attention to proper follow-up and data acquisition.

The surgical targeting of white matter is thus burdened by a tarnished history in the recent past, and any approach of this kind must be undertaken with the utmost care and strictest adherence to ethical guidelines. Psychosurgery does appear to have a role in the treatment of selected, intractable neuropsychiatric conditions (Anderson and Arciniegas, 2004), but it is difficult at present to envision a scenario in which a patient with dementia – related to white matter or any neuropathology – could be helped by such intervention. Surgical options for the treatment of WMD (existing and theoretical) are not intended to involve the ablation of tracts, but rather their protection or restoration.

Rehabilitative

The rehabilitation of neurobehavioral disorders generally falls under the heading of cognitive rehabilitation, also known as cognitive neurorehabilitation (Stuss, Winocur, and Robertson, 2008). Much uncertainty has surrounded this field since its inception, with abundant enthusiasm unmatched by solid data supporting efficacy, and often considerable cost. Indeed, many patients are drawn to this form of treatment by overly optimistic predictions of successful recovery. Recent evidence, however, has offered more compelling support for this type of intervention. Most of the work has been done on TBI and stroke, and in selected patients cognitive rehabilitation has been shown effective for the remediation of attention, memory, executive function, social cognition, aphasia, apraxia, and visuospatial skills (Cicerone et al., 2011). Cognitive rehabilitation typically involves a variety of individual, group, and computer-based sessions targeted to specific cognitive deficits, and the goal is to produce improvement on therapeutic measures and achieve real-world functional gains (Arciniegas, Wortzel, and Frey, 2013).

Cognitive rehabilitation targeted specifically to individuals with WMD and MCD has not been formally addressed. One inherent advantage of attempting to treat cognitive impairments in white matter disorders is that treatment does not encounter the major obstacle of many gray matter diseases in which neurodegeneration produces inexorable loss of neurons and synapses. Static, relapsing, or slowly progressive deficits are more typical of white matter disorders, and thus the opportunity for substantial restoration of white matter tracts is not illusory. Very little is known about whether the repair of damaged white matter tracts relevant to neurobehavioral competence can be enhanced by cognitive rehabilitation, but the question is an important one given the substantial morbidity produced by white matter disorders.

One of the appealing possibilities in this area is the exploitation of new understanding regarding the response of cerebral white matter to neuropathological insult. As discussed in Chapter 10, evidence has been presented that white matter may be reparable by intrinsic plasticity that can remyelinate axonal segments through activity-dependent myelination (Wake, Lee, and Fields, 2011). One of the mechanisms by which this phenomenon is thought to occur is via glutamatergic transmission at axo-oligodendroglial synapses, present within white matter, which leads to increased production of myelin basic protein and enhanced myelination of the distal axon. In essence, the greater the electrical activity through a given tract, the more extensive will be its myelination. If this process is found to be sufficiently common and widespread after neuropathological insult, a rationale could be established for procedures intended to engage and stimulate the brain's natural recovery system for the restoration of normal myelination and axonal function.

Studies in normal adults are beginning to shed light on the possibility of white matter repair as a result of behavioral interventions (Wang and Young, 2014). Box 11.1 lists some methods by which aspects of white matter structure have been suggested to be modifiable by environmental influences (Wang and Young, 2014). These methods will be familiar from the section on plasticity in Chapter 10, in which activities such as playing a musical instrument or speaking two languages were presented as capable of altering the structure of white matter. Such interventions have yet to be studied in the setting of rehabilitation after white matter pathology has been sustained, but they offer an intriguing new way to think about how brain repair might be accomplished, complementing emerging knowledge more relevant to gray matter such as synaptic plasticity and neurogenesis (Wang and Young, 2014).

Some of the more provocative investigations will serve to illustrate this work. Takeuchi and colleagues (2010) used DTI to show that young adults who

BOX 11.1 Behavioral interventions with the potential to alter white matter structure

- Playing a keyboard instrument
- Playing a string instrument
- Musical training
- Learning another language
- Working memory training
- Reasoning training
- Interactive mind–body training

received training in working memory had higher FA in the parietal white matter and the corpus callosum. A DTI study of students who took a course to prepare for the Law School Admissions Test showed that reasoning training resulted in decreased radial diffusivity in the frontoparietal white matter (Mackey, Whitaker, and Bunge, 2012). Another DTI study explored the alternative approach of mindfulness meditation, and in normal subjects who received a 4-week course of integrative mind–body training (IMBT), FA increased in the anterior cingulate region (Tang, Lu, and Fan, 2012). Such nonpharmacological interventions may thus find a place in the rehabilitation of patients who harbor damaged white matter.

Finally, an emerging area of therapeutics that can be classified as rehabilitative involves the use of external brain stimulation. This idea is again based on the notion of white matter plasticity, and the two most commonly used techniques, repetitive transcranial magnetic stimulation (rTMS) and transcranial direct current stimulation (tDCS), have most often been applied to the rehabilitation of motor function in stroke patients (Johansson, 2011). Investigators have also begun studying cognitive dysfunction, however, and rTMS, in particular, has been explored for the treatment of vascular dementia (Pennisi et al., 2011). While no clear indications for rTMS have been established, one study of nondemented patients with extensive leukoaraiosis did show that rTMS applied to the left dorsolateral prefrontal area resulted in improved executive function (Rektorova et al., 2005). The mechanism of this effect, if confirmed, is unclear, but one possibility is enhanced electrical conduction along white matter tracts. A study of tDCS in stroke patients documented improved white matter structure in parallel with functional motor improvement, and one possible mechanism was considered to be enhanced myelination (Zheng and Schlaug, 2015).

Psychiatric

In general, psychiatric treatment has for many years been based on behavioral and somatic therapies, either individually or in combination (Taber, Hurley, and Yudofsky, 2010). Behavioral therapy involves traditional psychotherapy, and more recently a variety of psychosocial interventions, the most promising of which appears to be cognitive-behavioral therapy (CBT), while somatic therapies rely mainly on medications (antidepressants, antipsychotics, benzodiazepines, anticonvulsants, stimulants, etc.) and rarely electroconvulsive therapy (Taber, Hurley, and Yudofsky, 2010). Whereas these modalities are of course widely employed for psychiatric and neurologic disorders with many underlying pathologies, their use in white matter disorders involving vascular compromise, trauma, and demyelination is well established (Taber, Hurley, and Yudofsky, 2010). Adherence to evidence-based medicine in all of these scenarios has been emphasized (Taber, Hurley, and Yudofsky, 2010), and with the increasing implementation of MRI in diagnosis and outcome assessment, steady improvements in psychiatric treatment can be expected for patients with many varieties of white matter disorder.

A major role of psychiatric treatment in WMD and MCD is in the area of drug addiction, as toxic leukoencephalopathy is an important sequel of the abuse of many drugs (Filley and Kleinschmidt-DeMasters, 2001; Rimkus et al., 2014). As there is no means yet known to foster the restitution of white matter after leukotoxic injury, prevention of further injury by addressing the primary addictive behavior is an important component of treatment. Although the extent to which white matter can recover with abstinence from leukotoxins is as yet unclear, some indications offer the hope that recovery can occur under certain circumstances. Inhalant abuse will serve as the prototype for this discussion.

Inhalant abuse is a largely unrecognized but distressingly prevalent form of substance abuse (Howard et al., 2011). Whereas exact figures are not available, it has been estimated that 9% of the United States population has tried an inhalant, and that as many as 50% of those who have done so are at risk for addiction (Howard et al., 2011). A frequently abused volatile substance, and the best-studied inhalant in terms of neurotoxicity, is toluene (methylbenzene), an organic hydrocarbon found in spray paint, glue, and other abusable substances (Filley, 2013). Long-term exposure to toluene is well known to cause WMD, as reviewed in Chapter 7. Treatment programs are rare in the United States (Howard et al., 2011), and the utility of intervention is not known. Highlighting the challenges posed by this problem, a study assessing treatment of inhalant-abusing boys found antisocial traits to be common both before and after 2 years of treatment (Sakai, Mikulich-Gilbertson, and Crowley, 2006).

However, if treatment can be instituted and abstinence achieved, it is possible that recovery of injured white matter may occur in some patients. A recent prospective study of Aboriginal inhalant abusers from Australia found complete recovery after 15 years of abstinence, although this group inhaled gasoline fumes and was not specifically exposed to toluene (Cairney et al., 2013). The outcome of toluene leukoencephalopathy after abstinence is not well understood. In the pre-MRI era, an optometrist developed cognitive dysfunction after inadvertent exposure to toluene and recovered completely once the exposure was recognized and stopped (Boor and Hurtig, 1977), and later a chemical salesman with accidental toluene exposure had complete cognitive recovery and substantial MRI improvement after toxin removal (Qureshi et al., 2009). More chronic exposure, unfortunately, may not permit such a good outcome, as an 18-month follow-up study of abstinent inhalant abusers disclosed clinical improvement in only 1 of 11 patients (Rosenberg et al., 1988).

Innovations in the treatment of major psychiatric diseases offer additional insights that may be relevant to the concepts of WMD and MCD. One such disease is depression, and a surgical procedure has attracted much interest. From a series of remarkable observations, the use of deep brain stimulation (DBS) has been demonstrated to be effective for intractable depression when applied to the subgenual cingulate white matter (Mayberg et al., 2005). The mechanism of action of DBS in depression is thought to involve modulation of activity within a network of frontal-limbic regions subserving mood regulation, and studies are underway to define the critical tracts mediating successful treatment (Riva-Posse et al., 2014). Whereas depression is not ordinarily considered a cognitive disorder, the presence of cognitive impairment in this illness might also prove to be amenable to the use of DBS.

In schizophrenia, another psychiatric disease in which cognition is often impaired, interesting data have appeared on the possible salutary effect of antipsychotic medication on white matter. An MRI study conducted among individuals with first-episode schizophrenia found that risperidone increased the volume of intracortical myelin in the frontal lobes, suggesting that dopamine receptor blockade with this drug, and possibly other antipsychotics, may promote brain myelination (Bartzokis et al., 2012). Schizophrenia is thought to be associated with a hyperdopaminergic state before the onset of psychosis, and dopamine activates glycogen synthase kinase-3 beta (GSK3β), an enzyme that retards brain myelination; it may be, therefore, that dopamine blockade enhances brain myelination (Bartzokis et al., 2012). The exact role of intracortical myelin in cognition – whether in schizophrenia or in any other clinical setting – is unknown, but the improvement in schizophrenia outcome that can be produced by risperidone (Keith, 2009) suggests that certain psychiatric treatments may exert beneficial effects on white matter that could address cognitive dysfunction. Support for this proposal comes from work on another atypical antipsychotic agent, quetiapine, which has been suggested as a potential treatment for MS based on preclinical observations that it has remyelinating and neuroprotective properties (Zhornitsky et al., 2013).

References

Akai K, Uchigasaki S, Tanaka U, Komatsu A. Normal pressure hydrocephalus: neuropathological study. Acta Pathol Jpn 1987; 37: 97–110.

Akiguchi I, Ishii M, Watanabe Y, et al. Shunt-responsive parkinsonism and reversible white matter lesions in patients with idiopathic NPH. J Neurol 2008; 255: 1392–1399.

Alperin N, Oliu CJ, Bagci AM, et al. Low-dose acetazolamide reverses periventricular white matter hyperintensities in NPH. Neurology 2014; 82: 1347–1351.

Anderson CA, Arciniegas DB. Neurosurgical interventions for neuropsychiatric syndromes. Curr Psychiatry Rep 2004; 6: 355–363.

Arciniegas D, Adler L, Topkoff J, et al. Attention and memory dysfunction after traumatic brain injury: cholinergic mechanisms, sensory gating, and a hypothesis for further investigation. Brain Inj 1999; 13: 1–13.

Arciniegas DB, Wortzel HS, Frey K. Rehabilitation and pharmacoptherapy of cognitive impairments. In: Arciniegas DB, Anderson CA, Filley CM, eds. *Behavioral neurology & neurospychiatry*. Cambridge: Cambridge University Press, 2013: 511–542.

Bartzokis G, Lu PH, Raven EP, et al. Impact on intracortical myelination trajectory of long acting injection versus oral risperidone in first-episode schizophrenia. Schizophr Res 2012; 140: 122–128.

Biffi A, Lucchini G, Rovelli A, Sessa M. Metachromatic leukodystrophy: an overview of current and prospective treatments. Bone Marrow Transplant 2008; 42 Suppl 2: S2–S6.

Biotti D, Esteban-Mader M, Diot E, et al. Clinical reasoning: a young woman with rapid mental deterioration and leukoencephalopathy. Neurology 2014; 83: e182–e186.

Birks J, Craig D. Galantamine for vascular cognitive impairment. Cochrane Database Syst Rev 2006; 4: CD004746.

Blasko I, Hinterberger M, Kemmler G, et al. Conversion from mild cognitive impairment to dementia: influence of folic acid and vitamin B12 use in the VITA cohort. J Nutr Health Aging 2012; 16: 687–694.

Boor JW, Hurtig HI. Persistent cerebellar ataxia after exposure to toluene. Ann Neurol 1977; 2: 440–442.

Cairney S, O' Connor N, Dingwall KM, et al. A prospective study of neurocognitive changes 15 years after chronic inhalant abuse. Addiction 2013; 108: 1107–1114.

Cardenas VA, Meyerhoff DJ, Studholme C, et al. Evidence for ongoing brain injury in human immunodeficiency virus–positive patients treated with antiretroviral therapy. J Neurovirol 2009; 15: 324–333.

Chatterjee A, Yapundich R, Palmer CA, et al. Leukoencephalopathy associated with cobalamin deficiency. Neurology 1996; 46: 832–834.

Cicerone KD, Langenbahn DM, Braden C, et al. Evidence-based cognitive rehabilitation: updated review of the literature from 2003 through 2008. Arch Phys Med Rehabil 2011; 92: 519–530.

Comi G. Effects of disease modifying treatments on cognitive dysfunction in multiple sclerosis. Neurol Sci 2010; 31(Suppl 2): S261–S264.

Del Bigio MR. Neuropathological changes caused by hydrocephalus. Acta Neuropathol 1993; 85: 573–585.

Del Bigio MR, da Silva MC, Drake JM, Tuor UI. Acute and chronic cerebral white matter damage in neonatal hydrocephalus. Can J Neurol Sci 1994; 21: 299–305.

Demaerschalk BM, Wingerchuk DM. Treatment of vascular dementia and vascular cognitive impairment. Neurologist 2007; 13: 37–41.

Deutsch MB, Mendez MF. Neurocognitive features distinguishing primary central nervous system lymphoma from other possible causes of rapidly progressive dementia. Cogn Behav Neurol 2015; 28: 1–10.

Dubois B, Slachevsky A, Litvan I, Pillon B. The FAB: a Frontal Assessment Battery at bedside. Neurology 2000; 55: 1621–1626.

Ehrenstein WH, Heister G, Cohen R. Trail Making Test and visual search. Arch Psychiatr Nervenkr 1982; 231: 333–338.

Ellingson BM, Cloughesy TF, Lai A, et al. Quantitative volumetric analysis of conventional MRI response in recurrent glioblastoma treated with bevacizumab. Neuro Oncol 2011; 13: 401–409.

Filippi CG, Sze G, Farber SJ, et al. Regression of HIV encephalopathy and basal ganglia signal intensity abnormality at MR imaging in patients with AIDS after the initiation of protease inhibitor therapy. Radiology 1998; 206: 491–498.

Filley CM. Toluene abuse and white matter: a model of toxic leukoencephalopathy. Psychiatr Clin North Am 2013; 36: 293–302.

Filley CM, Kleinschmidt-DeMasters BK. Toxic leukoencephalopathy. N Engl J Med 2001; 345: 425–432.

Filley CM, Kozora E, Brown MS, et al. White matter microstructure and cognition in non-neuropsychiatric systemic lupus erythematosus. Cogn Behav Neurol 2009; 22: 38–44.

Fischer JS, Priore RL, Jacobs LD, et al. Neuropsychological effects of interferon β-1-a in relapsing multiple sclerosis. Ann Neurol 2000; 48: 885–892.

Folstein MF, Folstein SE, McHugh PR. "Mini-Mental State": a practical method for grading the cognitive state of patients for the clinician. J Psychiatr Res 1975; 12: 189–198.

Giacino JT, Whyte J, Bagiella E, et al. Placebo-controlled trial of amantadine for severe traumatic brain injury. N Engl J Med 2012; 366: 819–826.

Goldman SA. Disease targets and strategies for the therapeutic modulation of endogenous neural stem and progenitor cells. Clin Pharmacol Ther 2007; 82: 453–460.

Gongvatana A, Harezlak J, Buchthal S, et al. Progressive cerebral injury in the setting of chronic HIV infection and antiretroviral therapy. J Neurovirol 2013; 19: 209–218.

Graber JJ, Sherman FT, Kaufmann H, et al. Vitamin B_{12}-responsive severe leukoencephalopathy and autonomic dysfunction in a patient with "normal" serum B_{12} levels. J Neurol Neurosurg Psychiatry 2010; 81: 1369–1371.

Graff-Radford NR. Normal pressure hydrocephalus. Neurol Clin 2007; 25: 809–832.

Grossman AW, Broderick JP. Advances and challenges in treatment and prevention of ischemic stroke. Ann Neurol 2013; 74: 363–372.

Gustafson L, Hagberg B. Recovery in hydrocephalic dementia after shunt operation. J Neurol Neurosurg Psychiatry 1978; 41: 940–947.

Hoogland ICM, Portegies P. HIV-associated dementia: prompt response to zidovudine. Neurol Clin Pract 2014; 4: 264–265.

Howard MO, Bowen SE, Garland EL, et al. Inhalant use and inhalant use disorders in the United States. Addict Sci Clin Pract 2011; 6: 18–31.

Jensen HB, Ravnborg M, Dalgas U, Stenager E. 4-Aminopyridine for symptomatic treatment of multiple sclerosis: a systematic review. Ther Adv Neurol Disord 2014; 7: 97–113.

Johansson BB. Current trends in stroke rehabilitation: a review with focus on brain plasticity. Acta Neurol Scand 2011; 123: 147–159.

Keith S. Use of long-acting risperidone in psychiatric disorders: focus on efficacy, safety and cost-effectiveness. Expert Rev Neurother 2009; 9: 9–31.

Klassen BT, Ahlskog JE. Normal pressure hydrocephalus: how often does the diagnosis hold water? Neurology 2011; 77: 1119–1125.

Kozora E, Arciniegas DB, Duggan E, et al. White matter abnormalities and working memory impairment in systemic lupus erythematosus. Cogn Behav Neurol 2013; 26: 63–72.

Krägeloh-Mann I, Groeschel S, Kehrer C, et al. Juvenile metachromatic leukodystrophy 10 years post transplant compared with a non-transplanted cohort. Bone Marrow Transplant 2013; 48: 369–375.

Krivit W, Peters C, Shapiro EG. Bone marrow transplantation as effective treatment of central nervous system disease in globoid cell leukodystrophy, metachromatic leukodystrophy, adrenoleukodystrophy, mannosidosis, fucosidosis, aspartylglucosaminuria, Hurler, Maroteaux-Lamy, and Sly syndromes, and Gaucher disease type III. Curr Opin Neurol 1999; 12: 167–176.

Lang C, Reiss C, Mäurer M. Natalizumab may improve cognition and mood in multiple sclerosis. Eur Neurol 2012; 67: 162–166.

Lee SP, Wu CS, Hsieh LC, et al. Efficacy of magnetic resonance diffusion tensor imaging and three-dimensional fiber tractography in the detection of clinical manifestations of central nervous system lupus. Magn Reson Imaging 2014; 32: 598–603.

Leinonen V, Koivisto AM, Savolainen S, et al. Post-mortem findings in 10 patients with presumed normal-pressure hydrocephalus and review of the literature. Neuropathol Appl Neurobiol 2012; 38: 72–86.

Leone P, Janson CG, Bilianuk L, et al. Aspartoacylase gene transfer to the mammalian central nervous system with therapeutic implications for Canavan's disease. Ann Neurol 2000; 48: 27–38.

Mackey AP, Whitaker KJ, Bunge SA. Experience-dependent plasticity in white matter microstructure: reasoning training alters structural connectivity. Front Neuroanat 2012; 6: 32.

Mayberg HS, Lozano AM, Voon V, et al. Deep brain stimulation for treatment-resistant depression. Neuron 2005; 45: 651–660.

McDowell S, Whyte J, D'Esposito M. Differential effect of a dopaminergic agonist on prefrontal function in traumatic brain injury patients. Brain 1998; 121: 1155–1164.

Meythaler JM, Brunner RC, Johnson A, Novack TA. Amantadine to improve neurorecovery in traumatic brain injury–associated diffuse axonal injury: a pilot double-blind randomized trial. J Head Trauma Rehabil 2002; 17: 300–313.

Miner ME. Acetazolamide treatment of progressive hydrocephalus secondary to intraventricular hemorrhage in a preterm infant. Childs Nerv Syst 1986; 2: 105–106.

Navia BA, Jordan BD, Price RW. The AIDS dementia complex: I. Clinical features. Ann Neurol 1986; 19: 517–524.

Navia BA, Cho E-S, Petito CK, Price RW. The AIDS dementia complex: II. Neuropathology. Ann Neurol 1986; 19: 525–535.

Orchard PJ, Tolar J. Transplant outcomes in leukodystrophies. Semin Hematol 2010; 47: 70–78.

Pennisi G, Ferri R, Cantone M, et al. A review of transcranial magnetic stimulation in vascular dementia. Dement Geriatr Cogn Disord 2011; 31: 71–80.

Pliskin NH, Hamer DP, Goldstein DS, et al. Improved delayed visual reproduction test performance in multiple sclerosis patients receiving interferon βeta-1-b. Neurology 1996; 47: 1463–1468.

Qureshi SU, Blanchette AR, Jawaid A, Schulz PE. Reversible leukoencephalopathy due to chronic unintentional exposure to toluene. Can J Neurol Sci 2009; 36: 388–389.

Rektorova I, Megova S, Bares M, Rektor I. Cognitive functioning after repetitive transcranial magnetic stimulation in patients with cerebrovascular disease without dementia: a pilot study of seven patients. J Neurol Sci 2005; 229–230: 157–161.

Rimkus C de M, Andrade CS, Leite C da C, et al. Toxic leukoencephalopathies, including drug, medication, environmental, and radiation-induced encephalopathic syndromes. Semin Ultrasound CT MR 2014; 35: 97–117.

Riva-Posse P, Choi KS, Holtzheimer PE, et al. Defining critical white matter pathways mediating successful subcallosal cingulate deep brain stimulation for treatment-resistant depression. Biol Psychiatry 2014; 76: 963–969.

Román GC, Salloway S, Black SE, et al. Randomized, placebo-controlled, clinical trial of donepezil in vascular dementia: differential effects by hippocampal size. Stroke 2010; 41: 1213–1221.

Rosenberg NL, Spitz MC, Filley CM, et al. Central nervous system effects of chronic toluene abuse – clinical, brainstem evoked response and magnetic resonance imaging studies. Neurotoxicol Teratol 1988; 10: 489–495.

Rudick RA, Cohen JA, Weinstock-Guttman B, et al. Management of multiple sclerosis. N Engl J Med 1997; 337: 1604–1611.

Sakai JT, Mikulich-Gilbertson SK, Crowley TJ. Adolescent inhalant use among male patients in treatment for substance and behavior problems: two-year outcome. Am J Drug Alcohol Abuse 2006; 32: 29–40.

Siddall OM. Use of methylphenidate in traumatic brain injury. Ann Pharmacother 2005; 39: 1309–1313.

Simon JH. From enhancing lesions to brain atrophy in relapsing MS. J Neuroimmunol 1999; 98: 7–15.

Solders M, Martin DA, Andersson C, et al. Hematopoietic SCT: a useful treatment for late metachromatic leukodystrophy. Bone Marrow Transplant 2014; 49: 1046–1051.

Stabler SP. Vitamin B_{12} deficiency. N Engl J Med 2013; 368: 149–160.

Stojsavljević N, Lević Z, Drulović J, Dragutinović G. A 44-month clinical-brain MRI follow-up in a patient with B_{12} deficiency. Neurology 1997; 49: 878–881.

Stuss DT, Winocur G, Robertson IH, eds. *Cognitive neurorehabilitation.* 2nd ed. Cambridge: Cambridge University Press, 2008.

Su S, Libman RB, Diamond A, Sharfstein S. Infratentorial and supratentorial leukoencephalopathy associated with vitamin B_{12} deficiency. J Stroke Cerebrovasc Dis 2000; 9: 136–138.

Taber KH, Hurley RA, Yudofsky SC. Diagnosis and treatment of neuropsychiatric disorders. Annu Rev Med 2010; 61: 121–133.

Takeuchi H, Sekiguchi A, Taki Y, et al. Training of working memory impacts structural connectivity. J Neurosci 2010; 30: 3297–3303.

Tang YY, Lu Q, Fan M, et al. Mechanisms of white matter changes induced by meditation. Proc Natl Acad Sci 2012; 109: 10570–10574.

Tenovuo O, Alin J, Helenius H. A randomized controlled trial of rivastigmine for chronic sequels of traumatic brain injury – what it showed and taught? Brain Inj 2009; 23: 548–558.

Thurnher MM, Schindler EG, Thurnher SA, et al. Highly active antiretroviral therapy for patients with AIDS dementia complex: effect on MR imaging findings and clinical course. AJNR 2000; 21: 670–678.

Tomimoto H, Ohtani R, Shibata M, Nakamura N, Ihara M. Loss of cholinergic pathways in vascular dementia of the Binswanger type. Dement Geriatr Cogn Disord 2005; 19: 282–288.

Tozzi V, Narciso P, Galgani S, et al. Effects of zidovudine in 30 patients with mild to end-stage AIDS dementia complex. AIDS 1993; 7: 683–692.

Tran KD, Ho A, Jandial R. Stem cell transplantation methods. Adv Exp Med Biol 2010; 671: 41–57.

Tullberg M, Hultin L, Ekholm S, et al. White matter changes in normal pressure hydrocephalus and Binswanger disease: specificity, predictive value and correlations to axonal degeneration and demyelination. Acta Neurol Scand 2002; 105: 417–426.

Tumani H., Uttner I. Influences on cognition by immunosuppression and immunomodulation in multiple sclerosis. J Neurol 2007; 254 Suppl 2: II69–II72.

Vanderver A, Tonduti D, Schiffmann R, et al. Leukodystrophy overview. In: Pagon RA, Adam MP, Ardinger HH, Wallace SE, Amemiya A, Bean LJH, Bird TD, Dolan CR, Fong CT, Smith RJH, Stephens K, eds. GeneReviews® [Internet]. Seattle: University of Washington, Seattle; 1993–2015. 2014 Feb 6.

Wake H, Lee PR, Fields RD. Control of local protein synthesis and initial events in myelination by action potentials. Science 2011; 333: 1647–1651.

Wang S, Young KM. White matter plasticity in adulthood. Neuroscience 2014; 276: 148–160.

Weinstein A, Schwid SI, Schiffer RB, et al. Neuropsychologic status in multiple sclerosis after treatment with glatiramer. Arch Neurol 1999; 56: 319–324.

Wilson RK, Williams MA. The role of the neurologist in the longitudinal management of normal pressure hydrocephalus. Neurologist 2010; 16: 238–248.

Wortzel HS, Arciniegas DB. Treatment of post-traumatic cognitive impairments. Curr Treat Options Neurol 2012; 14: 493–508.

Xu J, Cheng Y, Chai P, Lu Z, et al. White-matter volume reduction and the protective effect of immunosuppressive therapy in systemic lupus erythematosus patients with normal appearance by conventional magnetic resonance imaging. J Rheumatol 2010; 37: 974–986.

Zhang L, Plotkin RC, Wang G, et al. Cholinergic augmentation with donepezil enhances recovery in short-term memory and sustained attention after traumatic brain injury. Arch Phys Med Rehabil 2004; 85: 1050–1055.

Zheng X, Schlaug G. Structural white matter changes in descending motor tracts correlate with improvements in motor impairment after undergoing a treatment course of tDCS and physical therapy. Front Hum Neurosci 2015; 30: 9. 229.

Zhornitsky S, Wee Yong V, Koch MW, et al. Quetiapine fumarate for the treatment of multiple sclerosis: focus on myelin repair. CNS Neurosci Ther 2013; 19: 737–744.

Chapter 12

White matter and cognition: research perspectives

The prevailing view that cortical gray matter is the seat of higher functions has inspired a vast amount of research, and similar productivity can be imagined when white matter is considered with the same degree of interest. Many new directions can be imagined from thinking about the role of white matter in normal cognition, all of which implicate the pursuit of a better understanding of white matter as it participates in the architecture of cognitive operations. First, the normal neuroanatomy of myelinated systems in the brain is a topic of vigorous investigation. Next, the study of white matter connectivity in distributed neural networks is attracting steady interest as the operations of these networks become more securely understood. The contribution of cerebellar white matter to cognition merits discussion as support grows for the provocative idea that the cerebellum has neurobehavioral importance. Finally, the emerging role of inflammation as a general pathological phenomenon within white matter deserves comment.

Normal white matter anatomy

An important outcome of work on myelinated systems is that the normal white matter of the brain will be much better understood. Classic neuroanatomy, for all its elegance and detail, has left many questions unanswered about the origin, course, and termination of white matter tracts (Schmahmann and Pandya, 2006), especially for clinicians attempting to assign functions to specific connecting structures. Indeed, neurologists at present are accustomed to conceptualizing the white matter as an essentially homogeneous mass of myelinated tissue packed into large bundles that cannot be readily teased out one from another. New neuroimaging methods promise to address this issue with increasing sophistication. The steady improvement in technology, notably including increases in field strength of magnets used for magnetic resonance imaging (MRI), will also help clarify the nascent topic of intracortical myelin, long known from neuroanatomy but only now visible in vivo (Schmahmann and Pandya, 2006; Nieuwenhuys, 2013). At the same time, traditional neuroanatomic studies can be informed by clinical neuroimaging data, and useful insights will come forth whether the neuroimaging findings confirm the currently accepted neuroanatomy or present new information. A productive interplay can be developed between neuroimaging and neuroanatomy to refine knowledge of normal white matter (Schmahmann and Pandya, 2006; Mesulam, 2012; Catani et al., 2012a).

An instructive example of the application of combined neuroimaging and neuroanatomy can be seen in the recent discovery of the frontal aslant tract (Catani et al., 2012b). This short frontal connection, which links the supplementary motor area with Broca's area, was identified with MRI and then confirmed by postmortem dissection (Catani et al., 2012b). Subsequent study of patients with primary progressive aphasia demonstrated the importance of this tract in verbal fluency and grammar processing (Catani et al., 2013a). The recognition of the frontal aslant tract also clarifies the understanding of a related syndrome, transcortical motor aphasia, which was thought on the basis of computed tomography studies to involve a disruption of the connections between the supplementary motor area and the left perisylvian region (Freedman, Alexander, and Naeser, 1984). Thus new research on white matter anatomy confirmed with more advanced technology what had been previously suspected on clinical grounds.

The discovery of the frontal aslant tract exemplified how improved understanding of normal white matter anatomy will generate a more informed approach to the identification and interpretation of white matter lesions seen in clinical settings. Neurologists are well aware that it is at times not a trivial task to determine whether a given brain structure seen on neuroimaging is normal or abnormal.

Knowledge of normal tract anatomy will enhance the recognition of what white matter structure is indeed not normal. White matter tractography appears to be among the most exciting clinical applications of advanced neuroimaging, and diffusion tensor imaging (DTI) holds the most promise. In the tradition of Geschwind, DTI promises to expand the understanding of disconnection syndromes by directly demonstrating damaged tracts in vivo that can be implicated in a variety of neurobehavioral syndromes (Catani, 2006).

With further progress, it is not unduly fanciful to imagine that tractography of tracts large and small will soon be applied in the routine clinical practice of neurology and psychiatry. A general consensus holds that MRI scanners with higher magnetic field strength will be crucial in the evolution of this research (Filippi et al., 2014), and other technical advances can safely be assumed to appear in the near future. As the location, size, extent, degree of myelination, sites of origin and termination, and functional affiliations of specific tracts become more clear, lesions of individual tracts and in multiple tracts will be identifiable by noninvasive methods. Early and accurate identification of these lesions may allow prompt and effective treatment that can potentially avert the development of white matter dementia (WMD) or its predecessor, mild cognitive dysfunction (MCD).

A research topic that is likely to impact treatment is the role of white matter lesions in neurochemical systems relevant to cognition (Butt, Fern, and Matute, 2014). A number of neurotransmitters are found in the white matter, not only within the large tracts but also within the smaller fascicles of the cerebral cortex and deep gray matter (Butt, Fern, and Matute, 2014). Box 12.1 displays the major white matter neurotransmitters currently recognized. This topic is broad and largely beyond the scope of this book, but two implications are immediately apparent.

BOX 12.1 Neurotransmitter systems within brain white matter

- Cholinergic
- Glutamatergic
- Dopaminergic
- Serotonergic
- Adrenergic
- GABAergic
- Glycinergic
- Purinergic

First, because many neurotransmitters course through axons that emanate from subcortical neuronal cell bodies and ascend to the cortex, they are susceptible to disruption by a variery of white matter lesions. In this regard, an instructive example is the cholinergic system (Román, 2005). Acetylcholine is an essential neurotransmitter conveyed by projections from the basal forebrain to widespread areas of the cerebrum, and is involved in many aspects of attention and memory. Neuroanatomic studies have found that cholinergic projections course within areas of white matter that are vulnerable to white matter disorders (Selden et al., 1998), including leukoaraiosis (Swartz, Sahlas, and Black, 2003) and cerebral autosomal-dominant arteriopathy with subcortical infarcts and leukoencephalopathy (CADASIL; Mesulam, Siddique, and Cohen, 2003). It is therefore plausible that cholinergic augmentation may come to occupy an important position in the treatment of WMD and MCD. Such an approach is well known in the treatment of patients with Alzheimer's Disease (AD), but in this disease the cholinergic deficit results from neuronal loss in the basal forebrain and not because of damage to cholinergic fibers extending rostrally (Kim, Moon, and Han, 2013). Extension of this generic concept to other neurotransmtters coursing within the white matter may offer a wide range of pharmacological treatment opportunities.

Second, because white matter is characterized by the absence of neuronal cell bodies and traditional synapses, and neuron-to-neuron communication does not occur, white matter neurotransmitters are engaged in other forms of signaling such as axo-oligodendroglial transmission (Butt, Fern, and Matute, 2014). This phenomenon in turn contributes to white matter plasticity (Fields, 2010), as has been considered earlier and will be further discussed in the next chapter.

Other questions germane to the normal anatomy of white matter are also relevant. Although the large brain of *Homo sapiens* has acquired a substantial complement of myelinated axons that permits efficient signaling across large intracranial distances (Zhang and Sejnowski, 2000), a percentage of the cerebral axons is unmyelinated. In the rat, an estimate of 80% has been offered as the percentage of corpus callosum axons that is unmyelinated (Gravel, Sasseville, and Hawkes, 1990), suggesting that human brains may harbor a proportion of similar axons. Preliminary autopsy data from the human fornix indicate that myelinated fibers outnumber those that are unmyelinated (Ozdogmus et al., 2009), but a substantial percentage of human brain axons is likely to be found devoid of myelin. The function of these fibers, however, is not well understood, and their importance for neurobehavioral competence is similarly obscure. Some evidence exists for a selective vulnerability of unmyelinated axons to trauma, possibly because they lack the structural support and protection of circumferential myelin (Reeves et al., 2012). More data on the location, relative abundance, location, functional role, and specific vulnerability – or resistance – of these axons to disease, injury, or intoxication will prove illuminating.

Another area deserving investigation is the presence of myelinated fascicles in all layers of the cerebral cortex. The accomplishments of the Vogts in the early twentieth century as they labored with autopsied human brains to describe a myeloarchitecture of the cortex (Chapter 3) can provide a basis for similar studies today, but now with the assistance of powerful in vivo neuroimaging. Intriguing ideas are being advanced, including the somewhat counterintuitive notion that increased intracortical myelination – such as that found in the line of Gennari within the calcarine cortex – may actually inhibit synaptic plasticity (Glasser et al., 2014). Myelin in the cortex may thus serve a much different purpose than myelin elsewhere in the brain. Evidence now suggests that heavily myelinated sensorimotor cortices function to enhance highly evolved but relatively invariant sensory and motor activity, whereas lightly myelinated association cortices – which have greatly expanded in humans over evolution compared to higher primates – subserve critical higher functions that require more flexibility and hence synaptic plasticity (Glasser et al., 2014). Thus the possibility presents itself that myelin in large subcortical tracts enhances cognition by facilitating information transfer between gray matter regions within distributed neural networks, whereas myelin within the cortex has the opposite effect, and is in fact more useful in its absence for the optimal function of the cortex in cognitive operations.

Intracortical myelin also appears to play a role in the recently introduced effort to measure cortical thickness as a method of studying aging and dementia (Teipel et al., 2008). In the continuing search to find reliable biomarkers of various dementias, the assessment of cortical thickness has become a popular application of rapidly emerging neuroimaging technology. While synaptic and neuronal loss likely plays a major role in any reduction in cortical thickness observed in older individuals, age-related changes in gray matter volume are also thought to result in part from a decline in intracortical myelin (Kochunov et al., 2011). Recent MRI studies using a 7.0 T magnet in normal humans have succeeded in visualizing white matter fascicles within the auditory cortices (De Martino et al., 2014), an encouraging development that could lead to high-resolution imaging of intracortical myelin damage. The mechanisms and implications of myelin loss within the cortex are provocative but little understood, yet the possibility of a parallel decline in myelin within large tracts and in the cortex raises interesting questions about the processes of aging as well as many dementia syndromes.

White matter in distributed neural networks

Neuroanatomic investigations will in turn clarify the architecture of distributed neural networks, the central organizational feature of the brain as it subserves the wide array of cognitive and emotional operations that make up the human behavioral repertoire (Geschwind, 1965; Mesulam, 1990; Solar and Stoner, 2011). White matter is the connecting tissue between cortical and subcortical gray matter regions within and between the hemispheres, and recent data also point to the importance of white matter in networks involving the cerebellum (Schmahmann and Pandya, 2006). The concept of the connectome – "a comprehensive structural description of the network of elements and connections forming the human brain" – has recently been proposed to capture the spirit of this endeavor (Sporns, 2011; Van Essen et al., 2013), and mapping of human brain connectivity is underway (Toga et al., 2012; Ajilore et al., 2013; DiMartino et al., 2014). Large tracts, intracortical myelin, and white matter fascicles coursing through deep gray matter nuclei all warrant study.

In the practice of behavioral neurology as well as a host of research endeavors, distributed neural networks already serve to inform thinking on brain–behavior relationships. For the past 200 years, the localization of cognitive function has been a central interest of neuroscience, beginning with pioneering studies of nineteenth-century neuroscientists who first began considering the idea that specific functions could be associated with discrete regions of the brain

(Young, 1970). The first notable figure of this period was Franz Joseph Gall, an accomplished neuroanatomist who is unfortunately better known today as the progenitor of the discredited notion of phrenology. Before venturing with his colleague Johann Kaspar Spurzheim into the speculations of phrenology, which held that various mental faculties could be determined by palpation of bony irregularities of the skull that signified underlying brain areas, Gall conducted pioneering neuroanatomic studies that were far ahead of his time. Using dissections of human brains, Gall and Spurzheim emphasized the importance of the cerebral cortex in the organization of brain functions, and recognized the functional specialization of cortical regions (Schmahmann and Pandya, 2006). In addition, they identified white matter tracts linking cortical regions, dividing these tracts into projection and association fibers, a classification still in use today (Schmahmann and Pandya, 2006). Gall is thus a key figure in the history of systems neuroscience (Schmahmann and Pandya, 2006), and even the practice of phrenology can be interpreted as a flawed but influential harbinger of more legitimate brain–behavior correlations that would subsequently appear. Later in the nineteenth century came seminal observations on aphasia by Paul Broca (1861) and Karl Wernicke (1874), who not only established the foundation for the cortical localization of language but also introduced white matter connectivity as an integral component of the organization of language.

As time went on, the idea of distributed networks steadily gained ground as it was appreciated that a slavish one gyrus–one function correspondence was not supported by the accumulating data. The operations of cognition and emotion came to be seen as both localized and distributed, so that the behavior resulting from brain activity was widely represented in cerebral networks (Mesulam, 1990). Much of the knowledge gained in this endeavor was derived from the monkey, but the limitations of studying this animal as a model of human connectivity are apparent (Mesulam, 2012). However, from the study of human diseases and the application of advanced neuroimaging, a number of distributed neural networks were tentatively established (Mesulam, 1990; Catani et al., 2012a), all presumed to involve combinations of gray and white matter structures (Filley, 2012). These networks (Table 12.1) include one for arousal involving the rostral brain stem, thalamus, and cerebral cortex

Table 12.1 Distributed neural networks

Domain	Gray matter structures	Connecting tracts
Arousal	Reticular activating system Thalamus Cerebral cortex	Medial forebrain bundle Thalamocortical radiations
Spatial attention	Parietal lobe (right) Prefrontal cortex (right) Cingulate gyrus (right)	Superior occipitofrontal fasciculus (right) Cingulum (right)
Memory	Hippocampus Diencephalon Basal forebrain	Fornix Mammillothalamic tract
Language	Broca's area Wernicke's area	Arcuate fasciculus Extreme capsule
Visuospatial ability	Parietal lobe (right) Frontal lobe (right)	Superior occipitofrontal fasciculus (right)
Visual recognition	Temporal lobes Occipital lobes	Inferior occipitofrontal fasciculus
Executive function	Dorsolateral prefrontal cortices Parietal cortices	Superior occipitofrontal fasciculus
Emotions and personality	Temporolimbic system Orbitofrontal cortices	Medial forebrain bundle Uncinate fasciculus
Social cognition (salience network)	Anterior insula Orbitofrontal cortex Anterior cingulate	Inferior occipitofrontal fasciculus Cingulum
Resting state (default mode network)	Anterior cingulate Posterior cingulate Precuneus Medial temporal cortices	Cingulum

(Parvizi and Damasio, 2001), the medial temporal lobe–hippocampal network for declarative memory (Jang and Kwon, 2014), a spatial attention network with major hubs in the right parietal and frontal lobes (Bartolomeo, Thiebaut de Schotten, and Chica, 2012), a visuospatial network with right parietofrontal distribution (Parks and Madden, 2013), a visual recognition network involving bilateral occipitotemporal regions (Tavor et al., 2014), an executive function network with frontal and parietal hubs (Gold et al., 2010), the limbic system as it subserves basic aspects of emotions and personality (Catani, Dell'acqua, and Thiebaut de Schotten, 2013b), and, as was recognized with the use of functional neuroimaging including positron emission tomography (PET) and functional MRI (fMRI), the salience network mediating social cognition (Seeley et al., 2007) and the default mode network subserving resting brain activity (Raichle et al., 2001). As functional neuroimaging began to explore connectivity using coactivation of cortical regions, it was found, reassuringly, that structural connectivity generally mirrors that which is found using studies of cortical function (Damoiseaux and Greicius, 2009).

The idea of distributed neural networks that include both gray and white matter components has also helped revive the century-old concept of diaschisis (Feeney and Baron, 1986; Carrera and Tononi, 2014). The phenomenon, the idea of which was introduced by Constantin von Monakow (1914) to describe the remote effects of a focal brain lesion, is now being elucidated by modern neuroimaging modalities that can identify the tracts connecting the involved regions. Preliminary evidence in stroke patients, for example, suggests that gray matter lesions are associated with white matter damage that can lead to indirect effects on other regions that are structurally intact but connected to the area of infarction (Stenset et al., 2007; Bonilha et al., 2014). Further study of diaschisis in light of modern knowledge of distributed neural networks will prove illuminating.

The role of the cerebellum

One of the most provocative developments related to the growing emergence of white matter neurobiology is the newly recognized role of the cerebellum in cognition and emotion. Long considered a component of the brain with strong motor affiliations but little meaningful role in neurobehavioral function, the cerebellum began receiving attention in the 1980s as an underappreciated participant in distributed neural networks subserving higher function (Schmahmann, 1991). From detailed study of patients with cerebellar lesions including agenesis, developmental disorders, stroke, neoplasm, infection, and degeneration, it was recognized that whereas cerebellar dysfunction clearly produces impairments in motor coordination, patients may also develop a myriad of cognitive and emotional deficits (Schmahmann, 1991). With further study, a syndrome of disordered cognitive control and emotional regulation emerged, to be called the cerebellar-cognitive-affective syndrome (CCAS; Schmahmann and Sherman, 1998). A ubiquitous neurobehavioral manifestation of cerebellar lesions was conceptualized as nonmotor dysmetria, and the interesting term "dysmetria of thought" was proposed to capture the core feature of the CCAS (Schmahmann, 2004). In this syndrome, lesions of the anterior lobe of the cerebellum produce motor dysmetria, with its familiar manifestations in limb ataxia, speech impairment, and impaired eye movements, whereas damage to the lateral portion of the posterior lobes gives rise to cognitive dysfunction, and damage to the vermis (the limbic cerebellum) leads to affective disturbances (Schmahmann, 2004). These regional affiliations of the cerebellum have been validated by functional neuroimaging studies, as was demonstrated by a recent meta-analysis of relevant PET and fMRI studies (Stoodley and Schmahmann, 2009).

Implicit in these remarkable investigations has been the notion that the cerebellum is heavily interconnected with the cerebrum via many cerebro-cerebellar circuits, most prominently projecting to and from the frontal lobes (Schmahmann, 1991; Schmahmann and Sherman, 1998; Schmahmann, 2004, 2010). These connections have been known from classic neuroanatomic studies, but until recently were accorded little clinical importance by neurologists who were so impressed by the obvious phenomenology of ataxia and related motor deficits that investigation of possible neurobehavioral deficits with cerebellar disease was regarded as inconsequential. Yet as time went on and modern neuroimaging offered new insights, the existence of cerebral regions corresponding to specific cerebellar regions has become clear. Recent fMRI studies have shown, for example, that motor regions of the cerebellum are linked with sensorimotor areas of the cerebral cortex, whereas cognitive cerebellar regions are connected with frontal and parietal cortices (Stoodley, Valera, and Schmahmann, 2012). The elegance of these topographically specific connections strongly supports a role of the cerebellum in higher functions through direct white matter connectivity with the cerebral cortices.

As happens in all of neurology, further neuroanatomic study led to additional refinement of the concepts under study. Whereas it has been known since the work of Brodmann and others more than a century ago that the cerebral cortex has markedly variable cellular architecture that corresponds to the many distinct functions for which it is responsible, the cerebellar cortex has a uniform structure, implying that its basic work should be constant regardless of the operation involved. This neuroanatomic feature is the basis of the universal cerebellar transform, by which is meant the capacity of the cerebellum to modulate all the operations in which it participates, motor or neurobehavioral, in order to dampen oscillation around a homeostatic baseline and smooth out the performance achieved (Schmahmann, 2004).

The development of what might be called the behavioral neurology of the cerebellum is clearly reminiscent of the process that led to the focus on white matter that provides the background for this book. As with the white matter disorders, the recognition that the cerebellum has important neurobehavioral aspects underscores the fact that the key observations were not new, only hidden. In both cerebellar diseases and the white matter disorders, observations of cognitive and emotional disturbances existed for many decades before being formally characterized, and the work of earlier neurologists and psychiatrists was a harbinger of what has now become more clear. Clinicians many still find more obvious the motor deficits of patients with cerebellar lesions, but the data unequivocally show that more focused study of cognitive and affective aspects yields crucial information. As in the white matter disorders considered in this book, cerebellar lesions can be found to have important neurobehavioral consequences when these problems are specifically sought, and both lines of inquiry validate the centrality of brain connectivity in the operations of distributed neural networks.

Inflammation and white matter

Another emerging area of clinical and basic neuroscience is the investigation of brain inflammation as it relates to neurobehavioral function. The idea that inflammation in the brain exerts a deleterious effect on cognitive function is best supported in aging (Gorelick, 2010), and inflammatory mechanisms have recently been implicated in both neurodegenerative diseases such as AD (Bettcher and Kramer, 2014) and psychiatric disorders such as depression (Ownby, 2010). Laboratory investigation is also turning to the study of inflammatory pathophysiology, and experimental work is proceeding on topics such as stroke and traumatic brain injury (Baltan et al., 2014). With regard to the white matter, the pathophysiology of many known disorders, discussed in Chapter 6, includes a component of inflammation, and in some, such as systemic lupus erythematosus (SLE) and multiple sclerosis (MS), inflammation is directly involved in pathogenesis. Inflammation is also a common feature of aging, likely due both to upregulation of inflammation-associated genes (Lee, Weindruch, and Prolla, 2000) and to various environmental factors (Yaffe, 2007), and has been linked with atherosclerosis, cerebral ischemia, cognitive impairment, functional disability, frailty, and even mortality (Arfanakis et al., 2013). In light of these combined observations, which suggest that inflammation may exert important effects on white matter while not producing the overt clinical manifestations of diseases such as SLE or MS, the possible impact of systemic inflammation on brain white matter will now be considered.

As might be expected, the impact of subclinical inflammation on brain white matter is thought to be insufficient to cause grossly visible lesions on conventional MRI. Accordingly, the normal-appearing white matter (NAWM) has been examined, and most studies have used the diffusion tensor imaging parameter fractional anisotropy (FA) in combination with measures of systemic inflammation such as C-reactive protein (CRP) (Arfanakis et al., 2013; Gianaros et al., 2013; Bettcher et al., 2015) or interleukin-6 (Il-6) (Bettcher et al., 2014). These studies have typically shown that systemic inflammation appears to have an injurious effect on white matter microstructure (Arfanakis et al., 2013; Gianaros et al., 2013; Bettcher et al., 2014). While cognition has not been regularly examined in such studies, higher Il-6 levels were related to slower processing speed in one report (Bettcher et al., 2014). Moreover, in a prospective study in which the CRP of subjects declined over several years, FA improved significantly in frontoparietal and frontotemporal white matter tracts (Bettcher et al., 2015). Environmental determinants of systemic inflammation were specified in one study, which found that healthy adults from higher socioeconomic backgrounds had higher FA relative to disadvantaged individuals; this effect was in part mediated by lower CRP, and also by lower rates of cigarette smoking and adiposity (Gianaros et al., 2013).

These human studies on inflammation are all observational, and it is not known how systemic inflammation may exert its effects on white matter at the cellular or molecular level. The blood–brain barrier, while highly adept at preventing the ingress of pathogens into the brain, is not impermeable to various inflammatory mediators that arise from non-neural tissues (Sankowski, Mader, and Valdés-Ferrer, 2015), and a range of systemic inflammatory processes can thus find their way into the brain. One of the implications of this work is that brain inflammation may lead to neurodegeneration, a sequence increasingly accepted in MS, a disease characterized in many cases by early inflammation with enhancing MRI white matter lesions, followed later by neurodegeneration with brain atrophy (Sankowski, Mader, and Valdés-Ferrer, 2015). A plausible, although far from established, idea would thus be that systemic inflammation may trigger, or help potentiate, a neurodegenerative process through mechanisms that are not yet understood. Much remains to be learned about the precise role of brain inflammation, and in particular its effects on cognition, and the value of longitudinal studies to assess these relationships in the context of AD and all late-life disorders of cognition has been emphasized (Bettcher and Kramer, 2014). However, the detrimental effects of this form of pathology are well recognized in many known white matter disorders, and the evidence discussed earlier may expand our knowledge in important ways. If it is true that certain environmental influences increasing systemic inflammation harm white matter, a variety of medical and public health interventions can be considered with potentially major benefit for large numbers of individuals who do not yet suffer from any recognizable neurologic affliction.

References

Ajilore O, Zhan L, Gadelkarim J, et al. Constructing the resting state structural connectome. Front Neuroinform 2013; 7: 30.

Arfanakis K, Fleischman DA, Grisot G, et al. Systemic inflammation in non-demented elderly human subjects: brain microstructure and cognition. PLoS One 2013; 8: e73107.

Baltan S, Carmichael ST, Matute C, Xi G, Zhang JH, eds. *White matter injury in stroke and CNS disease.* New York: Springer, 2014.

Bartolomeo P, Thiebaut de Schotten M, Chica AB. Brain networks of visuospatial attention and their disruption in visual neglect. Front Hum Neurosci 2012; 6: 110.

Bettcher BM, Kramer JH. Longitudinal inflammation, cognitive decline, and Alzheimer's disease: a mini-review. Clin Pharmacol Ther 2014; 96: 464–469.

Bettcher BM, Watson CL, Walsh CM, et al. Interleukin-6, age, and corpus callosum integrity. PLoS One 2014; 9: e106521.

Bettcher BM, Yaffe K, Boudreau RM, et al. Declines in inflammation predict greater white matter microstructure in older adults. Neurobiol Aging 2015; 36: 948–954.

Bonilha L, Nesland T, Rorden C, et al. Mapping remote subcortical ramifications of injury after ischemic strokes. Behav Neurol 2014; 2014: 215380.

Broca P. Remarques sur la siège de la faculté du langage articule, suives d'une observation d'aphémie. Bulletin Societé Anatomique 1861; 36: 333–337, 398–407.

Butt AM, Fern RF, Matute C. Neurotransmitter signaling in white matter. Glia 2014; 62: 1762–1779.

Carrera E, Tononi G. Diaschisis: past, present, future. Brain 2014; 137: 2408–2422.

Catani M. Diffusion tensor magnetic resonance imaging tractography in cognitive disorders. Curr Opin Neurol 2006; 19: 599–606.

Catani M, Dell'acqua F, Bizzi A, et al. Beyond cortical localization in clinico-anatomical correlation. Cortex 2012a; 48: 1262–1287.

Catani M, Dell'acqua F, Vergani F, et al. Short frontal lobe connections of the human brain. Cortex 2012b; 48: 273–291.

Catani M, Mesulam M-M, Jakobsen E, et al. A novel frontal pathway underlies verbal fluency in primary progressive aphasia. Brain 2013a; 136: 2619–2628.

Catani M, Dell'acqua F, Thiebaut de Schotten M. A revised limbic system model for memory, emotion and behaviour. Neurosci Biobehav Rev 2013b; 37: 1724–1737.

Damoiseaux JS, Greicius MD. Greater than the sum of its parts: a review of studies combining structural connectivity and resting-state functional connectivity. Brain Struct Funct 2009; 213: 525–533.

De Martino F, Moerel M, Xu J, et al. High-resolution mapping of myeloarchitecture in vivo: localization of auditory areas in the human brain. Cereb Cortex 2014 Jul 3. [Epub ahead of print]

DiMartino A, Fair DA, Kelly C, et al. Unraveling the miswired connectome: a developmental perspective. Neuron 2014; 83: 1335–1353.

Feeney DM, Baron J-C. Diaschisis. Stroke 1986; 17: 817–830.

Fields RD. Neuroscience: change in the brain's white matter. Science 2010; 330: 768–769.

Filippi M, Charil A, Rovaris M, et al. Insights from magnetic resonance imaging. Handb Clin Neurol 2014; 122: 115–149.

Filley CM. *The behavioural neurology of white matter*. 2nd ed. New York: Oxford University Press, 2012.

Freedman M, Alexander MP, Naeser MA. Anatomic basis of transcortical motor aphasia. Neurology 1984; 34: 409–417.

Geschwind N. Disconnexion syndromes in animals and man. Brain 1965; 88: 237–294, 585–644.

Gianaros PJ, Marsland AL, Sheu LK, et al. Inflammatory pathways link socioeconomic inequalities to white matter architecture. Cereb Cortex 2013; 23: 2058–2071.

Glasser MF, Goyal MS, Preuss TM, et al. Trends and properties of human cerebral cortex: correlations with cortical myelin content. Neuroimage 2014; 93 Pt2: 165–175.

Gold BT, Powell DK, Xuan L, et al. Age-related slowing of task switching is associated with decreased integrity of frontoparietal white matter. Neurobiol Aging 2010; 31: 512–522.

Gorelick PB. Role of inflammation in cognitive impairment: results of observational epidemiological studies and clinical trials. Ann N Y Acad Sci 2010; 1207: 155–162.

Gravel C, Sasseville R, Hawkes R. Maturation of the corpus callosum of the rat: II. Influence of thyroid hormones on the number and maturation of axons. J Comp Neurol 1990; 291: 147–161.

Jang SH, Kwon HG. Perspectives on the neural connectivity of the fornix in the human brain. Neural Regen Res 2014; 9: 1434–1436.

Kim HJ, Moon WJ, Han SH. Differential cholinergic pathway involvement in Alzheimer's disease and subcortical ischemic vascular dementia. J Alzheimers Dis 2013; 35: 129–136.

Kochunov P, Glahn DC, Lancaster J, et al. Fractional anisotropy of cerebral white matter and thickness of cortical gray matter across the lifespan. Neuroimage 2011; 58: 41–49.

Lee CK, Weindruch R, Prolla TA. Gene-expression profile of the ageing brain in mice. Nat Genet 2000; 25: 294–297.

Mesulam M-M. Large-scale neurocognitive networks and distributed processing for attention, memory, and language. Ann Neurol 1990; 28: 597–613.

Mesulam M. The evolving landscape of human cortical connectivity: facts and inferences. Neuroimage 2012; 62: 2182–2189.

Mesulam M, Siddique T, Cohen B. Cholinergic denervation in a pure multi-infarct state: observations on CADASIL. Neurology 2003; 60: 1183–1185.

Nieuwenhuys R. The myeloarchitectonic studies on the human cerebral cortex of the Vogt-Vogt school, and their significance for the interpretation of functional neuroimaging data. Brain Struct Funct 2013; 218: 303–352.

Ownby RL. Neuroinflammation and cognitive aging. Curr Psychiatry Rep 2010; 12: 39–45.

Ozdogmus O, Cavdar S, Ersoy Y, et al. A preliminary study, using electron and light-microscopic methods, of axon numbers in the fornix in autopsies of patients with temporal lobe epilepsy. Anat Sci Int 2009; 84: 2–6.

Parks EL, Madden DJ. Brain connectivity and visual attention. Brain Connect 2013; 3: 317–338.

Parvizi J, Damasio A. Consciousness and the brainstem. Cognition 2001; 79: 135–160.

Raichle ME, MacLeod AM, Snyder AZ, et al. A default mode of brain function. Proc Natl Acad Sci 2001: 98: 676–682.

Reeves TM, Smith TL, Williamson JC, Phillips LL. Unmyelinated axons show selective rostrocaudal pathology in the corpus callosum after traumatic brain injury. J Neuropathol Exp Neurol 2012; 71: 198–210.

Román GC. Cholinergic dysfunction in vascular dementia. Curr Psychiatry Rep 2005; 7: 18–26.

Sankowski R, Mader S, Valdés-Ferrer SI. Systemic inflammation and the brain: novel roles of genetic, molecular, and environmental cues as drivers of neurodegeneration. Front Cell Neurosci 2015; 9: 28.

Schmahmann JD. An emerging concept: the cerebellar contribution to higher function. Arch Neurol 1991; 48: 1178–1187.

Schmahmann JD. Disorders of the cerebellum: ataxia, dysmetria of thought, and the cerebellar cognitive affective syndrome. J Neuropsychiatry Clin Neurosci 2004; 16: 367–378.

Schmahmann JD. The role of the cerebellum in cognition and emotion: personal reflections since 1982 on the dysmetria of thought hypothesis, and its historical evolution from theory to therapy. Neuropsychol Rev 2010; 20: 236–260.

Schmahmann JD, Sherman JC. The cerebellar cognitive affective syndrome. Brain 1998; 121: 561–579.

Schmahmann JD, Pandya DN. *Fiber pathways of the brain*. Oxford: Oxford University Press, 2006.

Seeley WW, Menon V, Schatzberg AF, et al. Dissociable intrinsic connectivity networks for salience processing and executive control. J Neurosci 2007; 27: 2349–2356.

Selden NR, Gitelman DR, Salamon-Murayama N, et al. Trajectories of cholinergic pathways within the cerebral hemispheres of the human brain. Brain 1998; 121: 2249–2257.

Solari SV, Stoner R. Cognitive consilience: primate non-primary neuroanatomical circuits underlying cognition. Front Neuroanat 2011; 5: 65.

Sporns O. The human connectome: a complex network. *Ann N Y Acad Sci* 2011; 1224: 109–125.

Stenset V, Grambaite R, Reinvang I, et al. Diaschisis after thalamic stroke: a comparison of metabolic and structural changes in a patient with amnesic syndrome. Acta Neurol Scand Suppl 2007; 187: 68–71.

Stoodley CJ, Schmahmann JD. Functional topography in the human cerebellum: a meta-analysis of neuroimaging studies. Neuroimage 2009; 44: 489–501.

Stoodley CJ, Valera EM, Schmahmann JD. Functional topography of the cerebellum for motor and cognitive tasks: an fMRI study. Neuroimage 2012; 59: 1560–1570.

Swartz RH, Sahlas DJ, Black SE. Strategic involvement of cholinergic pathways and executive dysfunction: does location of white matter signal hyperintensities matter? J Stroke Cerebrovasc Dis 2003; 12: 29–36.

Tavor I, Yablonski M, Mezer A, et al. Separate parts of occipito-temporal white matter fibers are associated with recognition of faces and places. Neuroimage 2014; 86: 123–130.

Teipel SJ, Meindl T, Grinberg L, et al. Novel MRI techniques in the assessment of dementia. Eur J Nucl Med Mol Imaging 2008; 35 Suppl 1: S58–S69.

Toga AW, Clark KA, Thompson PM, et al. Mapping the human connectome. Neurosurgery 2012; 71: 1–5.

Van Essen DC, Smith SM, Barch DM, et al. The WU-Minn Human Connectome Project: an overview. Neuroimage 2013; 80: 62–79.

von Monakow C. Diaschisis. (1914 article translated by Harris G). In: Pribram KH, ed. *Brain and behavior: I. Mood states and mind*. Baltimore: Penguin Press, 1969: 27–36.

Wernicke K. *Der aphasiche symptomencomplex*. Breslau: Cohn and Weigert, 1874.

Yaffe K. Metabolic syndrome and cognitive disorders: is the sum greater than its parts? Alzheimer Dis Assoc Disord 2007; 21: 167–171.

Young RM. *Mind, brain, and adaptation in the nineteeth century*. London: Oxford University Press, 1970.

Zhang K, Sejnowski TJ. A universal scaling law between gray matter and white matter of cerebral cortex. Proc Natl Acad Sci 2000; 97: 5621–5626.

Chapter

13 Therapeutic innovations

The treatment of white matter disorders, as discussed in Chapter 11, is naturally based on the specific neuropathology involved, and progress is being made on all of the categories of white matter disorder considered in this book. It is now relevant to consider newer proposals that may be relevant to all manner of myelin disorders. These ideas invoke two fundamental objectives: the rapidly growing potential for preventing white matter damage before it occurs, and the intriguing notion of restoring myelin.

Prevention of white matter damage

The concept of dementia has unfortunately come to carry with it a nihilistic connotation related to the unavailability of not only curative treatment but also effective prevention. Even as it is acknowledged that common degenerative dementias such as Alzheimer's Disease (AD) have no prospect of cure in the foreseeable future, it is equally frustrating that no preventive measures have been identified. But this dismal picture appears to be changing. Whereas effective drug treatment for AD and most of the dementias still remains elusive, substantial evidence in recent decades has led to the arresting notion that a significant proportion of the pathogenesis of the dementias may be based on preventable factors. In contradistinction to the strong emphasis on genetic mutations associated with some dementias, such as early-onset autosomal-dominant AD and Huntington's Disease (HD), a growing body of knowledge now points to modifiable risk factors that play an important role in the etiopathogenesis of dementia. Genetics surely plays a role in many of the dementias, but the environment to which the brain is exposed is also being recognized as important in the origin of these disabling diseases.

Studies of the epidemiology of dementia have recently led to the conclusion that up to one-half of AD and dementia cases worldwide may be related to potentially modifiable risk factors (Barnes and Yaffe, 2011). These factors include midlife hypertension, diabetes mellitus, smoking, abdominal obesity, physical inactivity, low educational attainment, and depression (Barnes and Yaffe, 2011). Observations of this kind have led to a major shift in thinking about the dementias that is now gaining momentum. Conventional reasoning has held that because some dementia is genetically mediated, other genetic mutations lurking among affected patients have simply not been identified, but it has become clear that genetics may not answer all the remaining questions about pathogenesis. The opportunities presented by such common problems as hypertension, diabetes, smoking, obesity, and depression are crucial for clinicians seeking to prevent dementia, and the challenge of improving educational attainment presents a similar opportunity for society in general.

Still more remarkable in recent years have been observations that dementia may be a less common problem than in the past, quite plausibly because of efforts to deal with the same modifiable risk factors identified from epidemiological work. Large-scale studies in the United States (Rocca et al., 2011), England (Matthews et al., 2013), and Sweden (Qiu et al., 2013) have all indicated a declining burden of dementia since the 1980s, generally attributed to improved treatment of heart disease and stroke, disorders to which all of the modifiable risk factors listed earlier contribute. Closely related to the more effective treatment of problems such as heart disease and stroke is the availability of health care and education that permit and promote preventive intervention. The decline in dementia rates just noted has been observed in industrialized countries where people have greater access to the kinds of medical and societal resources that allow treatment of diseases that are becoming recognized as risk factors for dementia. Thus an unexpected but welcome avenue for addressing the dementia epidemic has been revealed. Even for the most dreaded of the dementias – AD – the

BOX 13.1 Acquired factors associated with white matter damage

- Hypertension
- Diabetes
- Obesity
- Smoking
- Hypercholesterolemia
- Metabolic syndrome
- Physical inactivity
- Low education
- Trauma
- Toxic insult
- Depression
- Sleep disturbance
- Delirium

prospects for prevention in many cases appear to be much more optimistic than in past years (Qiu, Kivipelto, and von Strauss, 2009; Filley, 2015).

In parallel with this development, new findings in epidemiology have also made it abundantly clear that a substantial proportion of white matter injury can be linked to acquired factors. White matter development and maintenance are to some extent under genetic control, but to an increasingly impressive extent, influences from the external milieu of the brain are being identified as crucial for the health of myelinated systems. Box 13.1 lists the acquired factors that have been putatively linked with damage to brain white matter. Because cerebrovascular disease and traumatic brain injury (TBI) account for much morbidity and mortality and are largely or completely preventable, the majority of patients affected by the disorders reviewed in Chapter 6 can be seen as having cognitive dysfunction or dementia that is primarily determined by acquired factors. The associations being discovered are particularly apparent in aging, a time in life when decades of exposure to a host of potentially injurious factors may have taken their toll. As white matter has so greatly expanded in evolution, so has it become especially vulnerable to the ravages of cardiovascular disease, trauma, and toxic insults, all of which can accumulate over the many years of life increasingly made possible, at least in developed countries, by the advances of modern medicine.

These insights lead to a revised view of dementia broadly considered, as the current approach to the problem often tends to be reactive more than proactive, seeking cure more vigorously than prevention. Whereas clinical medicine, including neurology, is more focused on the treatment of pathology after it has occurred, a public health approach may prove to be effective for the prevention of dementia, and attention to highly prevalent white matter pathology that can lead to white matter dementia (WMD) may be central. As will be considered in detail, white matter may also be fundamental to the understanding of other dementing disorders, including AD and chronic traumatic encephalopathy (CTE).

When all the dementias are considered, much recent evidence indicates that the most important environmental contributor is cerebrovascular disease. For at least the past decade, cerebrovascular disease has emerged as a central etiopathogenic consideration not just for vascular dementia but also for AD (Breteler, 2000), and together these categories account for the vast majority of dementias. At the origin of each may be damage to brain white matter. If public health efforts were to be concentrated in one area alone to prevent dementia, it is likely that cerebrovascular disease would be the one selected. The initiative to foster the notion of "brain attack" in acute stroke as analogous to "heart attack" may find a parallel in the world of dementia: prevention of a vascular assault on the brain may have enormous long-term value in preventing dementia (Filley, 2015).

If cerebrovascular disease is the most important acquired contributor to dementia, it would seem eminently reasonable to assess the impact of measures aimed at cerebrovascular risk factors on the incidence of various types of dementia. Hypertension would be the most obvious problem to address, but studies examining treatment of diabetes mellitus, metabolic syndrome, obesity, smoking, hypercholesterolemia, and physical inactivity would also be warranted. The effect of treatment on atherosclerosis is essential as one step, and promising data are appearing. To cite one relevant recent publication, encouraging results from a prospective study of stroke patients showed that the majority of high-grade intracranial atherosclerotic plaques regressed or remained quiescent after 12 months of intensive medical therapy that included antiplatelet medication and control of hypertension, diabetes, and hyperlipidemia (Leung et al., 2015).

Surprisingly little, however, has been done to examine the impact of such interventions on the development of dementia. Several longitudinal, randomized controlled trials of antihypertensive treatment have been conducted, but the primary outcomes involved cardiac disease and stroke incidence, and dementia was regarded as a secondary outcome (Valenzuela et al., 2012). Interesting data have been obtained nonetheless. The most provocative study with regard to dementia was the Systolic Hypertension in Europe (SYST-EUR) study, a large multicenter randomized controlled trial of antihypertensive medications in which the primary drug was the calcium channel blocker nitrendipine. The SYST-EUR trial showed that after a period of about 4 years, the incidence of dementia was reduced by 55%, and that the beneficial effect was apparent for both vascular dementia and AD (Forette et al., 2002). Other large studies have examined the effects of antihypertensive medications on dementia incidence, but the SYST-EUR study is the only one to show that dementia can be prevented by this form of treatment (Valenzuela et al., 2012). Of note, because the negative studies used thiazides, β-blockers, and angiotensin-converting enzyme inhibitors as antihypertensive agents, nitrendipine may have a special role in this setting, combining beneficial vascular effects with additional neuroprotective properties (Forette et al., 2002; Valenzuela et al., 2012). Whatever the mechanism(s), however, the SYST-EUR trial is remarkable in that it remains the only study that has ever provided evidence that a medication of any kind can lower the incidence of AD.

None of these studies specifically examined the white matter, however, and it is therefore possible only to speculate about whether the observed preventive advantage could be ascribed to protection of white matter integrity. An interesting study of non-demented elders showed that those with untreated hypertension had significantly greater progression of MRI white matter hyperintensities over 3.5 years than those whose hypertension was controlled with treatment (Verhaaren et al., 2013). Cognition was not evaluated in this study, but the accumulation of white matter hyperintensities could be expected to impair cognitive function. Further studies of antihypertensive treatment for dementia prevention are clearly needed, including longitudinal MRI examination of the white matter in parallel with serial cognitive assessment (Prins and Scheltens, 2015).

A related topic of much interest is the effect of lifestyle modifications on the preservation of white matter integrity. Recent data derived from normal elders have disclosed that a 2-year program of diet, exercise, and vascular risk monitoring produced a significant advantage in cognitive function compared to control participants (Ngandu et al., 2015). With regard to white matter, diffusion tensor imaging (DTI) studies of community-dwelling seniors have revealed that high cardiorespiratory fitness is correlated with increased fractional anisotropy (FA) in their corpus callosum (Johnson et al., 2012), and that physical exercise is associated with reduced mean diffusivity (MD) in numerous white matter regions (Gons et al., 2013). The benefits of exercise on white matter are also evident in children, as more physically fit 9- and 10-year-olds have been found to have higher FA in the corpus callosum, corona radiata, and superior longitudinal fasciculus (Chaddock-Heyman et al., 2014). Beyond these cross-sectional observations, a longitudinal DTI study of elders who participated in a 1-year aerobic exercise program that involved walking for 40 minutes three times per week demonstrated improved white matter integrity in frontal and temporal white matter regions (Voss et al., 2013).

One explanation for these effects could be an increase in cerebral blood flow that helps maintain the microstructure of myelinated tracts (Valenzuela et al., 2012). Lifestyle modifications may also enhance white matter integrity by reducing systemic inflammation, which has been implicated as a contributor to cognitive impairment in the metabolic syndrome (Yaffe, 2007). A DTI study, for example, showed that white matter microstructure improved as the level of the serum inflammatory marker C-reactive protein (CRP) declined (Bettcher et al., 2015). A critical research question raised by these studies is whether improving white matter integrity with physical exercise also improves cognitive performance (Voss et al., 2013; Prins and Scheltens, 2015). Much indirect evidence suggests that this conclusion will indeed be forthcoming.

An area of investigation that has recently received much attention with regard to many aspects of health and disease is sleep medicine. In comparison to disorders that are manifest during wakefulness, sleep has long been relatively neglected, in neurology as well as other medical disciplines, but this situation is changing rapidly. Evidence is steadily growing that sleep disturbances can affect cognitive function, and damage to white matter may be involved. In obstructive sleep apnea (OSA), executive function is commonly affected, and treatment with nocturnal devices providing continuous positive airway pressure (CPAP) can lead to improvement in this domain (Bucks, Olaithe, and Eastwood, 2013). In view of the association of white matter hyperintensities with not only OSA (Kim et al., 2013) but also a wide range of sleep disorders (Cheng et al., 2013), an appropriate question is whether treatment of sleep disturbances would be efficacious because of its capacity to prevent or even reverse white matter lesions. In this regard, a recent study of patients with OSA used DTI to show that treatment with CPAP resulted in impressive reversal of white matter abnormalities that occurred in parallel with improvement in working memory, attention, and executive function (Castronovo et al., 2014). In view of the possibility that white matter ischemic lesions are pathogenetically linked with the cortical lesions of AD (as will be discussed in Chapter 14), it is also noteworthy that normal sleep appears to enhance the clearance of β-amyloid from the brain (Xie et al., 2013) and that elders who report shorter sleep duration and poorer sleep quality accumulate more cortical β-amyloid (Spira et al., 2013).

Data coming to light in the past few years have called attention to another, largely unexpected setting that increases the risk for white matter damage, and these findings could potentially permit effective prevention in some cases. These new data come from the intensive care unit (ICU), where patients with critical illnesses, often involving multiple organs, are admitted for comprehensive and sometimes invasive medical and surgical care. The syndrome of delirium, often known as acute confusional state and metabolic-toxic encephalopathy, is common is such patients, particularly those who are older. Recent findings have documented that critical illness with delirium can result in long-term cognitive impairment (Pandharipande et al., 2013), and that the duration of delirium in the ICU is associated with cerebral white matter disruption, as assessed by DTI, at the time of discharge and 3 months later (Morandi et al., 2012). The mechanism of such injury is not known, and may well be a multifactorial combination of vascular, metabolic, and toxic insults (Morandi et al., 2012), but the implications of these findings may be important for patients in whom white matter injury was not formerly suspected. Intensivist physicians are already working to mitigate the adverse cognitive effects of critical illness and delirium, and measures such as more judicious use of sedatives and other centrally active medications, improved sleep, and early mobilization may all prove helpful (Pandharipande et al., 2013).

Finally, prevention of white matter injury would also be vastly enhanced by more effective control of the problem of traumatic brain injury (TBI). A critical neuropathological feature of TBI is diffuse axonal injury (DAI), a white matter lesion that contributes to static encephalopathy after moderate or severe TBI, and may be fundamental to the pathogenesis of both AD and chronic traumatic encephalopathy (CTE). The prevention of static encephalopathy alone justifies vigorous effort, but if degenerative dementia were also reduced by such efforts, immeasurable benefit could be realized. In AD, the damage to axons and myelin from DAI may be one of the processes that leads to the cascade of normal reparative events that in some cases eventuates in the clinical syndrome of AD (Bartzokis, 2011), and in CTE, multiple concussions are postulated to lead in some individuals to progressive tauopathy years later (McKee et al., 2009). As TBI occurs in a wide range of settings, effective prevention clearly requires a major public health effort. The wider use of seat belts and helmets, more stringent officiating of contact sports, and similar measures in civilian life would prove invaluable, and of course the reduction of TBI by diminished engagement in military conflicts would be desirable for a host of reasons.

In summary, preventive medicine may offer major benefits in terms of avoiding primary damage to white matter that could underlie common dementia syndromes. Although much remains to be learned, many of the dementias have important origins in acquired risk factors that implicate white matter, and in view of these insights, medical and societal measures to protect white matter integrity are warranted. A complete understanding of these complex issues will require consideration of many factors, but because cerebrovascular disease and TBI are so prevalent around the world, efforts targeting these problems alone could have enormous value. To illustrate this point, Figure 13.1 illustrates in simplified form how acquired insults to white matter may be central to the etiopathogenesis of both AD and CTE. In the two chapters that follow, these emerging relationships will be taken up in greater detail.

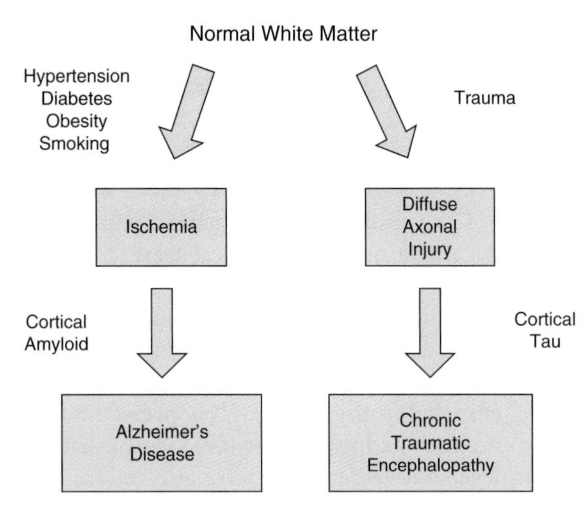

Figure 13.1 Simplified depiction of acquired factors implicated in the etiopathogenesis of two neurodegenerative diseases: Alzheimer's Disease and chronic traumatic encephalopathy.

Myelin repair

The idea that myelin in the brain may have some capacity to regenerate after its injury has long intrigued neurologists, and the often-disabling sequelae of demyelination in young adults with multiple sclerosis (MS) has stimulated the most interest (Lassmann et al., 1997; Franklin and Ffrench-Constant, 2008). More recently, thought has also been given to the repair of white matter ischemic and traumatic injuries (Salat, 2014; Shi et al., 2015). Interest in myelin repair has surged in other contexts as well, and the idea may have broad implications for the treatment of neurologic disease (Maki et al., 2013).

As a first point in this discussion, it is important to recognize that myelin repair occurs as a normal phenomenon in adulthood and aging. Although white matter volume declines in the aging process, as reviewed in Chapter 3, remyelination is evident in normal adulthood, and has been observed well into late life (Peters, 2009). Without this phenomenon, thought to be an ongoing response to oligodendrocyte stress and subsequent apoptotic death (Peters, 2009), the loss of white matter volume in aging would be even greater. The mechanism of remyelination in aging is thought to involve the differentiation of new oligodendrocytes from oligodendrocyte precursor cells (OPCs), also known as NG2 cells, which are scattered throughout the central nervous system (CNS) and constitute 5% of all glial cells (Levine, Reynolds, and Fawcett, 2001). In aging, the number of oligodendrocytes produced by this process of NG2 differentiation may increase by as much as 50% (Peters and Sethares, 2002). Given that oligodendrogenesis occurs under normal conditions, a natural assumption would be that the potential exists to facilitate this process for therapeutic benefit.

Vascular white matter disease is relevant in this context because myelin repair after vascular injury may be mediated by the formation of new oligodendrocytes. Recent laboratory investigations have demonstrated that oligodendrogenesis is stimulated by cerebral ischemia (Zhang, Chopp, and Zhang, 2013). Experimental studies have also suggested the possibility that several exogenous agents may be able to further enhance oligodendrogenesis after ischemia; one such drug is the familiar nonprescription drug aspirin (Chen et al., 2014), and others include erythropoietin, thymosin β4, cerberolysin, and sildenafil (Zhang, Chopp, and Zhang, 2013). In addition, myelin repair can conceivably be enhanced by angiogenesis within damaged white matter. This possibility is most relevant to stroke and related vascular white matter damage (Salat, 2014) but may also apply to TBI, in which microvascular injury regularly accompanies DAI (Xiong, Mahmood, and Chopp, 2010). Stimulation of angiogenesis has been observed with a diverse array of agents, including statins, sildenafil, erythropoietin, and various growth factors (Xiong, Mahmood, and Chopp, 2010), and the benefits of increasing perfusion to injured white matter by such treatments could be profound.

Turning to MS, remyelination would clearly be a direct means of addressing the fundamental pathology of this common disease. Remyelination is known to occur in MS, but the extent of effective repair of demyelinated axons is generally regarded as disappointingly modest (Franklin and Ffrench-Constant, 2008). Despite the repeated demonstration of the efficacy of remyelination in animal models of the disease, patients with MS are generally thought to gain clinical benefit only infrequently from this process (Franklin and Ffrench-Constant, 2008). Of interest, an exception to this rule may exist in the case of cortical remyelination. Recent evidence has indicated that remyelination in the cerebral cortex of MS patients is considerably more extensive than in lesions within large white matter tracts (Albert, Antel, and Brick, 2007; Chang et al., 2012). The result of this phenomenon may be the attenuation or abolition of cognitive deficits related to cortical lesions in MS, and robust cortical remyelination may help explain why the cognitive profile of MS more resembles other white matter disorders than cortical dementia such as AD (Chapter 7). However vigorous the remyelination of cortical versus subcortical lesions may be, the idea remains highly attractive, and investigation continues.

One line of inquiry considers the capacity of available immunotherapeutic agents for MS to enhance remyelination (Keough and Yong, 2013). Two of the existing drugs for this disease – glatiramer acetate and fingolimod, the first oral medication for MS – have been shown experimentally to have some potential for remyelination, but clinical data to support this capacity are at present lacking (Keough and Yong, 2013). The consensus view (Keough and Yong, 2013) is therefore that drugs specifically designed to enhance remyelination will be needed to complement the immunomodulation available through the existing MS armamentarium.

Looking ahead to new treatments, it is becoming clear that foundational to this work is the recognition that myelination is under the control of a wide range of molecular signals that could potentially be manipulated with beneficial result (Mitew et al., 2014). These signals are of two types: those that enhance myelination, and those that act to inhibit the process. Treatments for MS, and perhaps other white matter disorders in which remyelination is a goal, would therefore logically be aimed at either stimulating the factors that enhance myelination or inhibiting those that have the opposite effect. An agent that might stimulate remyelination, to cite but one example, is retinoic acid (Huang et al., 2011), and one intended to block the inhibition of remyelination is the anti-LINGO-1 antibody (Mi, Pepinsky, and Cadavid, 2013).

More recent information has introduced the idea that endogenous systems exist for the repair of white matter by potentiating the activity of normal oligodendrocytes. These systems may be restorative to white matter after damage of many varieties. One such system involves neuregulin, a protein growth factor that has been well recognized in the peripheral nervous system (PNS) and more recently in the central nervous system (CNS) as well (Hu et al., 2006). In the brain, neuregulin has been proposed to protect myelinated neurons in perinatal white matter injury (Dammann et al., 2008), and its contribution to myelination has been implicated in a variety of adult neuropsychiatric disorders (Mei and Nave, 2014). One key role of neuregulin appears to be its capacity to induce oligodendrocytes to remyelinate axons after white matter damage has been sustained (Lundgaard et al., 2013). Because neuregulin is activated by the enzyme β-secretase, also known as β-site APP cleaving enzyme (BACE), the generation of new myelin in response to injury may be accompanied by the formation of β-amyloid from its parent molecule amyloid precursor protein (APP) (Evin, Barakat, and Masters, 2010). Thus, because BACE has a dual mechanism, the restorative process of myelin repair may involve a simultaneously damaging accumulation of β-amyloid (Evin, Barakat, and Masters, 2010). As postulated by Bartzokis (2011), cortical β-amyloid may be a by-product of the continuous activation of neuregulin as it attempts to repair damaged myelin. The role of neuregulin with respect to both white matter repair and AD pathogenesis is thus of potentially great interest, and will be discussed further in the next chapter.

A related idea invokes the role of the apolipoprotein E (APOE) genotype in myelin repair, as it has been found that the APOE ε4 allele, with its associated protein ApoE ε4, is less effective in this process than the other common alleles ε2 or ε3. ApoE has many functions in the brain, among them the potentiation of β-amyloid formation, but its primary role is the transport of cholesterol, principally from astrocytes to neurons (Bu, 2009). The APOE ε2 and ε3 alleles may assist in myelin repair because they enhance the delivery of cholesterol and other lipids to damaged axons, whereas the ε4 allele may have the opposite effect (Bu, 2009). Recent DTI studies have in fact shown that the presence of the APOE ε4 allele exacerbates white matter injury related to vascular risk factors in older people, and accelerates cognitive decline (Wang et al., 2015) as assessed by the Mini-Mental State Examination (Folstein, Folstein, and McHugh, 1975). This genetic influence on myelin repair may also be relevant to AD. As again proposed by Bartzokis (2011), the APOE ε4 allele may predispose to AD by hindering cholesterol transport to myelin that has been damaged by vascular and other age-related insults. In contrast, the ε2 allele may be protective against AD because of more effective delivery of cholesterol to axons that enhances their repair (Bartzokis, 2011). This notion is supported by neuroimaging studies showing that cognitively normal

APOE ε4 carriers have (1) lower magnetic resonance imaging (MRI) white matter volume that correlates with slower processing speed (Ready et al., 2011), (2) decreased frontal white matter FA on DTI that correlates with lower executive function (Ryan et al., 2011), and (3) disrupted structural connectivity and diminished memory performance (Chen et al., 2015), whereas APOE ε2 carriers have higher FA in many white matter tracts (Chiang et al., 2012). The following chapter will consider in more detail the possible role of ineffective white matter repair in the pathogenesis of AD.

Stem cells

The idea of stem cell therapeutics has been attracting much attention in recent decades as a means of restoring normal function in the brain and spinal cord. The most obvious approach using stem cells is the targeting of damaged neurons, and the degenerative diseases offer many opportunities to test the efficacy of this strategy. Hence diseases such as Parkinson's Disease, HD, AD, and amyotrophic lateral sclerosis have been examined with regard to the possibility of replacing expiring or absent neurons with stem cells that can assume the function of the dysfunctional or lost cells (Lunn et al., 2011). The replacement cells could be implanted via grafting procedures or possibly delivered intravenously or intrathecally to the desired site in the brain. Whereas these exogenous stem cells have much promise in the treatment of diseases characterized by primary neuronal loss, the possibility also exists that endogenous stem cells can be exploited for the treatment of white matter disorders such as MS in which myelin damage is prominent (Franklin and Goldman, 2015). In this scenario, medical intervention would be intended to augment endogenous myelin repair mechanisms. Whereas the idea of using stem cells for treating neurologic disease has garnered most attention with respect to gray matter disease, stem cells may prove equally or even more efficacious for the treatment of white matter disorders (Maki et al., 2013; Braun and Jessberger, 2014).

The concept that neural stem cells could contribute to the prognosis of any neurologic disorder – originating in either gray or white matter – was not considered until recent years. For most of the history of neuroscience, it was firmly believed that neurologic and neurobehavioral functions are subserved by post-mitotic neurons, and recovery is solely a function of the activity of those neurons that remain intact after brain insult. Beginning in the 1960s, a remarkable series of observations has produced the steady accumulation of evidence indicating that neurogenesis – the generation of new neurons – actually does occur in the adult human brain (Ming and Song, 2011). Under normal conditions, these neurons are generated from precursor cells in two primary sites: the dentate gyrus of the hippocampus, and the subventricular zone adjacent to the lateral ventricle (Ming and Song, 2011). More recently, it was recognized that new glial cells are also generated in the adult human brain, and, in particular, OPCs that are widely distributed in the brain can differentiate into functional oligodendrocytes (Levine, Reynolds, and Fawcett, 2001). With the knowledge now accumulating on various stem cells, a new vista of opportunities has been revealed for improving the outcome of devastating disorders of cognition, many of which implicate white matter neuropathology.

Of the white matter disorders, MS, cerebral ischemia, the leukodystrophies, and periventricular leukomalacia have attracted the most attention as diseases that could be treated by stimulation of endogenous OPCs, the use of exogenous stem cells, or both (Goldman, Schanz, and Windrem, 2008; Ben-Hur, 2011; Zhang, Chopp, and Zhang, 2013; Vanderver et al., 2014; Chen et al., 2014). In the case of MS, in which remyelination is notoriously incomplete (Franklin and Ffrench-Constant, 2008), researchers have pondered the use of endogenous or exogenous stem cells as an approach to the long-elusive challenge of enhancing remyelination (Ben-Hur, 2011). From a clinical perspective, there are many obvious advantages of using the brain's existing precursor cells to repair myelin, and the idea that even a drug as familiar as aspirin (discussed previously) could be useful in enhancing oligodendrogenesis is most appealing. The relative simplicity and safety of stimulating endogenous brain cells to repair the white matter render this option preferable to the use of invasive methods – most notably intracerebral implantation of exogenous stem cells – that would entail more risk and expense. However, it has been pointed out that the typically feeble remyelination in MS is in part due to the axonal loss that occurs in many areas of demyelination, and because this process can occur early in MS, all options should be kept open (Ben-Hur, 2011). Indeed, an open-label study of intravenous and intrathecal mesenchymal stem cells in MS patients suggested clinical improvement without major side effects (Karussis et al., 2010).

Stem cell neurobiology, however, while surely exciting in ways that could not be imagined even a few decades ago, is still a field that is clearly in its formative stages, and much remains to be learned. In addition to ethical issues centering on the use of fetal tissue that dominated the field in its early years and at times still prove contentious, the technical challenges of this approach are far from trivial. Research will continue, and clinicians will await with interest the outcomes of many parallel investigations. The ultimate utility of stem cell therapeutics will likely depend not only on the details of how both endogeous and exogenous cells may be exploited, but also on the specific neuropathology and pathogenesis of the disorder being considered for treatment.

References

Albert M, Antel J, Brück W, Stadelmann C. Extensive cortical remyelination in patients with chronic multiple sclerosis. Brain Pathol 2007; 17: 129–138.

Barnes DE, Yaffe K. The projected effect of risk factor reduction on Alzheimer's disease prevalence. Lancet Neurol 2011; 10: 819–828.

Bartzokis G. Alzheimer's disease as homeostatic responses to age-related myelin breakdown. Neurobiol Aging 2011; 32: 1341–1371.

Ben-Hur T. Cell therapy for multiple sclerosis. Neurotherapeutics 2011; 8: 625–642.

Bettcher BM, Yaffe K, Boudreau RM, et al. Declines in inflammation predict greater white matter microstructure in older adults. Neurobiol Aging 2015; 36: 948–954.

Braun SM, Jessberger S. Adult neurogenesis and its role in neuropsychiatric disease, brain repair and normal brain function. Neuropathol Appl Neurobiol 2014; 40: 3–12.

Breteler MM. Vascular risk factors for Alzheimer's disease: an epidemiologic perspective. Neurobiol Aging 2000; 21: 153–160.

Bu G. Apolipoprotein E and its receptors in Alzheimer's disease: pathways, pathogenesis and therapy. Nat Rev Neurosci 2009; 10: 333–344.

Bucks RS, Olaithe M, Eastwood P. Neurocognitive function in obstructive sleep apnoea: a meta-review. Respirology 2013; 18: 61–70.

Castronovo V, Scifo P, Castellano A, et al. White matter integrity in obstructive sleep apnea before and after treatment. Sleep 2014; 37: 1465–1475.

Chaddock-Heyman L, Erickson KI, Holtrop JL, et al. Aerobic fitness is associated with greater white matter integrity in children. Front Hum Neurosci 2014; 8: 584.

Chang A, Staugaitis SM, Dutta R, et al. Cortical remyelination: a new target for repair therapies in multiple sclerosis. Ann Neurol 2012; 72: 918–926.

Chen J, Zuo S, Wang J, et al. Aspirin promotes oligodendrocyte precursor cell proliferation and differentiation after white matter lesion. Front Aging Neurosci 2014; 6: 7.

Chen Y, Chen K, Zhang J, et al. Disrupted functional and structural networks in cognitively normal elderly subjects with the APOE ε4 allele. Neuropsychopharmacology 2015; 40: 1181–1191.

Cheng CY, Tsai CF, Wang SJ, et al. Sleep disturbance correlates with white matter hyperintensity in patients with subcortical ischemic vascular dementia. J Geriatr Psychiatry Neurol 2013; 26: 158–164.

Chiang GC, Zhan W, Schuff N, Weiner MW. White matter alterations in cognitively normal apoE ε2 carriers: insight into Alzheimer resistance? AJNR 2012; 33: 1392–1397.

Dammann O, Bueter W, Leviton A, et al. Neuregulin-1: a potential endogenous protector in perinatal brain white matter damage. Neonatology 2008; 93: 182–187.

Evin G, Barakat A, Masters CL. BACE: therapeutic target and potential biomarker for Alzheimer's disease. Int J Biochem Cell Biol 2010; 42: 1923–1926.

Filley CM. Alzheimer's Disease prevention: new optimism. Neurol Clin Pract 2015; 5: 193–200.

Folstein MF, Folstein SE, McHugh PR. "Mini-Mental State": a practical method of grading the cognitive state of patients for the clinician. J Psychiat Res 1975; 12: 189–198.

Forette F, Seux ML, Staessen JA, et al. The prevention of dementia with antihypertensive treatment: new evidence from the Systolic Hypertension in Europe (Syst-Eur) study. Arch Intern Med 2002; 162: 2046–2052.

Franklin RJ, Ffrench-Constant C. Remyelination in the CNS: from biology to therapy. Nat Rev Neurosci 2008; 9: 839–855.

Franklin RJ, Goldman SA. Glia disease and repair-remyelination. Cold Spring Harb Perspect Biol 2015; 2015; 7 (7). pii: a020594.

Goldman SA, Schanz S, Windrem MS. Stem cell–based strategies for treating pediatric disorders of myelin. Hum Mol Genet 2008; 17: 876–883.

Gons RA, Tuladhar AM, de Laat KF, et al. Physical activity is related to the structural integrity of cerebral white matter. Neurology 2013; 81: 971–976.

Hu X, Hicks CW, He W, et al. Bace1 modulates myelination in the central and peripheral nervous system. Nat Neurosci 2006; 9: 1520–1525.

Huang JK, Jarjour AA, Nait Oumesmar B, et al. Retinoid X receptor gamma signaling accelerates CNS remyelination. Nat Neurosci 2011; 14: 45–53.

Johnson NF, Kim C, Clasey JL, et al. Cardiorespiratory fitness is positively correlated with cerebral white matter integrity in healthy seniors. Neuroimage 2012; 59: 1514–1523.

Karussis D, Karageorgiou C, Vaknin-Dembinsky C, et al. Safety and immunological effects of mesenchymal stem cell transplantation in patients with multiple sclerosis and amyotrophic lateral sclerosis. Arch Neurol 2010; 67: 1187–1194.

Keough MB, Yong VW. Remyelination therapy for multiple sclerosis. Neurotherapeutics 2013; 10: 44–54.

Kim H, Yun CH, Thomas RJ, et al. Obstructive sleep apnea as a risk factor for cerebral white matter change in a middle-aged and older general population. Sleep 2013; 36: 709–715B.

Lassmann H, Brück W, Lucchinetti C, Rodriguez M. Remyelination in multiple sclerosis. Mult Scler 1997; 3: 133–136.

Leung TW, Wang L, Soo YO, et al. Evolution of intracranial atherosclerotic disease under modern medical therapy. Ann Neurol 2015; 77: 478–486.

Levine JM, Reynolds R, Fawcett JW. The oligodendrocyte precursor cell in health and disease. Trends Neurosci 2001; 24: 39–47.

Lundgaard I, Luzhynskaya A, Stockley JH, et al. Neuregulin and BDNF induce a switch to NMDA receptor-dependent myelination by oligodendrocytes. PLoS Biol 2013; 11: e1001743.

Lunn JS, Sakowski SA, Hur J, Feldman EL. Stem cell technology for neurodegenerative diseases. Ann Neurol 2011; 70: 353–361.

Maki T, Liang AC, Miyamoto N, et al. Mechanisms of oligodendrocyte regeneration from ventricular-subventricular zone-derived progenitor cells in white matter diseases. Front Cell Neurosci 2013; 7: 275.

Matthews FE, Arthur A, Barnes LE, et al. A two-decade comparison of prevalence of dementia in individuals aged 65 years and older from three geographical areas of England: results of the Cognitive Function and Ageing Study I and II. Lancet 2013; 382: 1405–1412.

McKee AC, Cantu RC, Nowinski CJ, et al. Chronic traumatic encephalopathy in athletes: progressive tauopathy after repetitive head injury. J Neuropathol Exp Neurol 2009; 68: 709–735.

Mei L, Nave KA. Neuregulin-ERBB signaling in the nervous system and neuropsychiatric diseases. Neuron 2014; 83: 27–49.

Mi S, Pepinsky RB, Cadavid D. Blocking LINGO-1 as a therapy to promote CNS repair: from concept to the clinic. CNS Drugs 2013; 27: 493–503.

Ming GL, Song H. Adult neurogenesis in the mammalian brain: significant answers and significant questions. Neuron 2011; 70: 687–702.

Mitew S, Hay CM, Peckham H, et al. Mechanisms regulating the development of oligodendrocytes and central nervous system myelin. Neuroscience 2014; 276: 29–47.

Morandi A, Rogers BP, Gunther ML, et al. The relationship between delirium duration, white matter integrity, and cognitive impairment in intensive care unit survivors as determined by diffusion tensor imaging: the VISIONS prospective cohort magnetic resonance imaging study. Crit Care Med 2012; 40: 2182–2189.

Ngandu T, Lehtisalo J, Solomon A, et al. A 2 year multidomain intervention of diet, exercise, cognitive training, and vascular risk monitoring versus control to prevent cognitive decline in at-risk elderly people (FINGER): a randomised controlled trial. Lancet 2015; 385: 2255–2263.

Pandharipande PP, Girard TD, Jackson JC, et al. Long-term cognitive impairment after critical illness. N Engl J Med 2013; 369: 1306–1316.

Peters A. The effects of normal aging on myelinated nerve fibers in monkey central nervous system. Front Neuroanat 2009; 3: 11.

Peters A, Sethares C. Aging and the myelinated fibers in prefrontal cortex and corpus callosum of the monkey. J Comp Neurol 2002; 442: 277–291.

Prins ND, Scheltens P. White matter hyperintensities, cognitive impairment and dementia: an update. Nat Rev Neurol 2015; 11: 157–165.

Qiu C, Kivipelto M, von Strauss E. Epidemiology of Alzheimer's disease: occurrence, determinants, and strategies toward intervention. Dialogues Clin Neurosci 2009; 11: 111–128.

Qiu C, von Strauss E, Bäckman L, et al. Twenty-year changes in dementia occurrence suggest decreasing incidence in central Stockholm, Sweden. Neurology 2013; 80: 1888–1894.

Ready RE, Baran B, Chaudhry M, et al. Apolipoprotein E-e4, processing speed, and white matter volume in a genetically enriched sample of midlife adults Am J Alzheimers Dis Other Demen 2011; 26: 463–468.

Rocca WA, Petersen RC, Knopman DS, et al. Trends in the incidence and prevalence of Alzheimer's disease, dementia, and cognitive impairment in the United States. Alzheimers Dement 2011; 7: 80–93.

Ryan L, Walther K, Bendlin BB, et al. Age-related differences in white matter integrity and cognitive function are related to APOE status. Neuroimage 2011; 54: 1565–1577.

Salat DH. Imaging small vessel–associated white matter changes in aging. Neuroscience 2014; 276: 174–186.

Shi H, Hu X, Leak RK, Shi Y, et al. Demyelination as a rational therapeutic target for ischemic or traumatic brain injury. Exp Neurol 2015 Mar 24. [Epub ahead of print]

Spira AP, Gamaldo AA, An Y, et al. Self-reported sleep and β-amyloid deposition in community-dwelling older adults. JAMA Neurol 2013; 70: 1537–1543.

Valenzuela M, Esler M, Ritchie K, Brodaty H. Antihypertensives for combating dementia? A perspective on candidate molecular mechanisms and population-based prevention. Transl Psychiatry 2012; 2: e107.

Vanderver A, Tonduti D, Schiffmann R, et al. Leukodystrophy overview. In: Pagon RA, Adam MP, Ardinger HH, Wallace SE, Amemiya A, Bean LJH, Bird TD, Dolan CR, Fong CT, Smith RJH, Stephens K, eds. GeneReviews® [Internet]. Seattle: University of Washington, Seattle; 1993–2015. 2014 Feb 6.

Verhaaren BF, Vernooij MW, de Boer R, et al. High blood pressure and cerebral white matter lesion progression in the general population. Hypertension 2013; 61: 1354–1359.

Voss MW, Heo S, Prakash RS, et al. The influence of aerobic fitness on cerebral white matter integrity and cognitive function in older adults: results of a one-year exercise intervention. Hum Brain Mapp 2013; 34: 2972–2985.

Wang R, Fratiglioni L, Laukka EJ, et al. Effects of vascular risk factors and APOE ε4 on white matter integrity and cognitive decline. Neurology 2015; 84: 1128–1135.

Xie L, Kang H, Xu Q, et al. Sleep drives metabolite clearance from the adult brain. Science 2013; 342: 373–377.

Xiong Y, Mahmood A, Chopp M. Angiogenesis, neurogenesis and brain recovery of function following injury. Curr Opin Investig Drugs 2010; 11: 298–308.

Yaffe K. Metabolic syndrome and cognitive disorders: is the sum greater than its parts? Alzheimer Dis Assoc Disord 2007; 21: 167–171.

Zhang R, Chopp M, Zhang ZG. Oligodendrogenesis after cerebral ischemia. Front Cell Neurosci 2013; 7: 201.

Chapter 14

Alzheimer's Disease and white matter

The distinctions between categories of dementia made in this book buttress the view that the clinical features and neuropathological basis of Alzheimer's Disease (AD) differ markedly from those of white matter dementia (WMD). Indeed, the cognitive and emotional sequelae of cortical dysfunction offer a useful contrast to the neurobehavioral features associated with white matter involvement. These distinctions can serve not only to sharpen the clinical differentiation of various dementias, but also to better characterize the contributions of various brain components to the normal human behavioral repertoire. White matter and gray matter, in short, complement each other in the operations of cognition and emotion.

The entities of WMD and AD may not, however, be entirely separate. In light of a more nuanced perspective that includes the contribution of white matter, even the firmly entrenched view that AD is a cortical dementia at all stages of the illness may need revision. This potential revision is founded on the intriguing possibility that the neuropathology of AD may originate in cerebral white matter (Bartzokis, 2011). This arresting notion has prompted a turn toward considering the potential role of white matter in AD (Gold et al., 2012; Brickman et al., 2012b; Sachdev et al., 2013), and in particular requires a revision of conventional thinking regarding the classic histologic hallmarks of neuritic (amyloid) plaques and neurofibrillary tangles. In contrast to the conventional view that cortical amyloid and its oligomers are the primary toxic agents in the disease, the idea is emerging that amyloid may have a more complex role in the disease, perhaps even involving a protective effect in the early stages of AD etiopathogenesis.

Background

The problem of AD has been extensively recognized in recent decades as the aging of the population has become a central demographic feature of contemporary society. Aging is by far the strongest risk factor for AD, and the steady graying of the population implies an alarming increase in prevalence. The most common degenerative dementia, AD now afflicts some 5 million people in the United States alone, and by 2050 this number may reach 14 million (Thies et al., 2013). If no means to reverse or retard the clinical progression of the disease is found, the medical system and society as a whole will be faced with the formidable challenge of caring for increasing numbers of demented adults with multiple care needs not easily met. In this context, the need to find the cause and cure of AD is ever more urgent.

In the absence of a serendipitous discovery, finding effective treatment for AD will require an understanding of its etiology and pathogenesis. Yet this knowledge has proven remarkably elusive. A sobering comparison to the dementia of the acquired immunodeficiency syndrome (AIDS) can be aptly drawn: Despite AD being known for more than a century, there are still huge gaps in the understanding of its etiopathogenesis, preventive strategies, and effective pharmacotherapy, all of which are available for the dementia of AIDS despite its recognition as recently as the early 1980s.

AD does indeed present unique challenges as investigators grapple with unraveling its mysteries. In contrast to other pathological processes, both within the nervous system and elsewhere in the body, that involve recognizable gross or microscopic abnormalities such as ischemia, inflammation, neoplasia, and so on, the pathology of AD is fundamentally different. The disease is classified as neurodegenerative, like many other equally puzzling entities in neurology such as frontotemporal lobar degeneration, Parkinson's Disease, Huntington's Disease, and amyotrophic lateral sclerosis, and features the seemingly inexplicable disappearance of neurons. These diseases differ with respect to the location of neurons at risk, but all are similarly mysterious because there is in fact no neuropathological process that unequivocally accounts for the loss of cells. AD manifests a predilection for hippocampal and neocortical neurons, but the origin of the particular degenerative process at work in AD is as opaque as that of its companion degenerative diseases. The presence of neuritic plaques and neurofibrillary tangles has been a histologic clue motivating much work since Alois Alzheimer's first case came to light more than a century ago, but it is far from clear how these changes play a role in the etiopathogenesis of the disease.

The amyloid hypothesis

The search for the cause of AD has been dominated by a focus on the neuropathological hallmarks of the disease – commonly known simply as "plaques and tangles." That this should be so is not surprising in view of Alzheimer's initial observations in 1907: The striking preponderance of abundant and seemingly destructive plaques and tangles naturally directs attention to the neurobiology of these histologic findings. A major effort has been devoted to identifying the nature and importance of these cortical changes, and neuroscientists have tended to focus on either plaques or tangles as topics of primary investigation.

Neuritic plaques are extracellular collections of dystrophic neurites with a core of amyloid, an insoluble 42-amino acid protein known as ß-amyloid (ß-AP, or simply Aß) that is enzymatically cleaved from amyloid precursor protein (APP), its parent membrane-bound protein (Querfurth and LaFerla, 2010). In addition, Aß is also deposited in cerebral blood vessels in many cases, a condition known as cerebral amyloid angiopathy (CAA), and smaller amyloid oligomers are postulated to be toxic to cortical synapses (Querfurth and LaFerla, 2010; Koffie, Hyman, and Spires-Jones, 2011). Neurofibrillary tangles, in contrast, are intracellular collections of an abnormal protein called hyperphosphorylated tau (Querfurth and LaFerla, 2010). Both plaques and tangles are abundantly evident in autopsy cases of AD, and, somewhat facetiously, researchers in this field have come to be designated as either ß-APtists or tau-ists to signify their allegiance to one or the other histologic finding.

The majority of work on AD etiopathogenesis has been devoted to Aß, and the so-called amyloid hypothesis has come to dominate the field (Querfurth and LaFerla, 2010; Jack et al., 2010; Bateman et al., 2012). Although considerable work has been done and continues on tau metabolism (Iqbal, Liu, and Gong, 2014), current thinking favors the view that neurofibrillary tangles follow neuritic plaques in the neuropathological sequence that occurs in AD (Hardy and Selkoe, 2002; Querfurth and LaFerla, 2010). The intensity of focus on amyloid has considerable justification, as much evidence supports a prominent role of Aß in AD etiopathogenesis. The development of this idea merits consideration in some detail, as a tremendous effort to discover treatments for AD has followed its introduction.

The origin of the amyloid hypothesis of AD can be dated to 1984, when Aß was first sequenced post-mortem from meningeal blood vessels of AD patients (Glenner and Wong, 1984a), and from the brains of patients with AD as well as those with Down syndrome (DS) (Glenner and Wong, 1984b). A year later, the same protein was found to be the major constituent of neuritic plaques isolated from the brains of AD patients (Masters et al., 1985). As it was known that essentially all people with DS develop AD neuropathology if they live until age 50, investigation turned to the fact that DS features a third chromosome 21, and 1987 witnessed the discovery that the APP gene on this chromosome gives rise to Aß (Tanzi et al., 1987). These observations provided a significant insight into AD etiopathogenesis, implying that Aß is the pathogenic agent in both AD and DS, and that AD is likely to be strongly influenced by genetic factors.

As time went on, all of the known genetic risk factors for AD, including the three genes linked with autosomal-dominant familial AD (APP, presenilin-1, and presenilin-2), the trisomy 21 of DS, and the apolipoprotein E (APOE) ε4 genotype, are associated with excess Aß deposition (Hardy and Selkoe, 2002). If all of these genetic conditions lead to the accumulation of Aß, it is reasoned, then all AD may plausibly be caused by cortical amyloid toxicity (Hardy and Selkoe, 2002). This summary statement is the essence of the amyloid hypothesis, which was later somewhat modified to become the amyloid cascade hypothesis in view of neuropathological effects such as tau formation, neuronal loss, and synaptic destruction that are seen as a later result of Aß deposition (Hardy and Selkoe, 2002; Querfurth and LaFerla, 2010).

Although the amyloid hypothesis remains a proposal without proof, its plausibility has focused much attention on the development of neuroimaging technologies designed to provide visual evidence of the proteins that characterize AD. These methods involve positron emission tomography (PET) of the brain in combination with the intravenous injection of an agent that can bind to amyloid or tau, with the goal of noninvasively disclosing the location and extent of protein deposition in vivo. Most of the effort in this area has been devoted to amyloid imaging, and in 2004 the first human study appeared of the amyloid tracer Pittsburgh compound B (PiB) (Klunk et al., 2004). With further study, the amyloid ligand florbetapir was introduced, and in 2012 this agent was the first such ligand to be approved by the United States Food and Drug Administration as a diagnostic adjunct for AD (Vandenberge et al., 2013). Not to be outdone, investigators of neurofibrillary tangles have also been at work, and a tau ligand called T807 has recently been introduced as an injectable agent that can be used with PET to permit visualization of hyperphosphorylated tau in the living brain (Xia et al., 2013). Other tau ligands are also in development. Even though no therapeutic benefit has yet been shown by the use of amyloid and tau imaging, the imaging of protein aggregations in the AD brain is clearly a step forward.

The dominance of the amyloid hypothesis has motivated a quest to eradicate amyloid in the search for the long-sought cure for AD. The idea has strongly taken hold within the AD research community, motivating many multicenter clinical trials to cure the disease by eliminating amyloid from the AD brain. One of the most compelling reasons motivating these trials in humans came from work with transgenic mice that demonstrated significant attenuation of AD neuropathology with an active vaccine known as AN-1792 (Schenk et al., 1999). Human trials were rapidly organized and initiated, but unfortunately the appearance of meningoencephalitis in 6% of subjects who received AN-1792 forced the termination of the trial (Orgogozo et al., 2003), and no clinical benefit on the symptoms of AD could be demonstrated.

In response, efforts were then focused on the development of passive vaccination, and several anti-amyloid antibodies have been studied in large clinical trials. While these drugs have proven less toxic, the use of immunotherapeutic agents such as bapineuzumab (Salloway et al., 2014) and solaneuzumab (Doody et al., 2014) has not yet proven successful in treating AD. Moreover, the use of functional imaging with PET and amyloid tracers in these trials has shown that the cortical amyloid can in fact be reduced while still leaving the dementia of AD unaffected (Reitz, 2012). A major challenge to the amyloid hypothesis has thus been presented with mounting evidence that eradicating the putatively toxic protein has no effect on dementia (Hardy, 2009; Castellani and Smith, 2011; Reitz, 2012).

In considering how the amyloid hypothesis of AD can be misleading, it is important to begin with the fact that AD neuropathology has been typically documented only at autopsy, obviously late in the disease course. Although useful for many diagnostic and research purposes, the observations of terminal brain pathology prompt the question of what happens first in the disease. Perhaps some unrelated phenomena occur earlier in the individual's life, or upstream of the AD process seen at postmortem examination. Thus plaques and tangles may both be of lesser importance than commonly thought, or even epiphenomenal in etiopathogenesis. Indeed, it has been suggested that Aß and its relative APP may have a protective role, acting as damage-response proteins early in the course of AD (Hardy, 2009; Giuffrida et al., 2009; Castellani and Smith, 2011). The function of APP is not well understood, but evidence exists that this transmembrane glycoprotein has an important role in synapse formation and function, and thus may be protective rather than destructive (Hoe, Lee, and Pak, 2012). Moreover, Aß has been found to have anti-oxidant (Castellani and Smith, 2011) and anti-excitotoxic (Giuffrida et al., 2009) effects, implying that amyloid serves a physiological purpose in counteracting the oxidative stress known to occur in aging (Santos et al., 2013) and in AD (Parker, Parks, and Filley, 1994). A cogent argument can thus be made that (1) APP and Aß represent an active host response or adaptation to a previous and unrelated insult or multiple insults, and (2) plaques and tangles may be signatures of physiology and not pathology, meaning that APP, Aß, and tau are thus consequences of the AD pathogenesis rather than its cause (Castellani and Perry, 2014).

In this light, the widely accepted neurotoxicity of Aß may need to be reconsidered. Whereas cortical injury related to neuronal and synapse loss is likely a component of the pathophysiological cascade, Aß may have a more subtle role than has been assumed, particularly early in the course, when Aß may have beneficial properties in the mounting of a host response to prior insults (Castellani et al., 2008). Studies in mice, for example, have shown that traumatic brain injury (TBI) causes Aß accumulation (Tran et al., 2011), and in humans as young as 10 years of age TBI produces cortical Aß deposition within hours of injury (Roberts et al., 1994). These data have led to the notion that Aß deposition may be a normal acute-phase response to neuronal stress (Roberts et al., 1994; Castellani et al., 2008; Castellani et al., 2009).

Another important point germane to this discussion is that many cognitively normal elders who come to autopsy have been documented to harbor abundant plaques and tangles, often in sufficient amounts to justify the diagnosis of definite AD (Davis et al., 1999; Schmitt et al., 2000; Gandy and DeKosky, 2013). These observations clearly pose another obstacle to the amyloid hypothesis, and may again imply that the histologic changes in the cortex may in fact be beneficial in preventing the clinical syndrome of dementia. It may be that amyloid will be shown to have two roles, first serving as a protective agent in aging, and then acting as a destructive influence when the reparative process is overwhelmed.

The myelin model of Alzheimer's Disease

The many disappointments of the amyloid hypothesis have led clinicians and investigators to ask whether another research approach to the problem of AD may be warranted. Many conversations on AD pathogenesis now turn to the perceived need for a "new paradigm" in AD research that may refresh a struggling field with new ideas (Rapoport and Nelson, 2011). One of the insights that has generated thinking about such a new paradigm stems from the recognition that AD seems to be a uniquely human disease (Rapoport and Nelson, 2011; Bufill, Blesa, and Augustí, 2013). No other animal has been found to develop comparable amounts of brain amyloid and tau (Rapoport and Nelson, 2011), and even transgenic AD mouse models do not completely reproduce the human disease (Ashe and Zahs, 2010). The uniqueness of AD strongly suggests a search for what is singular about the human brain that would render it vulnerable to the AD process (Rapoport and Nelson, 2011). This question in turn raises the topic of evolution, which can shed much light on interspecies variation, and considerable evidence from comparative neuroanatomy exists to begin finding an answer. As reviewed in Chapter 3, one unique feature of the human brain is the salience of white matter, which has expanded in mammalian evolution to a greater extent than gray matter (Zhang and Sejnowski, 2000; Schoenemann, Sheehan, and Glotzer, 2005; Smaers et al., 2010), and is crucial to human cognitive abilities (Roth and Dicke, 2005; Bartzokis, 2011).

In this context, the "myelin model of AD" (Bartzokis, 2011) arises as a provocative alternative to the conventional wisdom that amyloid toxicity is central to AD etiopathogenesis. This hypothesis posits that the vulnerability of aging myelin to a host of insults such as ischemia, trauma, and iron excess may initiate a cascade of events culminating in dementia, and that plaques and tangles are markers of failed myelin repair rather than primary neuropathological lesions (Bartzokis, 2011). Normal aging is seen as a process involving the gradual accumulation of white matter insults for which compensatory responses implicating amyloid and tau can be effective only up to a certain point (Bartzokis, 2011). The slowing of cognition, mild executive dysfunction, and subtle attentional deficits of normal aging result from normal white matter changes, and AD develops only when the deposition of cortical amyloid and tau reaches a threshold level so that the characteristic amnesia, aphasia, apraxia, and agnosia become evident (Bartzokis, 2011).

The myelin model begins with the assumption that AD is a disease seen only in humans (Rapoport and Nelson, 2011; Bufill, Blesa, and Augustí, 2013). This specificity has proven a major obstacle to laboratory investigation of AD because animal models of the disease are in many respects inadequate. Transgenic mouse models, for example, in which the mice are manipulated to express brain amyloid, cannot be regarded as having AD because they typically lack the essential feature of neurodegeneration (Hall and Roberson, 2012). In other words, mice can be genetically manipulated to express abnormal brain protein, but this does not mean the animals have AD. In recognition of this limitation, the term "mouseheimer's" has been offered to describe the state of the brain that is produced in search of an AD animal model (Whitehouse, 2014). It should not be surprising, however, that a disease primarily affecting neurobehavioral function is confined to uniquely human regions of the brain. The greatly expanded cerebral cortex of *Homo sapiens* is one such region, and has been extensively examined as a target region for the neuropathology of AD. But the white matter is another such region, as it is most extensively developed in humans compared to other mammals (Zhang and Sejnowski, 2000; Bartzokis, 2011). An apt analogy to the Internet has been proposed, signifying that white matter subserves a critical integrative function uniquely related to human cognition (Bartzokis, 2011). In the myelin model of AD, the origin of AD neuropathology is to be found in the cerebral white matter.

Within this body of brain tissue, fertile soil comes to exist for the appearance of early neuropathology that could be the harbinger of the plaques and tangles that will follow. As discussed in Chapter 3, normal aging involves a decline in white matter volume (Bartzokis et al., 2001), sometimes referred to as white matter retrogenesis (Brickman et al., 2012a; Alves et al., 2015). With aging, therefore, the white matter becomes increasingly vulnerable to structural decline as a result of its normal developmental trajectory in late life (Bartzokis, 2011). Figure 14.1 displays the age-related white matter decline in humans that affects both major tracts and intracortical myelin (Bartzokis et al., 2001; Bartzokis, 2011). Many insults can affect these regions, particularly the large association and commissural tracts, and the most important of these insults are likely vascular in origin (Bartzokis, 2011; Salat, 2014). An important vulnerability of white matter derives from the fact that it is highly dependent on continuous energy supply; while oligodendrocytes require 2 to 3 times the energy of other brain cells for normal function, the white matter is supplied with less robust vascular supply from the relatively narrow penetrating arterioles that irrigate the deep structures of the cerebral hemispheres. Another insult to which white matter is uniquely vulnerable is the diffuse axonal injury (DAI) of TBI. Thus the two most common brain lesions acquired in the years before the usual age of AD onset – vascular disease followed by TBI – can both be seen as harbingers of AD through their impact on white matter: Stroke is firmly recognized as an AD risk factor (Gorelick et al., 2011), and moderate to severe TBI increases the risk of AD two- to fourfold (Plassman et al., 2000).

A key feature of this hypothesis is that amyloid may be toxic only late in the course of AD pathogenesis, after the early phase when it may in fact represent a protective response to insults such as ischemia, TBI, oxidative stress, and inflammation (Castellani et al., 2008; Catellani and Perry, 2014). Experimental work, for example, has shown that APP knockout mice have increased mortality in response to ischemia, suggesting that APP and its cleavage fragments have a protective role in response to this form of stress (Koike et al., 2012). Thus, for a time, the many insults of aging can be compensated for by the APP, Aß, and possibly other repair mechanisms, and only after a critical point is this capacity eroded to the point where cortical amyloid accumulates to a level at which it is neurotoxic. Tau pathology also develops (Querfurth and LaFerla, 2010), and by this time the progressive dementia of AD typically becomes apparent. Amyloid plaques and tau tangles are abnormal, but rather than be considered primary causes of dementia, they are better considered the late sequelae of a long struggle of the normal brain, over perhaps many decades, to stave

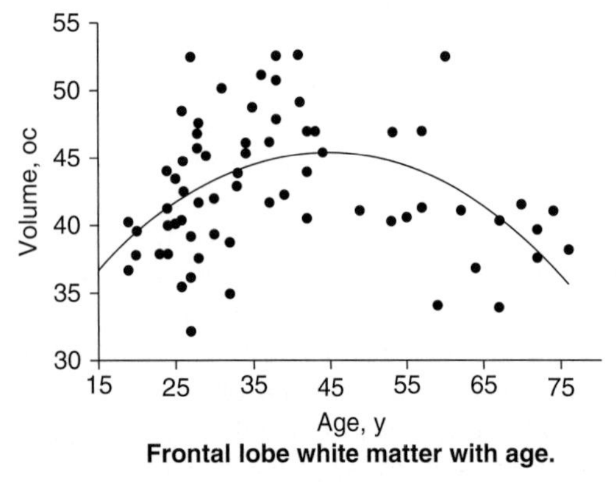

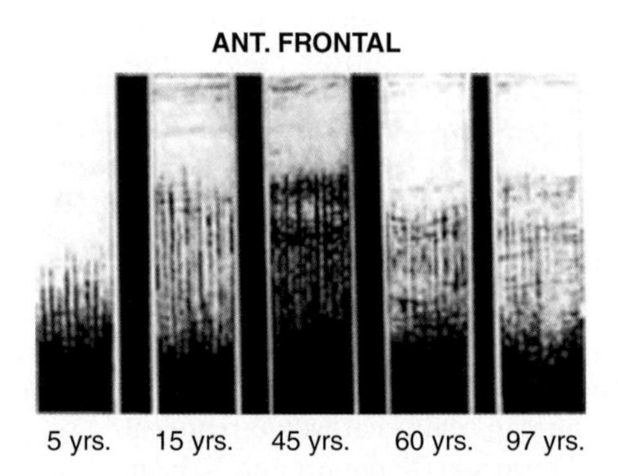

Figure 14.1 Diagrams illustrating the gradual loss of white matter with aging. The left panel shows the trajectory of MRI frontal lobe white matter volume, and the right panel depicts the myelin staining of intracortical white matter (from Bartzokis 2011).

off the many pathologies of aging that primarily beset the white matter.

Thus, in the myelin model, cortical involvement is important in AD, but not primary, and the deposition of abnormal proteins is downstream of the fundamental white matter neuropathology that has occurred many years before. When amyloid and tau accumulate to the point at which they do become toxic, protein deposition is accompanied by massive synapse loss and neuronal dropout in relevant cortical regions, and these phenomena are thought to be the basis for the clinical deficits of the disease (Terry et al., 1991; DeKosky, Scheff, and Styren, 1996; Coleman and Yao, 2003; Koffie, Hyman, and Spires-Jones, 2011).

Recent information has suggested that synapse loss may primarily result from the toxic effect of Aß oligomers, which are recognized to colocalize with neuritic plaques, and neuronal loss may follow through the toxic effects of hyperphosphorylated tau (Koffie, Hyman, and Spires-Jones, 2011). The subsequent clinical progression of AD to its terminal state may then be a result of unchecked protein propagation throughout the cerebral cortex. In this regard, Prusiner (2012) has raised the provocative idea that amyloid propagates much like a prion. This notion is compatible with the myelin model in that early insults to myelin may instigate the neuropathological cascade that eventually destroys the cerebral cortex via the progressive spread of amyloid and tau toxicity.

The prominence of white matter injury in the early pathogenesis of AD has been substantially supported by neuroimaging. This work has mainly been done with older persons who harbor ischemic white matter lesions. The deleterious cognitive impact of white matter hyperintensity progression has been often confirmed (Gunning-Dixon and Raz, 2000; Kloppenborg et al., 2014), and it appears that progression of periventricular white matter lesions can induce cortical atrophy (Kloppenborg et al., 2012). Compared with normal older people, those with both AD and mild cognitive impairment (MCI) have a greater number of white matter hyperintensities, reduced cerebral white matter volume, and widespread microstructural white matter disease as determined by diffusion tensor imaging (DTI) (Radanovic et al., 2013). Studies of older people have shown that white matter hyperintensity volume predicts the appearance of both MCI (Silbert et al., 2012) and AD (Brickman et al., 2012b), whereas hippocampal volume loss predicts neither. Studies such as these offer an emerging perspective that early white matter abnormalities related to common neuropathological processes may in some way drive the later cortical neuropathology of AD.

In view of considerable evidence that AD cortical neuropathology begins in the medial temporal regions, including the hippocampus and entorhinal cortex (Querfurth and LaFerla, 2010), direct examination of white matter in these areas has been particularly informative. The fornix has attracted much recent attention because of its critical position as the major efferent tract of the hippocampus (Oishi and Lyketsos, 2014; Nowrangi and Rosenberg, 2015), and this structure has special appeal as a potential early site of AD pathogenesis in view of the dominance of recent memory dysfunction as the usual presenting feature of the disease. Longitudinal study combining MRI and DTI in normal elders who converted to AD has indeed disclosed that the fornix may be vulnerable to deterioration before medial temporal gray matter is affected (Fletcher et al., 2014). The myelin model predicts that early white matter damage precedes cortical disease, and indeed the fornix is susceptible to many common forms of white matter pathology, including ischemia and TBI (Thomas, Koumellis, and Dineen, 2011). Typical small vessel disease of older adults as seen by MRI can damage the fornix (Moudgil et al., 2000), and DTI studies have documented delayed loss of forniceal white matter integrity after TBI (Adnan et al., 2013). Forniceal DTI changes have even been observed in presymptomatic carriers of familial AD mutations (Ringman et al., 2007). These studies add credence to the myelin model by documenting the neuropathological vulnerability of a key limbic tract that could explain the predilection of early AD for the medial temporal region.

The myelin model also sheds light on another long-recognized clinical feature of AD, which is that the disease is more common in women, even after accounting for the greater longevity of women compared to men in industrialized societies (Thies et al., 2013). Postmenopausal estrogen deficiency has been postulated as a risk factor of AD, although clinical trials with estrogen in women with AD have proven unsuccessful. Recent MRI studies of normal elders have shown that white matter hyperintensities are more common in women, which may mean that estrogen deficiency contributes to brain ischemia and the development of white matter lesions (de Leeuw et al., 2001;

Sachdev et al., 2009). Thus the higher prevalence of AD in women could be mediated by an increased risk for white matter hyperintensity development after menopause, which in turn leads to the etiopathogenetic sequence predicted by the myelin model.

Further perspective on this idea can be gleaned from considering the notion of MCI (Petersen et al., 1999) in more detail. This influential and much-studied condition has been widely regarded as a transitional stage between normal aging and AD, as many people with MCI do progress into dementia after variable intervals. If MCI is indeed the precursor of AD, and the amyloid hypothesis is correct, it would follow that plaques and tangles would be present in MCI but less abundantly so than in AD. Yet this is not always the case. Whereas many people with MCI do have AD changes, others do not, and indeed a host of other factors such as vascular pathology, Lewy body deposition, inflammation, oxidative stress, mitochondrial dysfunction, changes in genomic activity, and disrupted metabolic homeostasis can be found (Stephan et al., 2012). It thus appears that MCI is a heterogeneous condition that does little to support the amyloid hypothesis. Rather, MCI may more accurately be regarded as a pre-dementia state reflecting the brain in the midst of many diverse processes, with the clinical state representing the balance between the detrimental effects of these factors and the brain's capacity to withstand these insults.

In the myelin model, amyloid could be seen as one of the protective mechanisms employed by the brain – one that helps repair myelin and, in the course of doing so, leaves behind cortical amyloid as evidence that this process has occurred. Recent neuropsychological investigations of asymptomatic persons with AD neuropathology have been revealing in this context. In a study of asymptomatic people who died within 2 years of neuropsychological assessment, Monsell and colleagues (2014) found that those who were found to have AD changes displayed greater attentional and working memory deficits than those who had no AD changes. Whereas this finding could be interpreted as documenting the early effects of AD neuropathology in the cortex, it could alternatively be seen as evidence that the brain is responding to age-related damage to cerebral myelin. The latter interpretation would hold that attentional and working memory deficits in fact reflect white matter pathology, and the cortical amyloid is evidence of myelin repair.

When the dementia of AD ultimately sets in, the case can be made that the cortical synapse and neuronal loss reflect the damaging impact of progressive amyloid and tau deposition. From the perspective of the myelin model, it would follow that the clinical features of AD would result from the inability of the brain to continue myelin repair, and hence there develops an overwhelming accumulation of cortical amyloid and then tau. As this process is protracted, however, and may involve many years, it can be imagined that fluctuations in the neurotoxicity of these proteins occur as the disease progresses. An interesting idea has been suggested that the neuropathological alterations in the cortex may correspond to well-recognized clinical fluctuations of AD patients, reflecting a dynamic process of chronic protein intoxication that the brain can temporarily overcome (Palop, Chin, and Mucke, 2006). This notion may imply that even when cortical neuropathology is clinically eloquent, some opportunity for intervention may yet be possible (Palop, Chin, and Mucke, 2006).

The myelin model of AD is most pertinent to sporadic AD, which typically occurs in late life and implicates a wide range of environmental factors (Box 13.1). Yet the genetics of AD deserves attention in light of available data on the AD susceptibility gene APOE, early-onset familial AD, and DS. Remarkably, early white matter damage consistent with the myelin model can be implicated in all of these conditions. First, in contrast to the widely held assumption that the APOE ε4 genotype increases AD risk by enhancing Aß production, this allele may alternatively hinder myelin repair because of impaired cholesterol transport (Bartzokis, 2011). As discussed in the previous chapter, neuroimaging studies have shown that cognitively normal APOE ε4 carriers have lower MRI white matter volume that correlates with slower processing speed (Ready et al., 2011), decreased frontal white matter fractional anisotropy (FA) on DTI that correlates with lower executive function (Ryan et al., 2011), and disrupted structural connectivity together with diminished memory performance (Chen et al., 2015). In contrast, APOE ε2 carriers, who are presumably protected from the effects of white matter damage because of more efficient delivery of cholesterol and lipids to axons (Bartzokis, 2011), have higher FA in many white matter tracts (Chiang et al., 2012).

Next, mutations associated with familial AD may produce disease by virtue of inadequate myelination or myelin repair, and the deposition of cortical Aß may not be a crucial early event (Bartzokis, 2011). Supportive evidence for this notion comes from the DTI work of Ringman and colleagues (2007) documenting white matter changes in presymptomatic presenilin-1 and APP mutation carriers.

Finally, with regard to DS, it is of considerable interest that, despite developing AD pathology, some DS patients do not become demented (Tyrrell et al., 2001). Given this observation, one can imagine that Aß does not necessarily exert a pathogenic effect, and that damage to the brain white matter may be more critical. It has long been known that white matter hyperintensities are common in adults with DS, even before dementia occurs (Emerson et al., 1995), and may reflect vascular or other white matter insult. More recently, a provocative DTI study of adult DS patients with and without dementia found that frontal white matter integrity was diminished in those with dementia (Powell et al., 2014). These data merit particular attention in view of the observation that dementia in DS appears to be characterized by personality and behavior changes along with executive dysfunction, all securely associated with frontal lobe involvement (Ball et al., 2006). Thus it may be that the primary insult in DS leading to dementia is actually damage to white matter, which may then activate Aß deposition that reflects an attempt at brain repair after white matter injury.

When considered in its entirety, perhaps the most interesting implication of the model is a more refined view of amyloid in the complex etiopathogenesis of AD. Whereas plaques and tangles may be central to the pathology of AD, it is not clear that they hold the same position with respect to pathogenesis (Castellani and Perry, 2014). Rather than being seen as uniformly toxic, amyloid may be more usefully conceptualized as part of an adaptive or protective system to deal with encroaching changes of brain aging and the insults accumulated over a lifetime. In this context, it is appropriate to point out that while clinicians and neuroscientists are quite logically drawn to readily observable histologic hallmarks of a disease such as AD – much as they are to the clearly undesirable pathologies such as thrombosis, infection, and neoplasia – it is not at all clear that plaques and tangles have the same destructive impact on the brain as do the better-known pathologies with which medicine is well acquainted. The normal functions of APP and Aß remain unknown, and the assumption that the mere presence of neuritic plaques guarantees their pathogenicity in all cases is premature. Rather, it may be more accurate to consider a more diverse function of these proteins, even to a point where APP and Aß may be beneficial at some point in disease development and toxic only later.

Implications for prevention and treatment

The myelin model of AD offers a strikingly novel idea about how this devastating disease begins. If the model is correct, many new and important implications for prevention and treatment should be recognized. Two principal topics merit consideration in this light: (1) the prediction that the major clinical trials now underway for the treatment of AD are not likely to succeed, and may even be hazardous, and (2) the prospects for alternative treatment modalities that may hold more promise.

The continuing influence of the amyloid hypothesis has led to large-scale clinical trials in AD designed to rid the brain of amyloid. At present, this approach relies heavily on passive immunization with monoclonal antibodies that can clear presumably toxic Aß from the brain (Prins and Scheltens, 2013). Although amyloid-targeted therapies have uniformly failed to date, trials using such monoclonal antibodies as solaneuzumab are being conducted in AD, and even in elders with "preclinical AD" who have brain amyloid demonstrated by florbetapir PET but are cognitively normal (Prins and Scheltens, 2013). While the idea of removing Aß before dementia sets in has some plausibility, it is not clear that Aß is toxic in nondemented individuals, as it is well known that at least 25% of normal older people have sufficient brain amyloid at autopsy to qualify as having AD (Gandy and DeKosky, 2013).

Moreover, removing the protein at an early stage may actually be harmful because of interference with normal repair processes that are underway before dementia begins (Bartzokis, 2011; Castellani and Smith, 2011). Other concerns relate to the propensity of these agents to produce adverse neuroimaging findings, known as amyloid-related imaging abnormalities (ARIAs), that include vasogenic edema, microhemorrhages, hemosiderin deposition, and superficial siderosis (Prins and Scheltens, 2013). The etiology of these ARIAs is thought to be increased vascular permeability following clearance of amyloid from brain arterioles (Prins and Scheltens, 2013), and the use of agents with these risks is concerning, particularly in individuals who are clinically normal.

Another therapeutic approach to AD based on the amyloid hypothesis is the exploitation of ß-secretase inhibition (Vassar, 2014). ß-secretase, or, more specifically, the ß-site APP cleaving enzyme (BACE), is the enzyme initially involved in the generation of Aß from its parent molecule APP, and inhibition of this enzyme has been proposed as an AD treatment that could succeed by preventing the formation of Aß (Vassar, 2014). From the perspective of the myelin model, the important point regarding ß-secretase is that this enzyme also activates neuregulin, a protein growth factor important in the process of myelination (Xu et al., 2006). This topic was considered in Chapter 13 with respect to myelin repair, where it was pointed out that the promyelinative activity of neuregulin has been observed in the brain as well as in the peripheral nervous system (Hu et al., 2006; Pankonin et al., 2009). In the brain, neuregulin is concentrated in white matter astrocytes, and is elevated in the cerebrospinal fluid of AD patients (Pankonin et al., 2009), implying that it may be a response to ongoing myelin injury. The therapeutic inhibition of ß-secretase may thus produce the undesired effect of inhibiting myelin repair even as it helps reduce Aß formation. Therefore, if myelin repair is crucial to avert the onset of AD, the use of ß-secretase inhibitors may produce more harm than good by inhibiting neuregulin when it is most needed (Glabe, 2006; Figure 14.2). Furthermore, the control of acquired factors that damage white matter, to be considered later, could by itself reduce the generation of Aß because the brain has less need for the activation of neuregulin by ß-secretase.

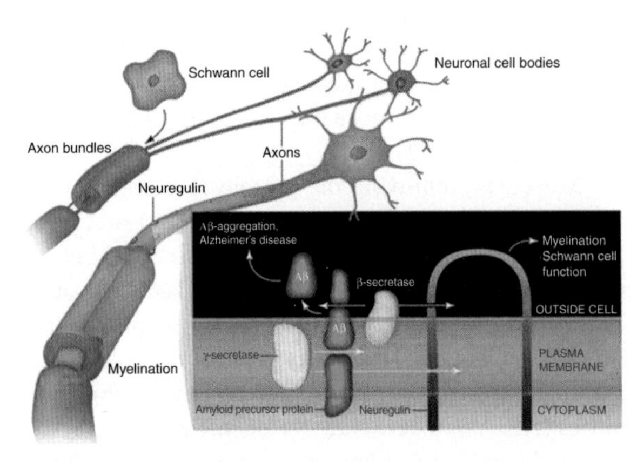

Figure 14.2 The dual action of ß-secretase: activation of neuregulin and generation of ß-amyloid (from Glabe, 2006).

These considerations naturally lead to a radically different approach to treatment of AD. Instead of striving to eradicate amyloid from the brain, clinicians may be well advised to recognize that this protein, and its downstream partner tau, can be seen as participating in an adaptive response to white matter injury, and efforts to prevent or repair this form of injury take precedence. The most effective treatment of AD may thus be the lifelong maintenance and protection of brain white matter. The eradication of amyloid may be useful in certain individuals at the point when the toxic effects of the protein begin to be clinically significant, but a more effective strategy could involve avoidance of white matter damage before any cortical protein deposition occurs. Both preventive and therapeutic strategies to achieve this objective can be imagined.

First, as the history of public health abundantly documents, prevention may be a most salutary intervention. Given the increasing recognition that AD is related to cardiovascular risk factors such as hypertension, diabetes, smoking, and obesity, and that TBI is another predisposing factor, opportunities for effective prevention are readily apparent (Qiu, Kivipelto, and von Strauss, 2009; Knopman and Roberts, 2010; Filley, 2015). In this regard, it has been proposed that AD should be considered a public health problem strongly related to preventable risk factors (Fotuhi, Hachinski, and Whitehouse, 2009). As these problems damage white matter before the appearance of the dementia of AD or even the signs of its precursor MCI, it is conceivable that early intervention using control of blood pressure and glucose, avoidance of tobacco, promotion of regular exercise and proper diet, and the wearing of seat belts and helmets may offer highly effective benefits with regard to preventing AD. As discussed in Chapter 13, a large European trial of hypertension control lasting about 4 years was able to show that dementia incidence was reduced by 55%, and, most important, this benefit was apparent not just for vascular dementia, but for AD as well (Forette et al., 2002). The fact that the only medication ever shown to lower the incidence of AD may exert a primary effect on white matter should serve as a stimulus for investigating this mechanism of action as a general preventive strategy.

Evidence for prevention of AD on a large scale has already begun to appear. Remarkably, several recent epidemiological studies from the United States and Europe have found a decline in the incidence and prevalence of dementia over the past two decades, and these statistics also include dementia related to AD (Larson, Yaffe, and Langa, 2013). These trends have been tentatively explained by the improving care of cardiovascular risk factors and access to education in industrialized nations (Larson, Yaffe, and Langa, 2013). One estimate holds that up to 50% of the worldwide burden of AD can be attributed to modifiable risk factors (Barnes and Yaffe, 2011). Thus the intervention of primary care and other physicians, combined with the institution of public health initiatives – all designed to address such factors as hypertension, diabetes, smoking, obesity, hyperlipidemia, physical inactivity, TBI, depression, sleep disorders, and cognitive inactivity – may bring about effective preventive measures for many cases of AD (Filley, 2015). Moreover, if the myelin model of AD is correct, other acquired insults to white matter may be identified and present additional opportunities for prevention.

As for treatment, it is assuredly the case that some people will still develop AD despite the best preventive efforts of medicine and society. In the context of the myelin model, this unfortunate event may occur for many reasons, including unavoidable medical disorders, accidental TBI, or a genetic predisposition in amyloid genes leading to excessive cortical amyloid deposition (Hardy, 2009). A significant component of genetic risk is also known in AD, clearly in early-onset disease (Howard and Filley, 2009), and to some extent in late-onset AD as well, with susceptibility conferred by the APOE ε4 allele, and other genetic effects that are being investigated with genome-wide association studies (Tosto and Reitz, 2013). These factors cannot be ignored, and it may be that therapies targeting amyloid or even tau may find a place in the therapeutic armamentarium for AD. Indeed, ongoing clinical trials with solaneuzumab and other similar antibodies may yet find success and offer solid support for the amyloid hypothesis.

Yet even when cortical proteins have accumulated and dementia has developed, attempts to enhance the endogenous repair capacities of the brain may still be effective. If damage to white matter precedes the appearance of plaques and tangles, this injury may continue throughout the disease, and efforts to repair white matter may be worth considering at any point in the disease course. In this regard, intriguing possibilities are raised by promising experimental results with the use of APOE-mimetic peptides (Sarantseva et al., 2009; Vitek et al., 2012) and neuregulin (Min et al., 2011; Woo et al., 2012), both of which may function to help repair white matter at an early stage of cognitive impairment, and prevent the excess deposition of amyloid that could lead to a less reversible state of cortical degeneration.

The myelin model of AD is of course hypothetical, and much remains to be done so that it may be confirmed or refuted. As the disease remains alarming because of its high prevalence and incurability, however, a new paradigm is eminently reasonable to consider. If the myelin hypothesis is correct, it may provide the long-sought answer to the scourge of AD, and the present goal of eradicating amyloid from the brain will be seen as a worthy but inadequate attempt to solve the problem.

References

Adnan A, Crawley A, Mikulis D, et al. Moderate-severe traumatic brain injury causes delayed loss of white matter integrity: evidence of fornix deterioration in the chronic stage of injury. Brain Inj 2013; 27: 1415–1422.

Alves GS, Oertel Knöchel V, Knöchel C, et al. Integrating retrogenesis theory to Alzheimer's disease pathology: insight from DTI-TBSS investigation of the white matter microstructural integrity. Biomed Res Int 2015; 2015: 291658.

Ashe KH, Zahs KR. Probing the biology of Alzheimer's disease in mice. Neuron 2010; 66: 631–645.

Ball SL, Holland AJ, Hon J, et al. Personality and behaviour changes mark the early stages of Alzheimer's disease in adults with Down's syndrome: findings from a prospective population-based study. Int J Geriatr Psychiatry 2006; 21: 661–673.

Barnes DE, Yaffe K. The projected effect of risk factor reduction on Alzheimer's disease prevalence. Lancet Neurol 2011; 10: 819–828.

Bartzokis G. Alzheimer's disease as homeostatic responses to age-related myelin breakdown. Neurobiol Aging 2011; 32: 1341–1371.

Bartzokis G, Beckson M, Lu PH, et al. Age-related changes in frontal and temporal lobe volumes in men: a magnetic resonance imaging study. Arch Gen Psychiatry 2001; 58: 461–465.

Bateman RJ, Xiong C, Benzinger TL, et al. Clinical and biomarker changes in dominantly inherited Alzheimer's disease. N Engl J Med 2012; 367: 795–804.

Brickman AM, Meier IB, Korgaonkar MS, et al. Testing the white matter retrogenesis hypothesis of cognitive aging. Neurobiol Aging 2012a; 33: 1699–1715.

Brickman AM, Provenzano FA, Muraskin J, et al. Regional white matter hyperintensity volume, not hippocampal atrophy, predicts incident Alzheimer Disease in the community. Arch Neurol 2012b; 69: 1621–1627.

Bufill E, Blesa R, Augustí J. Alzheimer's disease: an evolutionary approach. J Anthropol Sci 2013; 91: 135–157.

Castellani RJ, Lee HG, Zhu X, et al. Alzheimer disease pathology as a host response. J Neuropathol Exp Neurol 2008; 67: 523–531.

Castellani RJ, Lee HG, Siedlak SL, et al. Reexamining Alzheimer's disease: evidence for a protective role for amyloid-beta protein precursor and amyloid-beta. J Alzheimers Dis 2009; 18: 447–452.

Castellani RJ, Smith MA. Compounding artefacts with uncertainty, and an amyloid cascade hypothesis that is "too big to fail." J Pathol 2011; 224: 147–152.

Castellani RJ, Perry G. The complexities of the pathology-pathogenesis relationship in Alzheimer disease. Biochem Pharmacol 2014; 88: 671–676.

Chen Y, Chen K, Zhang J, et al. Disrupted functional and structural networks in cognitively normal elderly subjects with the APOE ε4 allele. Neuropsychopharmacology 2015; 40: 1181–1191.

Chiang GC, Zhan W, Schuff N, Weiner MW. White matter alterations in cognitively normal apoE ε2 carriers: insight into Alzheimer resistance? AJNR 2012; 33: 1392–1397.

Coleman PD, Yao PJ. Synaptic slaughter in Alzheimer's disease. Neurobiol Aging 2003; 24: 1023–1027.

Davis DG, Schmitt FA, Wekstein DR, Markesbery WR. Alzheimer neuropathologic alterations in aged cognitively normal subjects. J Neuropathol Exp Neurol 1999; 58: 376–388.

DeKosky ST, Scheff SW, Styren SD. Structural correlates of cognition in dementia: quantification and assessment of synapse change. Neurodegeneration 1996; 5: 417–421.

de Leeuw FE, de Groot JC, Achten E, et al. Prevalence of cerebral white matter lesions in elderly people: a population based magnetic resonance imaging study; the Rotterdam Scan Study. J Neurol Neurosurg Psychiatry 2001; 70: 9–14.

Doody RS, Thomas RG, Farlow M, et al. Phase 3 trials of solanezumab for mild-to-moderate Alzheimer's disease. N Engl J Med 2014; 370: 311–321.

Emerson JF, Kesslak JP, Chen PC, Lott IT. Magnetic resonance imaging of the aging brain in Down syndrome. Prog Clin Biol Res 1995; 393: 123–138.

Filley CM. Alzheimer's Disease prevention: new optimism. Neurol Clin Pract 2015; 5: 193–200.

Fletcher E, Carmichael O, Pasternak O, et al. Early brain loss in circuits affected by Alzheimer's Disease is predicted by fornix microstructure but may be independent of gray matter. Front Aging Neurosci 2014; 6: 106.

Forette F, Seux ML, Staessen JA, et al. The prevention of dementia with antihypertensive treatment: new evidence from the Systolic Hypertension in Europe (Syst-Eur) study. Arch Intern Med 2002; 162: 2046–2052.

Fotuhi M, Hachinski V, Whitehouse PJ. Changing perspectives regarding late-life dementia. Nat Rev Neurol 2009; 5: 649–658.

Gandy S, DeKosky ST. Toward the treatment and prevention of Alzheimer's disease: rational strategies and recent progress. Annu Rev Med 2013; 64: 367–383.

Giuffrida ML, Caraci F, Pignataro B, et al. Beta-amyloid monomers are neuroprotective. J Neurosci 2009; 29: 10582–10587.

Glabe C. Biomedicine: avoiding collateral damage in Alzheimer's disease treatment. Science 2006; 314: 602–603.

Glenner GG, Wong CW. Alzheimer's disease: initial report of the purification and characterization of a novel cerebrovascular amyloid protein. Biochem Biophys Res Commun 1984a; 120: 885–890.

Glenner GG, Wong CW. Alzheimer's disease and Down's syndrome: sharing of a unique cerebrovascular amyloid fibril protein. Biochem Biophys Res Commun 1984b; 122: 1131–1135.

Gold BT, Johnson NF, Powell DK, Smith CD. White matter integrity and vulnerability to Alzheimer's disease: preliminary findings and future directions. Biochim Biophys Acta 2012; 1822: 416–422.

Gorelick PB, Scuteri A, Black SE, et al. Vascular contributions to cognitive impairment and dementia: a statement for healthcare professionals from the American Heart Association/American Stroke Association. Stroke 2011; 42: 2672–2713.

Gunning-Dixon FM, Raz N. The cognitive correlates of white matter abnormalities in normal aging: a quantitative review. Neuropsychology 2000; 14: 224–232.

Hall AM, Roberson ED. Mouse models of Alzheimer's disease. Brain Res Bull 2012; 88: 3–12.

Hardy J. The amyloid hypothesis for Alzheimer's disease: a critical reappraisal. J Neurochem 2009; 110: 1129–1134.

Hardy J, Selkoe DJ. The amyloid hypothesis of Alzheimer's disease: progress and problems on the road to therapeutics. Science 2002; 297: 353–356.

Hoe HS, Lee HK, Pak DT. The upside of APP at synapses. CNS Neurosci Ther 2012; 18: 47–56.

Howard KL, Filley CM. Advances in genetic testing for Alzheimer's disease. Rev Neurol Dis 2009; 6: 26–32.

Hu X, Hicks CW, He W, et al. Bace1 modulates myelination in the central and peripheral nervous system. Nat Neurosci 2006; 9: 1520–1525.

Iqbal K, Liu F, Gong CX. Alzheimer disease therapeutics: focus on the disease and not just plaques and tangles. Biochem Pharmacol 2014; 88: 631–649.

Jack CR Jr, Knopman DS, Jagust WJ, et al. Hypothetical model of dynamic biomarkers of the Alzheimer's pathological cascade. Lancet Neurol 2010; 9: 119–128.

Kloppenborg RP, Nederkoorn PJ, Grool AM, et al. Cerebral small-vessel disease and progression of brain atrophy: the SMART-MR study. Neurology 2012; 79: 2029–2036.

Kloppenborg RP, Nederkoorn PJ, Geerlings MI, van den Berg E. Presence and progression of white matter hyperintensities and cognition: a meta-analysis. Neurology 2014; 82: 2127–2138.

Klunk WE, Engler H, Nordberg A, et al. Imaging brain amyloid in Alzheimer's disease with Pittsburgh Compound-B. Ann Neurol 2004; 55: 306–319.

Knopman DS, Roberts R. Vascular risk factors: imaging and neuropathologic correlates. J Alzheimers Dis 2010; 20: 699–709.

Koffie RM, Hyman BT, Spires-Jones TL Alzheimer's disease: synapses gone cold. Mol Neurodegener 2011; 6: 63.

Koike MA, Lin AJ, Pham J, et al. APP knockout mice experience acute mortality as the result of ischemia. PLoS One 2012; 7: e42665.

Larson EB, Yaffe K, Langa KM. New insights into the dementia epidemic. N Engl J Med 2013; 369: 2275–2277.

Masters CL, Simms G, Weinman NA, et al. Amyloid plaque core protein in Alzheimer disease and Down syndrome. Proc Natl Acad Sci 1985; 82: 4245–4249.

Min SS, An J, Lee JH, et al. Neuregulin-1 prevents amyloid β-induced impairment of long-term potentiation in hippocampal slices via ErbB4. Neurosci Lett 2011; 505: 6–9.

Monsell SE, Mock C, Hassenstab J, Roe CM, et al. Neuropsychological changes in asymptomatic persons with Alzheimer disease neuropathology. Neurology 2014; 83: 434–440.

Moudgil SS, Azzouz M, Al-Azzaz A, et al. Amnesia due to fornix infarction. Stroke 2000; 31: 1418–1419.

Nowrangi MA, Rosenberg PB. The fornix in mild cognitive impairment and Alzheimer's disease. Front Aging Neurosci 2015 Jan 21; 7: 1.

Oishi K, Lyketsos CG. Alzheimer's disease and the fornix. Front Aging Neurosci 2014; 6: 241.

Orgogozo JM, Gilman S, Dartigues JF, et al. Subacute meningoencephalitis in a subset of patients with AD after Abeta42 immunization. Neurology 2003; 61: 46–54.

Palop JJ, Chin J, Mucke L. A network dysfunction perspective on neurodegenerative diseases. Nature 2006; 443: 768–773.

Pankonin MS, Sohi J, Kamholz J, Loeb JA. Differential distribution of neuregulin in human brain and spinal fluid. Brain Res 2009; 1258: 1–11.

Parker WD Jr, Parks J, Filley CM, Kleinschmidt-DeMasters BK. Electron transport chain defects in Alzheimer's disease brain. Neurology 1994; 44: 1090–1096.

Petersen RC, Smith GE, Waring SC, et al. Mild cognitive impairment: clinical characterization and outcome. Arch Neurol 1999; 56: 303–308.

Plassman BL, Havlik RJ, Steffens DC, et al. Documented head injury in early adulthood and risk of Alzheimer's disease and other dementias. Neurology 2000; 55: 1158–1166.

Powell D, Caban-Holt A, Jicha G, et al. Frontal white matter integrity in adults with Down syndrome with and without dementia. Neurobiol Aging 2014; 35: 1562–1569.

Prins ND, Scheltens P. Treating Alzheimer's disease with monoclonal antibodies: current status and outlook for the future. Alzheimers Res Ther 2013; 5: 56.

Prusiner SB. Cell biology: a unifying role for prions in neurodegenerative diseases. Science 2012; 336: 1511–1513.

Qiu C, Kivipelto M, von Strauss E. Epidemiology of Alzheimer's disease: occurrence, determinants, and strategies toward intervention. Dialogues Clin Neurosci 2009; 11: 111–128.

Querfurth HW, LaFerla FM. Alzheimer's disease. N Engl J Med 2010; 362: 329–344.

Radanovic M, Pereira FR, Stella F, et al. White matter abnormalities associated with Alzheimer's disease and mild cognitive impairment: a critical review of MRI studies. Expert Rev Neurother 2013; 13: 483–493.

Rapoport SI, Nelson PT. Biomarkers and evolution in Alzheimer disease. Prog Neurobiol 2011; 95: 510–513.

Ready RE, Baran B, Chaudhry M, et al. Apolipoprotein E-e4, processing speed, and white matter volume in a genetically enriched sample of midlife adults. Am J Alzheimers Dis Other Demen 2011; 26: 463–468.

Reitz C. Alzheimer's disease and the amyloid cascade hypothesis: a critical review. Int J Alzheimers Dis 2012; 2012: 369808.

Ringman JM, O'Neill J, Geschwind D, et al. Diffusion tensor imaging in preclinical and presymptomatic carriers of familial Alzheimer's disease mutations. Brain 2007; 130: 1767–1776.

Roberts GW, Gentleman SM, Lynch A, et al. Beta amyloid protein deposition in the brain after severe head injury: implications for the pathogenesis of Alzheimer's disease. J Neurol Neurosurg Psychiatry 1994; 57: 419–425.

Roth G, Dicke U. Evolution of the brain and intelligence. Trends Cogn Sci 2005; 9: 250–257.

Ryan L, Walther K, Bendlin BB, et al. Age-related differences in white matter integrity and cognitive function are related to APOE status. Neuroimage 2011; 54: 1565–1577.

Sachdev PS, Parslow R, Wen W, et al. Sex differences in the causes and consequences of white matter hyperintensities. Neurobiol Aging 2009; 30: 946–956.

Sachdev PS, Zhuang L, Braidy N, Wen W. Is Alzheimer's a disease of the white matter? Curr Opin Psychiatry 2013; 26: 244–251.

Salat DH. Imaging small vessel-associated white matter changes in aging. Neuroscience 2014; 276: 174–186.

Salloway S, Sperling R, Fox NC, et al. Two phase 3 trials of bapineuzumab in mild-to-moderate Alzheimer's disease. N Engl J Med 2014; 370: 322–333.

Santos RX, Correia SC, Zhu X, et al. Mitochondrial DNA oxidative damage and repair in aging and Alzheimer's disease. Antioxid Redox Signal 2013; 18: 2444–2457.

Sarantseva S, Timoshenko S, Bolshakova O, et al. Apolipoprotein E-mimetics inhibit neurodegeneration and restore cognitive functions in a transgenic Drosophila model of Alzheimer's disease. PLoS One 2009; 4: e8191.

Schenk D, Barbour R, Dunn W, et al. Immunization with amyloid-beta attenuates Alzheimer-disease-like pathology in the PDAPP mouse. Nature 1999; 400: 173–177.

Schmitt FA, Davis DG, Wekstein DR, et al. "Preclinical" AD revisited: neuropathology of cognitively normal older adults. Neurology 2000; 55: 370–376.

Schoenemann PT, Sheehan MJ, Glotzer LD. Prefrontal white matter volume is disproportionately larger in humans than in other primates. Nat Neurosci 2005; 8: 242–252.

Silbert LC, Dodge HH, Perkins LG, et al. Trajectory of white matter hyperintensity burden preceding mild cognitive impairment. Neurology 2012; 79: 741–747.

Smaers JB, Schleicher A, Zilles K, Vinicius L. Frontal white matter volume is associated with brain enlargement and higher structural connectivity in anthropoid primates. PLoS One 2010; 5: e9123.

Stephan BC, Hunter S, Harris D, et al. The neuropathological profile of mild cognitive impairment (MCI): a systematic review. Mol Psychiatry 2012; 17: 1056–1076.

Tanzi RE, Gusella JF, Watkins PC, et al. Amyloid beta protein gene: cDNA, mRNA distribution, and genetic linkage near the Alzheimer locus. Science 1987; 235: 880–884.

Terry RD, Masliah E, Salmon DP, et al. Physical basis of cognitive alterations in Alzheimer's disease: synapse loss is the major correlate of cognitive impairment. Ann Neurol 1991; 30: 572–580.

Thies W, Bleiler L, Alzheimer's Association. 2013 Alzheimer's disease facts and figures. Alzheimers Dement 2013; 9: 208–245.

Thomas AG, Koumellis P, Dineen RA. The fornix in health and disease: an imaging review. Radiographics 2011; 31: 1107–1121.

Tosto G, Reitz C. Genome-wide association studies in Alzheimer's disease: a review. Curr Neurol Neurosci Rep 2013; 13: 381.

Tran HT, LaFerla FM, Holtzman DM, Brody DL. Controlled cortical impact traumatic brain injury in 3xTg-AD mice causes acute intra-axonal amyloid-β accumulation and independently accelerates the development of tau abnormalities. J Neurosci. 2011; 31: 9513–9525.

Tyrrell J, Cosgrave M, McCarron M, et al. Dementia in people with Down's syndrome. Int J Geriatr Psychiatry 2001; 16: 1168–1174.

Vandenberghe R, Adamczuk K, Dupont P, et al. Amyloid PET in clinical practice: its place in the multidimensional space of Alzheimer's disease. Neuroimage Clin 2013; 2: 497–511.

Vassar R. BACE1 inhibitor drugs in clinical trials for Alzheimer's disease. Alzheimers Res Ther 2014; 6: 89.

Vitek MP, Christensen DJ, Wilcock D, et al. APOE-mimetic peptides reduce behavioral deficits, plaques and tangles in Alzheimer's disease transgenics. Neurodegener Dis 2012; 10: 122–126.

Whitehouse PJ. The end of Alzheimer's disease – from biochemical pharmacology to ecopsychosociology: a personal perspective. Biochem Pharmacol 2014; 88: 677–681.

Woo RS, Lee JH, Kim HS, et al. Neuregulin-1 protects against neurotoxicities induced by Swedish amyloid precursor protein via the ErbB4 receptor. Neuroscience 2012; 202: 413–423.

Xia CF, Arteaga J, Chen G, et al. [(18)F]T807, a novel tau positron emission tomography imaging agent for Alzheimer's disease. Alzheimers Dement 2013; 9: 666–676.

Zhang K, Sejnowski TJ. A universal scaling law between gray matter and white matter of cerebral cortex. Proc Natl Acad Sci 2000; 97: 5621–5626.

Chapter 15

Chronic traumatic encephalopathy and white matter

The possibility that Alzheimer's Disease (AD) may originate in the white matter was discussed in the previous chapter, but a similar and equally novel idea can be considered for another dementia syndrome, one that exclusively implicates long-term sequelae of traumatic brain injury (TBI). In recent years, the entity chronic traumatic encephalopathy (CTE) has been described mainly in professional athletes and combat veterans who were exposed to multiple episodes of mild TBI during their careers. Not only are certain athletes proposed to be at risk for CTE, but military personnel exposed to repeated concussions and blast injuries may present a larger group of individuals who may develop progressive and incurable dementia as a result of combat. CTE is very similar, if not identical, to the older entity of dementia pugilistica, adding some credibility to the idea, but CTE is a highly controversial topic, and much remains unknown about the relationship between repetitive mild TBI and dementia. One perspective that may prove helpful in this area, however, is a focus on white matter as the primary site of injury from which later neuropathology develops. Accordingly, this chapter will take up the possibility that the common white matter lesion known as diffuse axonal injury (DAI) could lead to a form of degenerative dementia as a late sequel of earlier brain damage. To begin a discussion of this rapidly evolving area, a review of concussion serves as a necessary introduction.

Concussion

Until recently, concussion and the area of TBI in general were to a large extent ignored by the medical profession, so much so that TBI was referred to as a "silent epidemic" (Goldstein, 1990). This era of relative neglect has now been replaced by a time of rapidly growing interest, and concussion – by far the most common form of TBI – is being investigated with special vigor. One lingering issue, however, is the problem of exactly what constitutes a concussion, and unfortunately a lack of consensus persists (Levin and Diaz-Arrastia, 2015). For the purposes of this chapter, a concussion will be considered a typically reversible alteration of mental status induced by physical trauma (Filley, 2011). It is worth pointing out that the trauma of concussion differs from that implied by the psychiatric diagnosis of posttraumatic stress disorder, in which the trauma is purely psychological. Concussion has been proposed to be a milder form of a larger category called mild TBI (mTBI), implying that mTBI features structural brain injury whereas concussion involves a functional disturbance, but no substantial difference between mTBI and concussion has been definitively established (Levin and Diaz-Arrastia, 2015), and the two terms will be used synonymously in this account.

Many physicians have been taught that loss of consciousness, surely an obvious manifestation of altered mental status, is required for concussion, but it has become clear that this syndrome can occur with preserved consciousness (Kelly et al., 1991). Indeed, most concussions do not involve loss of consciousness, and, more often, affected individuals experience an alteration of mental status manifested by symptoms of confusion and amnesia. Whereas this refinement in understanding reflects a deeper understanding of concussion, it does complicate the clinical diagnosis, and because no neuroimaging or other biomarker exists for concussion, the lack of objective assessment measures has been a significant obstacle to accurate diagnosis.

In view of the inherent subjectivity of clinical diagnosis, and in recognition of the range of clinical severity that can occur, the Colorado Medical Society Guidelines of 1991, which specifically dealt with sports concussion, defined levels of injury and the actions that should be taken if such injuries are detected (Kelly et al., 1991). These guidelines relied

Table 15.1 Levels of concussion severity as described in the Colorado Medical Society Guidelines for the Management of Concussion in Sports

Grade 1	Grade 2	Grade 3
Confusion without amnesia, no loss of consciousness	Confusion with amnesia, no loss of consciousness	Loss of consciousness

From Kelly et al. (1991)

Table 15.2 Classification of traumatic brain injury severity

Criteria	Mild	Moderate	Severe
Loss of consciousness	0–30 mins	> 30 mins, < 24 hrs	> 24 hrs
Alteration of consciousness (confusion, amnesia)	< 24 hrs	> 24 hrs	> 24 hrs
Posttraumatic amnesia	0–1 day	> 1 day, < 7 days	> 7 days
GCS score (best available in first 24 hours)	13–15	9–12	3–8
Structural imaging	Normal	Normal or abnormal	Normal or abnormal

Adapted from Management of Concussion/mTBI Working Group, VA/DoD Clinical Practice Guideline for Management of Concussion/Mild Traumatic Brain Injury (mTBI), 2009

on a classification of concussion into three grades, based on the specific identification of confusion, amnesia, and loss of consciousness (Table 15.1).

This important advance soon led to improved standardization of concussion diagnosis in all settings where this injury occurs (ACRM, 1993). In turn, these developments have helped clarify the classification of TBI at all levels of severity, and the assessment of military personnel with TBI has been particularly important in recent years. Table 15.2 presents criteria currently employed by the United States Veterans Administration and Department of Defense to diagnose not only concussion but also the less common moderate and severe forms of TBI. The use of mild, moderate, and severe categories of TBI now has widespread acceptance, and has enhanced both the care of head-injured patients and research on this major area of behavioral neurology.

Concussion is remarkably prevalent, with an estimated 42 million worldwide mTBI episodes occurring yearly (Gardner and Yaffe, 2015). In the United States, concussion occurs in civilians most often as a result of motor vehicle accidents, sporting events, falls, and assaults, and in military personnel because of direct head blows from various insults including missiles, other objects, and blast waves from nearby explosions. As a general clinical rule, the great majority of patients with concussion experience complete recovery within weeks or a few months (Alexander, 1995; Cassidy et al., 2014). A small number are troubled by persistent complaints that indicate what has been called the postconcussion syndrome (McAllister and Arciniegas, 2002; Cassidy et al., 2014). The largely benign prognosis of concussion has long been a reassuring assumption for all concerned, and while long-term cognitive sequelae have been linked with moderate and severe TBI (Gardner and Yaffe, 2015), there is no convincing epidemiological evidence for dementia after a single episode of mTBI (Godbolt et al., 2014).

Against this background, however, concussion in sports has recently generated a flurry of attention because of new data suggesting the possibility of long-term cognitive effects from repetitive mTBI in American professional athletes engaged in contact sports (Omalu et al., 2005; Omalu et al., 2006; McKee et al., 2009). This idea has precedent in the study of professional boxing in the twentieth century (Roberts, 1969; Corsellis, Bruton, and Freeman-Browne, 1973; Unterharnscheidt, 1995), but American football, ice hockey, soccer, baseball, and other sports have all come under recent scrutiny. The notion that concussion in sport is trivial in most cases – with the expectation that the player, often a young and highly eager pugilist or contestant, would simply shake off the injury and resume participation in the bout or contest – is now being widely contested. While it has been known for some time that concussion can have a catastrophic short-term outcome, such as death from the second impact syndrome (Kelly et al., 1991), mTBI may pose other, more insidious hazards. The issue of repetitive mTBI has been central in these investigations, as it is clear that concussion can occur hundreds of times in a single season (Cobb et al., 2013). As work in this area proceeded, military personnel with dementia putatively attributed to repetitive mTBI were also identified, immediately expanding the implications of the idea (McKee et al., 2009; Levin and Diaz-Arrastia, 2015). Thus the presumably benign nature of concussion is being reconsidered, and this form of injury is being vigorously investigated as a possible source of dementia later in life.

Moreover, concern is mounting that repeated "subconcussive" injuries may also contribute to cumulative cognitive effects far beyond the time of injury (Levin and Diaz-Arrastia, 2015). Subconcussive injury is postulated to be a form of cranial injury in which no clinical features can be documented, but in which brain damage is nevertheless sustained (Bailes et al., 2013). This kind of injury has been suspected in both athletes (Bailes et al., 2013) and military personnel (Taber et al., 2015), and may be far more common than concussion, thus posing a largely unappreciated threat to brain health. The importance of subconcussive blows remains uncertain, however, as neuropsychological studies in athletes have not demonstrated any convincing relationship between subconcussive events and cognitive change (Belanger, Vanderploeg, and McAllister, 2015). Concern about an unrecognized epidemic is unwarranted because the study of subconcussive injury is clearly in its infancy (Bailes et al., 2013), but this issue deserves attention as it may expand the scope of trauma-related cognitive impairment.

Dementia pugilistica

The typically favorable prognosis of those who sustain concussion is likely attributable to the resilience of the normal brain, as humans are routinely subject to minor head blows but do not then develop dementia. More vexing is the question of repeated concussive injury, such as occurs most clearly in the course of certain activities such as boxing. The medical community has long recognized a dementia syndrome in boxers, whose regrettable objective in the ring is nothing less than to inflict TBI upon one another.

In 1928, the term "punch drunk" was applied to the altered cognition and staggering gait that often afflicted pugilists who came to medical attention (Martland, 1928). This descriptor was later replaced by the less pejorative term dementia pugilistica (Millspaugh, 1937), and an association was observed between repeated bouts with head injury and neurobehavioral decline in subsequent years. In both syndromes, a progressive dementia in boxers was recognized, although specific information about this syndrome was slow to accumulate.

The most detailed clinical study of dementia pugilistica was presented by Roberts (1969), who examined former British boxers and found a wide spectrum of deficits such as dysarthria, dysequilibrium, corticospinal signs, ataxia, gait disorder, parkinsonism, and, of course, dementia. The most comprehensive neuropathological study of this disorder was published in 1973, and an autopsy series of 15 ex-boxers concluded that this condition could be distinguished from other degenerative dementias (Corsellis, Bruton, and Freeman-Browne, 1973). Core features of the disease were cerebral atrophy, cavum septum pellucidum, forniceal atrophy, thinning of the corpus callosum, demyelination and loss of Purkinje cells in the cerebellum, and neurofibrillary tangles in the substantia nigra and cerebral cortices, most prominently of the medial temporal lobes (Corsellis, Bruton, and Freeman-Browne, 1973). Of particular interest was the typical paucity of neuritic plaques (Corsellis, Bruton, and Freeman-Browne, 1973).

For many decades after 1928, the understanding prevailed among neurologists, but not necessarily among advocates of boxing, that dementia pugilistica was a progressive disorder of boxers that featured cognitive dysfunction, as well as pyramidal, extrapyramidal, and cerebellar characteristics (Roberts, 1969; Corsellis, Bruton, and Freeman-Browne, 1973; Unterharnscheidt, 1995). But as a similar syndrome came to be recognized in athletes previously engaged in contests other than the "manly art of self-defense" and in individuals exposed to military combat, a new direction of research was organized that focused on the late effects of repetitive mTBI.

Chronic traumatic encephalopathy

The popularity of contact sports in the United States and other countries has grown steadily for many years, and with it an expanded focus on the medical consequences of these often highly injurious contests. Sport is a peacetime endeavor, however, and equally significant is the problem of concussion in the military, as has been clear from study of the recent conflicts in the Middle East. Not only has mTBI in the traditional sense of closed head injury been distressingly common in these wars, but the newer wound of blast injury related to explosions near to combatants has achieved widespread recognition (Ling et al., 2009; Magnuson, Leonessa, and Ling, 2012). Blast injury is in many respects closely related to concussion, and as currently understood, the immediate, subacute, and long-term consequences of these injuries appear to be similar.

As discussed earlier, a recent development evolving from the study of concussion in sports and the military is the proposal that a chronic dementing disorder can result from repeated concussions, or possibly even subconcussive blows to the head. Much uncertainty is apparent in this field, as it is unclear, to list but two questions, how common this syndrome may be and how many impacts may be necessary for its development; but major concerns have arisen because of the possibility of dementia occurring after what has been considered to be head blows that usually portend no long-term deleterious effects (Godbolt et al., 2014).

The term CTE was first used in 1949 by the British neurologist Macdonald Critchley, who suggested that not just boxers were susceptible to long-standing neurologic decline from repetitive brain injuries (Critchley, 1949). Although the literatures on CTE and dementia pugilistica cannot be interpreted as proving identity in all respects, it is likely that these conditions are two examples of the same fundamental process.

The first modern case of CTE was described in 2005 in a retired National Football League (NFL) player who was found unexpectedly at autopsy to have numerous diffuse amyloid plaques and less frequent neurofibrillary tangles (Omalu et al., 2005). A second case, again in a retired NFL player, appeared the following year, and featured neurofibrillary tangles but no amyloid deposition (Omalu et al., 2006). As both players clearly had long-term repetitive concussive brain injury, the idea began to take shape that American football can lead to encephalopathy similar to that of dementia pugilistica in boxers. With further study, and more athletes coming to postmortem analysis, the prominence of neurofibrillary tangles was increasingly recognized, and CTE came to be recognized as a progressive dementia with prominent tauopathy that is postulated to occur as a consequence of repetitive mTBI (McKee et al., 2009; McKee et al., 2013; McKee et al., 2015). As time went on, CTE was also recognized in college and high school football players, amateur athletes in boxing and hockey, and military veterans (McKee et al., 2013; McKee et al., 2015), expanding the implications of the syndrome to a far wider population than those engaged in professional sport.

The clinical phenomenology of CTE is thought to include both cognitive dysfunction and behavioral changes. Clinical features include memory loss, personality change, disinhibition, aggressiveness, depression, suicidality, parkinsonism, ataxia, gait disorder, and impaired olfaction (Gavett, Stern, and McKee, 2011). In a study of autopsy-verified cases of CTE, cognitive dysfunction had been present in nearly all, but, in comparison to an older group, a younger group of patients manifested greater depression and behavioral changes such as irritability, anger, impulsivity, and paranoia (Stern et al., 2013). The clinical similarity of CTE to frontotemporal dementia (FTD) has been noted by many neurologists, and an unequivocal distinction between these two similar entities remains to be established. In addition to many neurobehavioral similarities between CTE and FTD, another potential link comes from the observation that amyotrophic lateral sclerosis (ALS) can occur with both diseases (Ng, Rademakers, and Miller, 2015). Whereas CTE by definition features multiple premorbid brain injuries and also differs from FTD by the longer duration of disease, lasting decades in many cases (McKee et al., 2013), the frequent neuropathological finding of TAR DNA-binding protein 43 (TDP-43) in CTE (McKee et al., 2013) does suggest a possible pathogenetic link to FTD. A particularly distressing clinical aspect of CTE is the high risk of suicide, which is thought to result from severe depression in many individuals. The mood disorder of CTE has often culminated in the suicide of affected persons, some of whom have donated their brains to science in an effort to help researchers learn more of the disorder.

The incidence of CTE is not known, as population-based studies have not been conducted. Whereas it is possible that a large number of CTE cases will be found to result from repetitive mTBI, it is equally plausible that most individuals who sustain this form of injury are unscathed by any late neurobehavioral deterioration. A recent autopsy case series of six retired professional football players with multiple concussions and cognitive impairment found AD, ALS, and Parkinson's Disease, but no CTE (Hazrati et al., 2013. The only meaningful epidemiological data regarding repetitive mTBI derive from the study of boxers mentioned previously (Roberts, 1969), among whom 17% had neurologic deficits that were plausibly attributable to boxing. In general, the longer the fighter had been engaged in boxing, the greater was the likelihood that these deficits were present (Roberts, 1969). However, the substantial number of athletes, military personnel, and others at risk presents the worrisome possibility that CTE may be far more common than currently appreciated. The specter of CTE is still more ominous if subconcussive blows are in fact determined to be injurious (Bailes et al., 2013).

Whereas these concerns are legitimate, it needs to be kept in mind that not all individuals who have sustained repetitive head impact develop CTE; stated another way, exposure to head impacts is a necessary but not sufficient condition for the occurrence of CTE (Baugh et al., 2014). An alarmist view – that essentially all humans are at risk for CTE because life without some form of a blow to the head at some time is unimaginable – is clearly unjustified based on the available data. Indeed, the incidence of CTE may well be significantly moderated by factors such as a protective genotype, cognitive reserve, and endogenous reparative capacity of the brain. Much remains to be learned of the long-term of impact of TBI, and appropriate concern has been raised about the potential of "catastrophizing" the effects of concussion (Wortzel, Brenner, and Arciniegas, 2013), but the idea of CTE is important and deserves much further study.

The role of white matter dysfunction in CTE, our major topic, is intriguing. The vulnerability of white matter to TBI is of course well known, as both macroscopic (Strich, 1970) and microscopic (Adams et al., 1982) lesions in the cerebral white matter have been recognized for many years. To illustrate, Figure 15.1 shows an autopsied brain after TBI with DAI in the corpus callosum. The accumulation of many such injuries over an extended period of time leads to the reasonable proposition that dementia can be a long-term sequel. With respect to the development of CTE many years after repetitive mTBI, neuropathological study has naturally concentrated on findings such as cerebral atrophy and the deposition of proteins such as tau, TDP-43, and amyloid, but as white matter is unmistakenly affected in TBI, injury to myelinated systems may be primary (Bigler, 2013). Indeed, the largest published CTE study to date found tau pathology in 68 of 85 subjects with repetitive mTBI, but all 68 had some degree of white matter change as well, ranging from axonal varicosities to widespread myelin and axonal loss with tract atrophy (McKee et al., 2013).

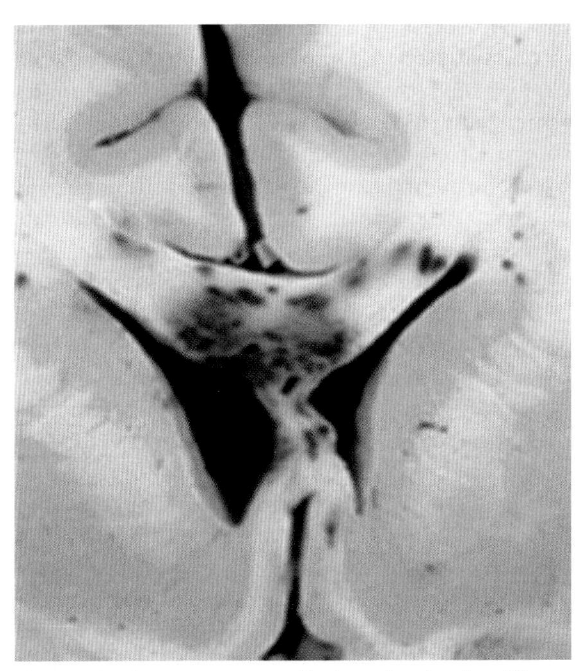

Figure 15.1 Postmortem coronal brain section showing diffuse axonal injury (DAI) in the corpus callosum after TBI (from Sharp DJ, Scott G, and Leech R, 2014).

Neuroradiologists have endeavored to find white matter changes in the acute phase of mTBI, but this task has proven difficult, and even the more recent and promising MRI sequences such as gradient echo (GRE) and susceptibility-weighted imaging (SWI) likely miss many areas of DAI. Thus conventional neuroimaging cannot yet provide conclusive answers as to whether and in what way white matter changes influence the progression from concussion to CTE. However, intriguing new data in the chronic phase of TBI have found that white matter damage may actually progress in subsequent years while gray matter injury remains stable (Bigler, 2013). For example, the longest follow-up MRI study of severe TBI to date has shown that the corpus callosum continues to lose volume at 8 years postinjury while the hippocampus does not (Tomaiuolo et al., 2012). One component of this selective white matter injury may be ongoing inflammation, as reactive microglia in association with white matter degeneration have been documented as long as 18 years after moderate or severe TBI (Johnson et al., 2013).

Diffusion tensor imaging (DTI) may hold the most promise in the study of long-term effects of TBI (Shenton et al., 2012). Recent DTI studies extending to 4 years after TBI have shown volume loss in multiple association tracts and the corpus callosum, but not gray matter (Farbota et al., 2012). Similarly, data have been presented to support the role of DAI within white matter as a contributor to subcortical volume loss (Leunissen et al., 2014). Other studies have shown that diffuse white matter injury is present in nondemented older athletes who had sports-related concussions, and that cognitive deficits are associated with these abnormalities (Tremblay et al., 2014). The onset of mood disorder after TBI was highlighted by a recent DTI study of retired professional football players documenting a correlation between microstructural abnormalities of frontal white matter tracts and depressive symptoms (Strain et al., 2013). DTI has also been used to investigate blast injury, and veterans with a history of blast injury had widespread reduction in white matter fractional anisotropy compared to those who had not sustained this form of injury (Taber et al., 2015). In this study, some blast-exposed subjects had had no symptoms of concussion, implying that blast exposure may induce subconcussive injury (Taber et al., 2015). A similar conclusion was drawn from a controlled prospective study of high school hockey and football players, who were found to have white matter changes at the end of the season that could be attributed to subconcussive blows and not to concussion (Bazarian et al., 2014).

It is clear that the older literature on dementia pugilistica finds a close counterpart in the more recent writings on CTE. Both conditions are progressive dementing disorders that share many clinical and neuropathological features (Roberts, 1969; Corsellis, Bruton, and Freeman-Browne, 1973; McKee et al., 2009; McKee et al., 2013; McKee et al., 2015). The neuropathological hallmark of each is widespread cortical tau deposition, while cortical amyloid accumulates in less than half of the reported cases (Corsellis, Bruton, and Freeman-Browne, 1973; McKee et al., 2013). In CTE, the tau neuropathology has been the basis for designating the disorder as a progressive tauopathy, and indeed the prominence of this protein at autopsy is striking. Yet this interpretation of the neuropathology of CTE may require revision when the larger picture of this disorder is taken into account.

Diffuse axonal injury and tauopathy

The assumption that the protein deposits in cortical regions are the most important neuropathological aspect of CTE appears to reflect the corticocentric bias of neuroscience. Recent reviews highlight the intracellular cortical tau aggregates making up neurofibrillary tangles as the hallmark of CTE, yet the same reviews state that axonal pathology within white matter is present in all cases (Mez, Stern, and McKee, 2013; McKee et al., 2015). From these statements it may quite logically be questioned why tau is the hallmark lesion of CTE while white matter injury is not. The ready visibility of tangles in brains where these findings are unexpected no doubt exerts a powerful influence. Moreover, the strong precedence of amyloid plaques being accepted as a core feature of the AD brain likely colors judgment as well. However, as DAI is well known in TBI, qualifies as a neuropathological feature common to all degrees of TBI severity, and regularly appears in TBI brains in the absence of tau, it is at least as plausible that white matter injury is the hallmark feature of CTE while tau is a downstream phenomenon. It is to this intriguing possibility we now turn.

To begin, tau is a normal brain protein, and is in fact concentrated in white matter areas. The majority of tau is found in axons, where it functions to stabilize microtubules and maintain normal axonal transport (Shahani and Brandt, 2002). In the brain, this phenomenon critically underlies normal axonal physiology and supports the operations of distributed neural networks. Because of its location within axons that may extend over one meter in length (Stokin and Goldstein, 2006), tau is highly vulnerable to injury. Autopsy examination after severe TBI in humans has found that, among several abnormal proteins, phosphorylated tau accumulates within injured axons and neuronal cell bodies in association with DAI (Uryu et al., 2007), and studies in mice have yielded comparable results (Tran et al., 2011). The acceleration and deceleration forces associated with DAI in mTBI are thought to exert a similar effect, causing microtubular tau to become hyperphosphorylated and aggregate within neurofibrillary tangles, where it is presumably neurotoxic (McKee et al., 2009).

All CTE cases studied thus far, from the mildest to the most severe, display DAI (McKee et al., 2013; McKee et al., 2015). While this lesion is not likely to have long-term clinical sequelae if it is mild and has been only rarely sustained, the possibility emerges that repeated DAI as a result of repetitive mTBI leads to overwhelming disruption of normal tau metabolism and subsequent progressive tauopathy with dementia. Tauopathy may therefore be a late result of the repeated white matter injury that may occur during an athlete's or a soldier's career. The propensity for the deposition of other proteins to be activated by TBI (Uryu et al., 2007) may depend on genetic factors that modify the relative risk of one dementia versus another. But all these proteins may be deposited as a result of upstream white matter injury in TBI.

An important question can be raised as to why single episodes of mTBI do not result in CTE. Most concussions, as reviewed earlier, resolve spontaneously, and, if they do not, psychological factors are usually found to be responsible. In this light, the interesting observation has been made that hyperphosphorylated tau may serve a protective role (Castellani et al., 2008). This aggregated protein is found in many normal brains, can exist for decades without apparent ill effect, and has both anti-oxidant and anti-apoptotic properties (Castellani et al., 2008). Perhaps the hyperphosphorylation of tau that occurs with DAI serves as a repair mechanism, assisting in the recovery process from concussion. Repetitive mTBI, in contrast, may overwhelm the capacity of this endogenous repair mechanism, and trigger a progressive tauopathy in which hyperphosphorylated tau becomes toxic to the cerebral cortex. Although more work is needed to substantiate this idea, tau may be a marker of brain repair in a manner similar to the proposed role played by amyloid in AD that was presented in Chapter 14.

A fascinating study in support of tauopathy as a sequel of DAI has recently been conducted with the brains of individuals subjected to prefrontal leucotomy. This procedure was one of several psychosurgical operations commonly performed for the treatment of severe psychiatric illness in the mid-twentieth century (Anderson and Arciniegas, 2004), and offers a unique opportunity to study the delayed effects of white matter injury. In all of the brains examined from six patients with schizophrenia who had undergone prefrontal leucotomy and then survived another 40 years, abnormal tau was selectively found in frontal cortical areas adjacent to the leucotomy lesion sites (Edgerton et al., 2014). The tau collections were found at the depths of cortical sulci in a manner closely resembling the distribution of tau in CTE (Edgerton et al., 2014). Because prefrontal leucotomy can be considered a single episode of severe DAI, the late appearance of tauopathy in cortical areas related to the white matter lesion may serve as a dramatic example of the prolonged development of tauopathy that occurs in repetitive mTBI with DAI.

A helpful clinical development in CTE has been the possibility that tau can be seen in the living brain. Although the neuroimaging of tau in the brain has lagged somewhat behind that of amyloid, efforts to develop a ligand for this protein have been initiated, and the agent T807 has recently been introduced as a means of visualizing tau when used in combination with positron emission tomography (PET) (Xia et al., 2013). If there is merit to the idea that repetitive DAI in the cerebral white matter is the triggering event for what may become CTE in vulnerable individuals, tau imaging may prove conclusive by virtue of its capacity to enable the longitudinal study of injured persons at the time of TBI and for years or decades thereafter. The spread of tau pathology from injured axons outward to the cerebral cortices and other regions could be tracked and correlated with a variety of clinical, MRI, and neuropsychological data over protracted periods. In contrast to AD, in which the onset of disease remains an unresolved conundrum, the onset of CTE can potentially be regarded as the time of the first mTBI event, and with improved case recognition and follow-up – now apparent both in the world of sports and in the military – the prospects of following the evolution of tauopathy are favorable if T807 is found to be a suitable agent, or another more suitable ligand with this capacity is identified.

As it seems likely that a only small percentage of injured persons develops CTE, and a long latency between repetitive mTBI and CTE is typical (McKee et al., 2009), many other factors may be operative in the pathogenesis of this disease. In addition to the traumatic injuries sustained, it is important to consider the influence of brain and cognitive reserve, the capacity of the white matter to repair itself, comorbid medical problems, and the role of many genetic factors, some still to be discovered. The number and the severity of blows to the head are variables that can be meaningfully studied with improved clinical evaluation. Brain and cognitive reserve may well influence the effects of TBI, and preliminary work has appeared (Randolph, Karantzoulis, and Guskiewicz, 2013). An intriguing factor may be the variable capacity of the brain to repair itself, and, following the myelin model discussed in Chapter 14, tauopathy in CTE may be another example of inadequate myelin repair (Bartzokis, 2011). Comorbid medical problems such as cardiovascular disease and alcohol abuse are likely to be important. Genetics may also explain why some brains may be better able to withstand the effects of repeated concussion with DAI. Most obviously, the potential role of the APOE ε4 genotype in hampering myelin repair may be relevant (Bartzokis, 2011), but preliminary observations of the influence of APOE status have been inconclusive thus far (McKee et al., 2009).

If DAI causes tau disruption in damaged axons and then secondary tauopathy, how does the abnormal protein become so distributed so widely across the brain? It seems increasingly clear that TBI, through the mechanism of DAI, disrupts axonal structure and function in a manner that can lead to long-term neurodegeneration in at least some individuals (Johnson, Stewart, and Smith, 2013). If the deposition of abnormal amounts of protein occurs, which in the case of CTE means tau pathology, it must be understood how this protein arrives at cortical regions to produce the more clinically apparent problems in cognition and behavior.

In this context, the issue of protein propagation has lately become a central concern of human neurobiology. Tau likely spreads via multiple mechanisms throughout the brain, as has been shown in animal models (Le et al., 2012). The idea has even been advanced that tau in CTE is actually a prion, behaving in a manner similar to pathologic proteins known to be involved in rapidly progressive dementias such as Creutzfeldt-Jakob disease (Prusiner, 2012). But the spread of tauopathy after mTBI may not be as rapid as that seen in typical prion diseases. The study of leucotomized schizophrenics discussed previously (Edgerton et al., 2014) sheds some light on this issue by suggesting that tauopathy can develop as long as 40 years after acute axonal injury.

CTE thus remains a pivotal but controversial proposal with many implications regarding the relationship of white matter injury to degenerative dementia. In light of its uncertain pathogenesis, a comprehensive recent review of CTE tellingly includes the statements that (1) axonal injury and white matter atrophy are constant features of the disease, (2) hyperphosphorylated tau is a known sequel of DAI in experimental animal studies, and (3) hyperphosphorylated tau may spread interneuronally via prion-like tau misfolding (McKee et al., 2015). It may be that the idea of white matter injury being the *primum movens* of CTE is in fact gaining momentum. Further investigation, ideally involving longitudinal white matter imaging, identification of tau with PET, and neuropathological study when possible, may lead to the conclusion that the dementia and tauopathy of CTE are in fact the late consequences of early and repeated DAI in individuals who were exposed to repetitive mTBI.

References

ACRM (American Congress of Rehabilitation Medicine) Mild Traumatic Brain Injury Committee of the Head Injury Interdisciplinary Special Interest Group. Definition of mild traumatic brain injury. J Head Trauma Rehabil 1993; 8: 86–87.

Adams JH, Graham DI, Murray LS, Scott G. Diffuse axonal injury due to nonmissile head injury in humans: an analysis of 45 cases. Ann Neurol 1982; 12: 557–563.

Alexander MP. Mild traumatic brain injury: pathophysiology, natural history, and clinical management. Neurology 1995; 45: 1253–1260.

Anderson CA, Arciniegas DB. Neurosurgical interventions for neuropsychiatric syndromes. Curr Psychiatry Rep 2004; 6: 355–363.

Bailes JE, Petraglia AL, Omalu BI, et al. Role of subconcussion in repetitive mild traumatic brain injury. J Neurosurg 2013; 119: 1235–1245.

Bartzokis G. Alzheimer's disease as homeostatic responses to age-related myelin breakdown. Neurobiol Aging 2011; 32: 1341–1371.

Baugh CM, Robbins CA, Stern RA, McKee AC. Current understanding of chronic traumatic encephalopathy. Curr Treat Options Neurol 2014; 16: 306.

Bazarian JJ, Zhu T, Zhong J, et al. Persistent, long-term cerebral white matter changes after sports-related repetitive head impacts. PLoS One 2014; 9: e94734.

Belanger HG, Vanderploeg RD, McAllister T. Subconcussive blows to the head: a formative review of short-term clinical outcomes. J Head Trauma Rehabil 2015 Apr 29. [Epub ahead of print]

Bigler ED. Traumatic brain injury, neuroimaging, and neurodegeneration. Front Hum Neurosci 2013; 7: 395.

Cassidy JD, Cancelliere C, Carroll LJ, et al. Systematic review of self-reported prognosis in adults after mild traumatic brain injury: results of the International Collaboration on Mild Traumatic Brain Injury Prognosis. Arch Phys Med Rehabil 2014; 95 (3 Suppl): S132–S151.

Castellani RJ, Nunomura A, Lee HG, et al. Phosphorylated tau: toxic, protective, or none of the above. J Alzheimers Dis 2008; 14: 377–383.

Cobb BR, Urban JE, Davenport EM, et al. Head impact exposure in youth football: elementary school ages 9–12 years and the effect of practice structure. Ann Biomed Eng 2013; 41: 2463–2473.

Corsellis JA, Bruton CJ, Freeman-Browne D. The aftermath of boxing. Psychol Med 1973; 3: 270–303.

Critchley M. Punch-drunk syndromes: the chronic traumatic encephalopathy of boxers. In: *Hommage à Clovis Vincent*. Paris: Maloine, 1949.

Edgerton S, Shively S, Mufson E, et al. Single episode axonal injury can lead to tau pathology resembling chronic traumatic encephalopathy. J Neuropathol Exp Neurol 2014; 73: 588–589.

Farbota KD, Sodhi A, Bendlin BB, et al. Longitudinal volumetric changes following traumatic brain injury: a tensor-based morphometry study. J Int Neuropsychol Soc 2012; 18: 1006–1018.

Filley CM. *Neurobehavioral anatomy*. 3rd ed. Boulder: University of Colorado Press, 2011.

Gardner RC, Yaffe K. Epidemiology of mild traumatic brain injury and neurodegenerative disease. Mol Cell Neurosci 2015; 66: 75–80.

Gavett BE, Stern RA, McKee AC. Chronic traumatic encephalopathy: a potential late effect of sport-related concussive and subconcussive head trauma. Clin Sports Med 2011; 30: 179–188.

Godbolt AK, Cancelliere C, Hincapié CA, et al. Systematic review of the risk of dementia and chronic cognitive impairment after mild traumatic brain injury: results of the International Collaboration on Mild Traumatic Brain Injury Prognosis. Arch Phys Med Rehabil 2014; 95 (3 Suppl): S245–S256.

Goldstein, M. Traumatic brain injury: a silent epidemic. Ann Neurol 1990; 27: 327.

Hazrati LN, Tartaglia MC, Diamandis P, et al. Absence of chronic traumatic encephalopathy in retired football players with multiple concussions and neurological symptomatology. Front Hum Neurosci 2013; 7: 222.

Johnson VE, Stewart JE, Begbie FD, et al. Inflammation and white matter degeneration persist for years after a single traumatic brain injury. Brain 2013; 136: 28–42.

Johnson VE, Stewart W, Smith DH. Axonal pathology in traumatic brain injury. Exp Neurol 2013; 246: 35–43.

Kelly JP, Nichols JS, Filley CM, et al. Concussion in sports: guidelines for the prevention of catastrophic outcome. J Am Med Assoc 1991; 266: 2867–2869.

Le MN, Kim W, Lee S, et al. Multiple mechanisms of extracellular tau spreading in a non-transgenic tauopathy model. Am J Neurodegener Dis 2012; 1: 316–333.

Leunissen I, Coxon JP, Caeyenberghs K, et al. Subcortical volume analysis in traumatic brain injury: the importance of the fronto-striato-thalamic circuit in task switching. Cortex 2014; 51: 67–81.

Levin HS, Diaz-Arrastia RR. Diagnosis, prognosis, and clinical management of mild traumatic brain injury. Lancet Neurol 2015; 14: 506–517.

Ling G, Bandak F, Armonda R, et al. Explosive blast neurotrauma. J Neurotrauma 2009; 26: 815–825.

Magnuson J, Leonessa F, Ling GS. Neuropathology of explosive blast traumatic brain injury. Curr Neurol Neurosci Rep 2012; 12: 570–579.

Martland, HS. Punch drunk. J Am Med Assoc 1928; 91: 1103–1107.

McAllister TW, Arciniegas D. Evaluation and treatment of postconcussive symptoms. NeuroRehabilitation 2002; 17: 265–283.

McKee AC, Cantu RC, Nowinski CJ, et al. Chronic traumatic encephalopathy in athletes: progressive tauopathy after repetitive head injury. J Neuropathol Exp Neurol 2009; 68: 709–735.

McKee AC, Stein TD, Nowinski CJ, et al. The spectrum of disease in chronic traumatic encephalopathy. Brain 2013; 136: 43–64.

McKee AC, Stein TD, Kiernan PT, Alvarez VE. The neuropathology of chronic traumatic encephalopathy. Brain Pathol 2015; 25: 350–364.

Mez J, Stern RA, McKee AC. Chronic traumatic encephalopathy: where are we and where are we going? Curr Neurol Neurosci Rep 2013; 13: 407.

Millspaugh JA. Dementia pugilistica (punch drunk). U S Nav Med Bull 1937; 35: 297–303.

Ng AS, Rademakers R, Miller BL. Frontotemporal dementia: a bridge between dementia and neuromuscular disease. Ann N Y Acad Sci 2015; 1338: 71–93.

Omalu BI, DeKosky ST, Minster RL, et al. Chronic traumatic encephalopathy in a National Football League player. Neurosurgery 2005; 57: 128–134.

Omalu BI, DeKosky ST, Hamilton RL, et al. Chronic traumatic encephalopathy in a National Football League player: part II. Neurosurgery 2006; 59: 1086–1092.

Prusiner SB. Cell biology: a unifying role for prions in neurodegenerative diseases. Science 2012; 336: 1511–1513.

Randolph C, Karantzoulis S, Guskiewicz K. Prevalence and characterization of mild cognitive impairment in retired National Football League players. J Int Neuropsychol Soc 2013; 19: 873–880.

Roberts AH. *Brain damage in boxers: a study of the prevalence of traumatic encephalopathy among ex-professional boxers*. London: Pitman Medical & Scientific Publishing, 1969.

Shahani N, Brandt R. Functions and malfunctions of the tau proteins. Cell Mol Life Sci 2002; 59: 1668–1680.

Sharp DJ, Scott G, Leech R. Network dysfunction after traumatic brain injury. Nat Rev Neurol 2014; 10: 156–166.

Shenton ME, Hamoda HM, Schneiderman JS, et al. A review of magnetic resonance imaging and diffusion tensor imaging findings in mild traumatic brain injury. Brain Imaging Behav 2012; 6: 137–192.

Stern RA, Daneshvar DH, Baugh CM, et al. Clinical presentation of chronic traumatic encephalopathy. Neurology 2013; 81: 1122–1129.

Stokin GB, Goldstein LS. Axonal transport and Alzheimer's disease. Annu Rev Biochem 2006; 75: 607–627.

Strain J, Didehbani N, Cullum CM, et al. Depressive symptoms and white matter dysfunction in retired NFL players with concussion history. Neurology 2013; 81: 25–32.

Strich SJ. Lesions in the cerebral hemispheres after blunt head injury. J Clin Pathol Suppl (R Coll Pathol) 1970; 4: 166–171.

Taber KH, Hurley RA, Haswell CC, et al. White matter compromise in veterans exposed to primary blast forces. J Head Trauma Rehabil 2015; 30: E15–E25.

Tomaiuolo F, Bivona U, Lerch JP, et al. Memory and anatomical change in severe non missile traumatic brain injury: 1 vs. 8 years follow-up. Brain Res Bull 2012; 87: 373–382.

Tran HT, LaFerla FM, Holtzman DM, Brody DL. Controlled cortical impact traumatic brain injury in 3xTg-AD mice causes acute intra-axonal amyloid-β accumulation and independently accelerates the development of tau abnormalities. J Neurosci 2011; 31: 9513–9525.

Tremblay S, Henry LC, Bedetti C, et al. Diffuse white matter tract abnormalities in clinically normal ageing retired athletes with a history of sports-related concussions. Brain 2014; 137: 2997–3011.

Unterharnscheidt F. A neurologist's reflections on boxing: V. Conclude remarks. Rev Neurol 1995; 23: 1027–1032.

Uryu K, Chen XH, Martinez D, et al. Multiple proteins implicated in neurodegenerative diseases accumulate in axons after brain trauma in humans. Exp Neurol 2007; 208: 185–192.

Wortzel HS, Brenner LA, Arciniegas DB. Traumatic brain injury and chronic traumatic encephalopathy: a forensic neuropsychiatric perspective. Behav Sci Law 2013; 31: 721–738.

Xia CF, Arteaga J, Chen G, et al. [(18)F]T807, a novel tau positron emission tomography imaging agent for Alzheimer's disease. Alzheimers Dement 2013; 9: 666–676.

Chapter 16

Beyond corticocentrism

Community-based studies of large numbers of older people using magnetic resonance imaging (MRI) scans of the brain have shown that the great majority of these individuals have some degree of white matter hyperintensity (Ylikoski et al., 1995; Wen and Sachdev, 2004), most evident in the frontal lobes (Launer, 2004), and most likely on an ischemic basis (Debette and Markus, 2010; Erten-Lyons et al., 2013). Moreover, many other people of younger age – including adolescents, children, and even infants – have similarly located lesions of many diverse etiologies (Filley, 2012). Still more impressively, a great many more individuals of all ages harbor microstructural lesions when newer techniques are used to view their white matter (Filley, 2012). To add to the complexity of this field, even the gray matter of the cerebral cortex and deep nuclei are being reconsidered with respect to disruptions within the fine strands of myelinated fibers coursing within these regions (Grydeland et al., 2013; Schmahmann and Pandya, 2008). All of these observations imply that neuropathological changes in brain white matter are being far better appreciated.

With the increasing awareness that a host of neurobehavioral effects can be associated with structural changes in white matter (Fields, 2008; Schmahmann et al., 2008; Inzitari et al., 2009; Debette and Markus, 2010; Filley, 2012), it is apparent that the corticocentric view of brain–behavior relationships is beginning to yield to a more inclusive perspective. The subcortical gray matter first attracted attention in this regard, stimulating an effort that proved foundational in the characterization of dementia (Albert, Feldman, and Willis, 1974; McHugh and Folstein, 1975), and this work set the stage for further study examining how white matter can be conceptualized (Filley et al., 1989; Lafosse et al., 2007). Advances in MRI have opened up a wide vista of new opportunities to study the entire brain, and advancing beneath the cortex to pursue its connectivity is proving not only feasible but highly informative with regard to behavior and its disturbances. In this light, the syndrome of white matter dementia (WMD) merits continued attention (Filley et al., 1988; Filley, 1998; Schmahmann et al., 2008).

WMD has now existed as a theoretical construct for nearly 30 years, and its utility as an organizational concept appears to be expanding. WMD, and its more recent companion mild cognitive dysfunction (MCD), are not disease-specific diagnoses, and neither incidence nor prevalence data are available for either syndrome, but steadily mounting evidence for the role of white matter in cognition helps support their legitimacy. As a measure of how much this area has grown since the coining of the term WMD (Filley et al., 1988), a PubMed search in early 2015 disclosed that the term "white matter dementia" found only 211 citations from 1837 through 1987, whereas 4,235 citations appeared from 1988 through 2015 (Figure 16.1).

Since the idea of WMD was conceived, not only has the Human Connectome Project been vigorously launched (Sporns, 2011; Wang et al., 2015), but textbooks devoted to various dimensions of white

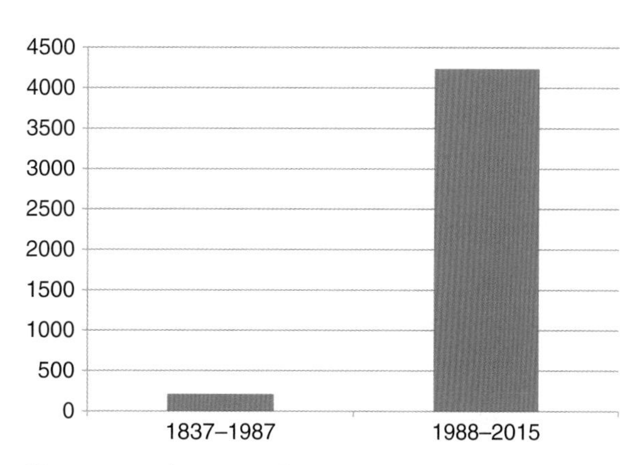

Figure 16.1 White matter dementia citations on PubMed before 1988 (211) and after (4,235).

matter and cognition have begun to appear, including an atlas of human brain connections as determined by diffusion tensor imaging (DTI) tractography (Catani and Thiebaut de Schotten, 2012) and a detailed account of pathophysiological mechanisms affecting white matter in a wide range of disorders (Baltan et al., 2014). White matter is clearly receiving more attention in the study of dementia (Ropper, Samuels, and Klein, 2014), and this development is apparent not only in the context of disorders primarily affecting white matter, but also in the study of other problems such as Alzheimer's Disease (AD; Bartzokis, 2011) and chronic traumatic encephalopathy (CTE; McKee et al., 2013).

Connectivity and cognition: the function of white matter

The role of white matter in human behavior is surely a vast and imposing topic. While many in neuroscience and cognitive neurology are deterred from the study of white matter because its role is considered merely supportive and the cerebral cortex mediates the higher functions, such a view is incomplete. The simple fact that about half the human brain is made up of white matter immediately compels respect for what has long been overlooked in the study of cognition and emotion (Filley, 2010). Moreover, as discussed in Chapter 3, white matter has expanded more in evolution than cortical gray matter (Zhang and Sejnowski, 2000), an observation that has helped foster the current view that the human brain owes its singular capacities not only to its large number of neurons (Rushton and Ankney, 2009) but also to the connectivity conferred by myelination (Roth and Dicke, 2005). The impressive evolutionary expansion of myelinated tracts, especially those intimately involved with the frontal lobes (Zhang and Sejnowski, 2000; Schoenemann, Sheehan, and Glotzer, 2005; Smaers et al., 2010), offers an important clue that the behavioral neurosciences will discover only partial understanding by focusing on the cerebral cortex alone.

Clinically, beyond the useful generalization that white matter facilitates the operations of distributed neural networks, in most cases the specific neurobehavioral details of tract function are yet to be worked out. Excepting such large tracts as the corpus callosum, neuroradiologists in clinical practice are usually unable to identify specific white matter connections so that the neurobehavioral effects of lesions can be observed. Whereas myelination clearly increases conduction velocity and improves network efficiency, white matter tracts will be increasingly found to carry out more specific functions in the panoply of cognitive and emotional operations, contributing to behavior by virtue of their location within networks dedicated to cognitive and emotional functions. White matter participates as an essential neuroanatomic component of cortical and subcortical structures linked in reciprocal relationships enabling the phenomena of cognition and emotion (Parvizi, 2009). Thus a myelinated connection will be uniquely contributory not because of its myelination alone but also because of its position within a network devoted to a given operation such as memory, language, or executive function. In this regard, white matter adheres perfectly to the neurobehavioral dictum that the location of the structure predicts its function. Moreover, by implication, the location of neuropathology determines the nature of the clinical deficit. Elucidation of the details of white matter connectivity will thus steadily expand the understanding of how the brain mediates singularly human capacities and their dissolution in neuropathological states (Filley, 2012).

The study of dementia in the context of white matter can be seen as one aspect of the broader issue of how white matter contributes to the higher functions of the human brain. WMD is a concept intended primarily to underscore the crucial part played by myelinated systems in higher function, not to instantiate an immutable diagnostic category that will be clearly distinguishable by clinical evaluation. If the idea of WMD, together with the related construct of MCD, encourages investigation of the means by which the brain exploits its exquisite connectivity to facilitate the myriad operations of human behavior, its purpose will have been well served.

A useful summary statement is that white matter subserves the essential function of information transfer in the brain as a complement to the information processing of gray matter. No doubt exists that the elaborate mechanisms of synaptic function within gray matter enable the extraordinary processes that have been linked with higher functions such as memory acquisition, and conceptualized in terms such as long-term potentiation. Equally vital are the pathways that link gray matter regions into coherent functional networks that permit the rapid and efficient activity of integrated cognitive and emotional operations (Mesulam, 1990; Catani, 2006; Wang et al., 2015).

The study of white matter and cognition also informs the long and only tenuously resolved debate in cognitive neuroscience regarding holism versus localizationism. If white matter is important in the operations of human behavior, does it function as an equipotential whole, or are individual tracts associated with specific functions? This question was raised in past eras with respect to the cerebral cortex in the controversy about whether the cortex mediates cognition in an undifferentiated manner, as Karl Lashley and Henry Head would contend, or contains specific regions invariantly dedicated to specific functions, as argued by Franz Joseph Gall and later Paul Broca. The debate has been tentatively settled by the recognition that while individual cortical regions are indeed seen as important, and focal syndromes do occur with focal damage, the entire cortex shares a certain commonality of function, and diffuse degeneration such as that seen with AD leads to widespread cognitive dysfunction. In the case of white matter, it is likely that the same solution to this debate will obtain; that is, whereas the entirety of white matter can be seen as important in the overall syndrome of WMD, certain regions can be seen as important for specific functions (Filley, 2011).

The key concept that helps resolve both debates is the idea of distributed neural networks, the collections of gray and white matter structures devoted to individual neurobehavioral functions (Mesulam, 1990). Disruption of these networks, whether involving gray or white matter, leads either to an isolated syndrome such as aphasia or executive function, or to a more pervasive syndrome of impairment such as AD or WMD. The challenges of understanding these networks are not to be met by stale arguments about holism versus localizationism, but by acknowledging that both focal and diffuse syndromes can be produced by brain disease, and that the contributions of both gray and white matter involvement must be included for a complete account.

Disconnection and leukocentrism

In 1965, Norman Geschwind famously championed the notion of disconnection, and made it clear that white matter deserves attention in the neuroscientific study of human behavior (Geschwind, 1965). His paper can thus be seen as inaugurating an era of leukocentrism. The years following this work have gradually but unequivocally demonstrated the prescience of his ideas. Geschwind was intrigued with specific connections made within the brain, and the neurobehavioral effects of disconnecting lesions. Realizing that gray matter regions as well as white matter tracts could act as relay stations within cerebral networks, he chose to focus more on cortical structures and less on white matter. Indeed, the term "white matter" appears only infrequently in his 1965 paper, and not a single diagram or illustration of brain connectivity appears in this work of well over 100 pages. But white matter tracts were clearly a part of his thinking, even if the details of their anatomy and pathology were often obscure. The cognitive effects of selective tract disruption were included in his views of the brain and behavior, as they had been in the previous century by many European neurologists.

After Sigmund Freud was largely responsible for turning neuroscientific attention away from the localization of behavior in the early twentieth century, Geschwind restored interest in brain–behavior relationships with a spirited reconsideration of the brain and its connectivity. He viewed this focus as critical to the understanding of behavior, since studying a patient without knowing the state of the brain, as Freud had made the standard approach for many decades of the twentieth century, would inevitably be insufficient. As Geschwind wrote a decade after the appearance of his disconnection paper, "It must be realized that every behavior has an anatomy" (Geschwind, 1975).

As more information has been gathered in the age of neuroimaging, however, the simultaneous involvement of many tracts has been found to be much more common than isolated tract disruption. Indeed, with some notable exceptions, it is rare in clinical neurology to encounter a single, well-defined white matter lesion that can be usefully studied with regard to its cognitive effects. Instead, clinicians are regularly confronted by patients in whom many lesions are simultaneously apparent. The consequences of such multifocal involvement immediately complicate the analysis of clinical effects, but a concerted effort from the neuroscientific community to take on this task cannot be avoided. Just as the effects of cortical disease, broadly envisioned, are routinely considered in the approach to dementia, so too should white matter disease be included in the discussion. In short, the idea of leukocentrism – which was at first founded on the study of isolated tracts, their lesions, and their clinical consequences – now implicates the entirety of white matter in the brain. One of the ways this diffuse form of white matter involvement is being studied is with respect to the major psychiatric diseases (Walterfang et al., 2005; Haroutunian et al., 2014), itself a worthy endeavor that may reveal major insights into mental illness. The task of this book, however, has been to show how this line of investigation unavoidably leads directly to the study of dementia.

The clinical and research benefits of investigating WMD may be substantial, and far more apparent than can be demonstrated at present. The diagnosis of many patients with white matter disorders affecting cognition can be enhanced, particularly if the precursor syndrome of MCD proves useful in identifying those with early involvement. Treatment, involving existing and many evolving modalities, will continue to advance, and the opportunity to treat at the early stage of MCD may substantially improve outcome. Research will be invigorated by a host of innovations that consider the white matter as the primary site of neuropathology, and as a tissue in which specifically targeted therapeutic interventions may be transformative. One of the key areas that will assume increasing importance is the role of intracortical white matter, as these small fascicles have not received the attention devoted to the larger tracts coursing within and between the hemispheres and to and from more caudal brain regions. Many insights are likely from the investigation of this largely unexplored field.

Study of the concepts of WMD and its companion MCD may also reveal new ways of conceptualizing major neurobehavioral disorders that are either idiopathic or poorly understood. AD is the most obvious example of how a leukocentric perspective may radically restructure the field and inform new efforts to detect the initial neuropathological insult and devise new and more effective treatments. Meanwhile, CTE is an example of a disease in which the initial insult is known but the details of pathogenesis later in the course are not clear. In both diseases, the role of protein misfolding and interneuronal propagation, intensely investigated as phenomena with potentially widespread relevance to a host of neurodegenerative processes (Prusiner, 2012), may in fact become clarified as a later effect of some primary process determined largely by acquired factors well before the onset of clinical symptoms. In contrast to what is thought typically to be a stochastic process, by which proteopathies develop as a random occurrence (Prusiner, 2012), the spread of deleterious proteins to various regions around the brain may often be found to relate to common and potentially reversible factors mediated through white matter pathology such as hypertension and traumatic brain injury. Meanwhile, from the world of neuropsychiatry, schizophrenia and autism stand out as examples of highly prevalent and disabling disorders in which an interpretation involving the fundamental disturbance as a connectopathy may be illuminating.

In short, leukocentrism offers the exhilarating prospect of a new way of thinking about the brain and behavior. What is the logic of ignoring one half of the brain in thinking about cognition? Is the greater enlargement of white matter compared to gray in evolution to be disregarded? Surely a cardiology that considers only the left side of the heart to be important, for example, would not long prove productive. There is much to be learned by investigation based on curiosity about how a leukocentric approach can be instructive. To invoke one example, it has recently been recognized that plasticity in the white matter may be an important foundation of learning and memory (Fields, 2010).

Still more intriguingly, the phenomenon of creativity, an area of cognitive performance widely cherished but imposingly difficult to study, has been investigated using DTI, and significant relationships have been disclosed between creativity as measured by a divergent thinking test and fractional anisotropy in a number of association tracts and the corpus callosum (Takeuchi et al., 2010). Given the widely held view that creativity generally involves the conjoining of seemingly unrelated concepts into a novel synthesis (Austin, 1978; Heilman, 2005), it would follow that studying brain connectivity via white matter tracts is a promising approach to understanding this cognitive capacity. A related and fascinating observation is that Albert Einstein's brain features a corpus callosum that is notably thicker than those of age-matched control brains, particularly in posterior callosal regions connecting the parietal lobes (Men et al., 2014), which have also been found to be exceptionally well developed in this creative genius (Witelson, Kigar, and Harvey, 1999). Could it be that the universally exalted capacity of creativity will be found to depend critically on the integrity of tracts interconnecting gray matter regions and enabling the formation of novel insights by enhancing the physical integration of disparate neural ensembles?

The notion that white matter tracts operate as integrative structures allowing for cooperation between gray matter regions is appealing indeed, and may inform the study of many questions in cognitive neuroscience that are not readily answered by a reductionistic focus on one or another cortical zone. Corticocentrism should of course not be put aside, consigning gray matter to the same fate that white matter has endured. But it should be combined with its leukocentric counterpart, allowing the fully integrated study of all the brain in the performance of its impressive operations.

Reflections on the study of white matter and cognition

In the course of examining the contributions of white matter to cognitive function, it becomes abundantly clear that this project involves not just clinical but also basic neuroscience. While the concepts of WMD and MCD surely provoke a broad range of clinical implications – prevention, diagnosis, prognosis, and treatment – they also require an understanding of the fundamental aspects of white matter as a component of the brain. These approaches, which can be considered top-down and bottom-up respectively, serve best when complementing each other, and the most thorough understanding derives from considering the tissue in which neuropathology arises as well as the clinical phenomenology produced.

Extending beyond the corticocentric perspective of much contemporary neuroscience, the study of white matter and cognition offers the invigorating prospect of uniquely furthering the pursuit of brain–behavior relationships. As described in Chapter 5, the process of integrative review (Grimes and Schulz, 2002; Whittemore et al., 2014) based mainly on the lesion method of behavioral neurology (Damasio, 1984) offers a legitimate means of exploring how a major component of the brain contributes to the operations of human behavior. As a medical concept, WMD qualifies as a topic of applied science (Davis, 2000), as it is anticipated that understanding the clinical syndrome will lead to interventions that can alter the outcome of human beings at risk for or enduring the clinical effects of white matter disorders. The practical applications of this perspective may have far-reaching implications in terms of medical care and public policy intended to reduce the human suffering produced by white matter disorders.

Importantly, however, the study of WMD can also be used to infer the structure and function of normal white matter, thus serving the essential goal of basic science, which is to understand the natural world (Davis, 2000). Indeed, the distinction between basic and applied science is often not clear (Davis, 2000), and in the study of dementia as well as other related syndromes, behavioral neurology has in fact flourished at the interface of these endeavors. The clinical task of caring for people who are facing the cognitive consequences of brain disorders necessarily involves the integration of basic neuroscience, and the two approaches complement and reinforce each other. The medical imperative of helping people cope with potentially devastating conditions has comfortably coexisted with the scientific goal of understanding the brain through detailed examination of the effects of its disorders on normal structure and function.

The relationship of the WMD concept to basic neuroscience has a special distinction in that the vast complexity of human cognition must be considered. It is not possible to fully understand the complexities of human behavior by only using experimental paradigms specific to isolated mental operations, and understanding the entire organism must ultimately be incorporated in a complete account. As a critical component of the brain that directs the organism's behavior, white matter as a whole demands focused study. As imposing as it may seem, this task is unavoidable.

Basic science necessarily involves reductionistic investigation in the laboratory, where a tightly defined problem can be isolated, described, and modeled as a basis for understanding a larger system. It is of course indisputable that enormous advances have been made in science by the use of reductionism, and many more are sure to follow. To call upon an example from the neurosciences, the histologic study of the brain, with its identification of abnormal proteins and the like, does indeed serve to inform the study of brain–behavior relationships (Mesulam, 2012) in concert with sophisticated neuroanatomic (Schmahmann and Pandya, 2006) and neuroimaging (Catani and Thiebaut de Schotten, 2012) studies that contribute to mapping brain connectivity. Similarly, it is crucial to appreciate from a neuropathological perspective, for example, that axonal damage in white matter substantially worsens the prognosis compared to lesions in which only myelin is damaged (Trapp et al., 1998; Medana and Esiri, 2003).

However, when the primary objective is the study of the impressive spectrum of cognitive operations, human beings in their extraordinary complexity must be the central focus of investigation (Damasio, 1984; Bear, 1997). This approach falls squarely within the realm of systems biology (Villoslada et al., 2009), an emerging field that adopts an integrative strategy to understand higher-level operating principles of living organisms (Villoslada et al., 2009). Systems biology, based on the notion of biological networks in which emergent properties can be derived from a consideration of both structure and dynamics (Villoslada et al., 2009), is ideally suited to inform the investigation of white matter as it functions to subserve human behavior in health and is altered in disease (Haroutunian et al., 2014).

Experimental laboratory studies focused on specific molecular, genetic, or pharmacological aspects of human behavior are not enough. Indeed, the classic reductionistic approach to biomedical investigation, while doubtless adding important information, has not produced comprehensive understanding of the pathogenesis and effective treatment of highly prevalent and threatening disorders such as AD (Villoslada et al., 2009). Many clinicians also tout the value of the meta-analysis, in which numerous quantitative investigations are rigorously combined by sophisticated statistical manipulation, but this too falls short in some respects.

Rather, it is critical to understand the cerebral origins of behavioral dysfunction by assembling the sequelae of structural damage from many common and uncommon disorders, and then seeking to combine these data into a coherent clinical syndrome with wide generalizability. Cataloguing and synthesizing the cognitive effects of white matter dysfunction can thus be seen as basic science as much as examining the impact of a gene mutation, a viral infection, or an inflammatory cascade. The reductionistic approach that has so dominated recent neurobiological investigation must be complemented by a systems approach founded on the principle that the whole is more than the sum of its parts (Villoslada et al., 2009).

As the two parallel inquiries – top-down and bottom-up – proceed in what will ideally be a mutually useful collaboration, the distinction between basic and clinical research in neuroscience becomes indistinct and increasingly irrelevant. To illustrate, the fact that the amyloid plaque is a *feature* of AD does not mean that it is an *explanation*, and the elucidation of the etiopathogenesis of AD may well demand a broader systems biology approach that considers the neural networks in which the disease first begins. The same reasoning can be applied to the problem of CTE, in which the neuropathological observation of cortical tau deposition may be a function of events affecting brain connectivity many years before symptoms even appear. As much as can be learned about one or another isolated protein, a reductionistic focus on these molecules may fail to identify the larger picture needed to understand a difficult problem. This broadly synthetic way of thinking has inspired and sustained the integrative review over many years underlying this monograph and its closely related predecessor (Filley, 2012).

Much remains to be accomplished, and many long-cherished ideas about the role of the cerebral cortex in higher functions will require a fresh look and critical reevaluation. The notion of the connectome not only highlights neuroscientific efforts in this quest over many centuries but also helps organize systematic study of the structure and function of normal and abnormal white matter with respect to cognition (Geschwind, 1965; Sporns, 2011; Catani et al., 2013). Considering the contributions of white matter to cognition and its decline significantly expands the study of human mentation that is the essence of behavioral neurology.

References

Albert ML, Feldman RG, Willis AL. The “subcortical dementia” of progressive supranuclear palsy. J Neurol Neurosurg Psychiatry 1974; 37: 121–130.

Austin JH. *Chase, chance, and creativity*. New York: Columbia University Press, 1978.

Baltan S, Carmichael ST, Matute C, Xi G, Zhang JH, eds. *White matter injury in stroke and CNS disease*. New York: Springer, 2014.

Bartzokis G. Alzheimer’s disease as homeostatic responses to age-related myelin breakdown. Neurobiol Aging 2011; 32: 1341–1371.

Bear DM. Interictal behavior in temporal lobe epilepsy. In: Schacter S, Devinsky O, eds. *Behavioral neurology and the legacy of Norman Geschwind*. Philadelphia: Lippincott-Raven, 1997: 213–222.

Catani M. Diffusion tensor magnetic resonance imaging tractography in cognitive disorders. Curr Opin Neurol 2006; 19: 599–606.

Catani M, Thiebaut de Schotten M. *Atlas of human brain connections*. New York: Oxford University Press, 2012.

Catani M, Thiebaut de Schotten M, Slater D, Dell'acqua F. Connectomic approaches before the connectome. Neuroimage 2013; 80: 2–13.

Damasio AR. Behavioral neurology: research and practice. Semin Neurol 1984; 4: 117–119.

Davis BD. The scientist's world. Microbiol Mol Biol Rev 2000; 64: 1–12.

Debette S, Markus HS. The clinical importance of white matter hyperintensities on brain magnetic resonance imaging: systematic review and meta-analysis. BMJ 2010; 26; 341: c3666.

Erten-Lyons D, Woltjer R, Kaye J, et al. Neuropathologic basis of white matter hyperintensity accumulation with advanced age. Neurology 2013; 81: 977–983.

Fields RD. White matter in learning, cognition and psychiatric disorders. Trends Neurosci 2008; 31: 361–370.

Fields RD. Neuroscience: change in the brain's white matter. Science 2010; 330: 768–769.

Filley CM. The behavioral neurology of cerebral white matter. Neurology 1998; 50: 1535–1540.

Filley CM. White matter: organization and functional relevance. Neuropsychol Rev 2010; 20: 158–173.

Filley CM. White matter: beyond focal disconnection. Neurol Clin 2011; 29: 81–97.

Filley CM. *The behavioral neurology of white matter*. 2nd ed. New York: Oxford University Press, 2012.

Filley CM, Franklin GM, Heaton RK, Rosenberg NL. White matter dementia: clinical disorders and implications. Neuropsychiatry Neuropsychol Behav Neurol 1988; 1: 239–254.

Filley CM, Heaton RK, Nelson LM, et al. A comparison of dementia in Alzheimer's Disease and multiple sclerosis. Arch Neurol 1989; 46: 157–161.

Geschwind N. Disconnexion syndromes in animals and man. Brain 1965; 88: 237–294, 585–644.

Geschwind N. The borderland of psychiatry and neurology: some common misconceptions. In: Blumer D, Benson DF, eds. *Psychiatric aspects of neurologic disease*. Vol. 1. New York: Grune and Stratton, 1975: 1–8.

Grimes DA, Schulz KF. Descriptive studies: what they can and cannot do. Lancet 2002; 359: 145–149.

Grydeland H, Walhovd KB, Tamnes CK, et al. Intracortical myelin links with performance variability across the human lifespan: results from T1- and T2-weighted MRI myelin mapping and diffusion tensor imaging. J Neurosci 2013; 33: 18618–18630.

Haroutunian V, Katsel P, Roussos P, et al. Myelination, oligodendrocytes, and serious mental illness. Glia 2014; 62: 1856–1877.

Heilman KM. *Creativity and the brain*. New York: Taylor and Francis, 2005.

Inzitari D, Pracucci G, Poggesi A., et al. Changes in white matter as determinant of global functional decline in older independent outpatients: three year follow-up of LADIS (leukoaraiosis and disability) study cohort. BMJ 2009; 6 339: b2477.

Lafosse JM, Corboy JR, Leehey MA, et al. MS vs. HD: can white matter and subcortical gray matter pathology be distinguished neuropsychologically? J Clin Exp Neuropsychol 2007; 29: 142–154.

Launer LJ. Epidemiology of white matter lesions. Top Magn Reson Imaging 2004; 15: 365–367.

McHugh PR, Folstein MF. Psychiatric syndromes of Huntington's chorea. In: Benson DF, Blumer D, eds. *Psychiatric aspects of neurologic disease*. Vol. 1. New York: Grune and Stratton, 1975: 267–286.

McKee AC, Stein TD, Nowinski CJ, et al. The spectrum of disease in chronic traumatic encephalopathy. Brain 2013; 136: 43–64.

Medana IM, Esiri MM. Axonal damage: a key predictor of outcome in human CNS diseases. Brain 2003; 26: 515–530.

Men W, Falk D, Sun T, et al. The corpus callosum of Albert Einstein's brain: another clue to his high intelligence? Brain 2014; 137: e268.

Mesulam M-M. Large-scale neurocognitive networks and distributed processing for attention, language, and memory. Ann Neurol 1990; 28: 597–613.

Mesulam M. The evolving landscape of human cortical connectivity: facts and inferences. Neuroimage 2012; 62: 2182–2189.

Parvizi J. Corticocentric myopia: old bias in new cognitive sciences. Trends Cogn Sci 2009; 13: 354–359.

Prusiner SB. Cell biology: a unifying role for prions in neurodegenerative diseases. Science 2012; 336: 1511–1513.

Ropper AH, Samuels MA, Klein JP. *Adams and Victor's principles of neurology*. 10th ed. New York: McGraw-Hill, 2014.

Roth G, Dicke U. Evolution of the brain and intelligence. Trends Cogn Sci 2005; 9: 250–257.

Rushton JP, Ankney CD. Whole brain size and general mental ability: a review. Int J Neurosci 2009; 119: 691–731.

Schmahmann JD, Pandya DN. *Fiber pathways of the brain*. Oxford: Oxford University Press, 2006.

Schmahmann JD, Pandya DN. Disconnection syndromes of basal ganglia, thalamus, and cerebrocerebellar systems. Cortex 2008; 44: 1037–1066.

Schmahmann JD, Smith EE, Eichler FS, Filley CM. Cerebral white matter: neuroanatomy, clinical neurology, and neurobehavioral correlates. Ann NY Acad Sci 2008; 1142: 266–309.

Schoenemann PT, Sheehan MJ, Glotzer LD. Prefrontal white matter volume is disproportionately larger in humans than in other primates. Nat Neurosci 2005; 8: 242–252.

Smaers JB, Schleicher A, Zilles K, Vinicius L. Frontal white matter volume is associated with brain enlargement and higher structural connectivity in anthropoid primates. PLoS One 2010; 5: e9123.

Sporns O. The human connectome: a complex network. Ann N Y Acad Sci 2011; 1224: 109–125.

Takeuchi H, Taki Y, Sassa Y, et al. White matter structures associated with creativity: evidence from diffusion tensor imaging. Neuroimage 2010; 51: 11–18.

Trapp BD, Peterson J, Ransohoff RM, et al. Axonal transection in the lesions of multiple sclerosis. N Engl J Med 1998; 338: 278–285.

Villoslada P, Steinman L, Baranzini SE. Systems biology and its application to the understanding of neurological diseases. Ann Neurol 2009; 65: 124–139.

Walterfang M, Wood SJ, Velakoulis D, et al. Diseases of white matter and schizophrenia-like psychosis. Aust N Z J Psychiatry 2005; 39: 746–756.

Wang Z, Dai Z, Gong G, et al. Understanding structural-functional relationships in the human brain: a large-scale network perspective. Neuroscientist 2015; 21: 290–305.

Wen W, Sachdev P. The topography of white matter hyperintensities on brain MRI in healthy 60- to 64-year-old individuals. Neuroimage 2004; 22: 144–154.

Whittemore R, Chao A, Jang M, et al. Methods for knowledge synthesis: an overview. Heart Lung 2014; 43: 453–461.

Witelson SF, Kigar DL, Harvey T. The exceptional brain of Albert Einstein. Lancet 1999; 353: 2149–2153.

Ylikoski A, Erkinjuntti T, Raininko R, et al. White matter hyperintensities on MRI in the neurologically nondiseased elderly: analysis of cohorts of consecutive subjects aged 55 to 85 years living at home. Stroke 1995; 26: 1171–1177.

Zhang K, Sejnowski TJ. A universal scaling law between gray matter and white matter of cerebral cortex. Proc Natl Acad Sci 2000; 97: 5621–5626.

Index

Note: Italicized page numbers indicate a table or box on the designated page

acetazolamide, in NPH treatment, 72, 145
acquired factors in white matter disorders, 163, *163*
acute confusional state. *See* delirium
acute disseminated encephalomyelitis, 58
acute toxic leukoencephalopathy, 97
ADC. *See* AIDS-dementia complex
addiction disorders
- inhalant abuse, 148
- possible white matter derangement in, 38, 105
- toxic leukoencephalopathy and, 148

adolescent dementia, 37
adrenoleukodystrophy, 51, 76, 77, 145–146
age-associated memory impairment, 121
agnosia
- in AD, 29, 59, 175
- amnesia in, 29
- in BD, 48
- intracortical myelin damage and, 109
- in subcortical dementia, 30
- tau and, 175

AIDS (acquired immunodeficiency syndrome), 65. *See also* human immunodeficiency virus (HIV) infection
- articulation deficits in, 105
- dementia in, comparison with AD, 172
- history, 144
- white matter dysfunction in, 66

AIDS-dementia complex (ADC), 65
- ART treatment, 67, 144
- memory retrieval deficit in, 103
- myoclonus in, 106
- neuropsychological deficits in, 66
- normal procedural memory in, 106
- relatively preserved language in, 66
- treatment, 65, 144
- visuospatial function and, 66
- white matter changes in, 65, 144

AIDS encephalopathy, 65
Akiguchi, I., 146
Albert, Martin, 30, 96
alexia without agraphia, 6
Alzheimer, Alois, 2, 27, 28, 46
Alzheimer's Disease (AD). *See also* neuritic plaques/neurofibrillary tangles
- accepted neuropathology of, 1–2, 3
- age range of onset, 37
- aging risk factors, 172
- amnesia in, 29, 59, 103
- amyloid hypothesis of, 173–175, 178, 179, 180
- BD comparison, 46, 47, 142
- brain/cognitive reserve studies, 137–138
- brain inflammation in, 121, 158
- challenges for investigators, 172
- cholinergic augmentation in, 154
- cognitive deficit patterns in, 59
- concussions and, 188
- cortical damage in, 28, 29, 36, 177
- corticocentric diagnostic bias, 46
- corticospinal dysfunction and, 128
- diffuse axonal injury in, 165
- drug trials/failures, 174
- early onset, 37, 181
- early-onset autosomal dominant, 162
- early-onset familial, 33, 178
- epidemiological studies, 137, 162
- exercise as preventive measure, 180
- FTLD's comparison with, 29
- genetic influence of myelin repair, 167
- genetic mutations in, 33, 162
- HD, distinctions from, 30–31
- higher prevalence in women, 177–178
- historical background of, 2, 27, 28
- hypertension risk factors, 162, 164
- language impairment in, 100, 102
- late onset, 181
- MCI as precursor to, 123–124
- modifiable risk factors, 162
- MRI studies, findings, 108
- MS comparison, 100, 102, 105, 138, 167
- MS comparison studies, 100
- myelin alteration in, 22
- myelin model of, 175–179, 180, 181, 191
- NAWM abnormalities in, *119*
- NPH comparison, 101–102
- PD, distinctions from, 30–31, 96
- prevention/treatment implications, 179–181
- procedural memory preservation in, 106
- research on genetic basis of, 33
- sleep/β-amyloid clearance, 165
- sporadic AD, 178
- stem cell therapeutics potential, 168
- symptoms/diagnostic criteria of, 28–29
- SYST-EUR trial findings, 164
- TBI association, 57, 176
- transgenic mice trials, 174, 175
- vascular disease with, 32, 176
- white matter and, 172–181
- WMD similarities, 172
- WMH in, 177

amantadine, in TBI, 143
aminoacidurias, *74*
4-aminopyridine, in MS treatment, 144
amnesia
- in AD, 29, 59, 103
- in concussions, *186*
- in DAI, 56
- forgetfulness *vs.*, 31
- intracortical myelin damage and, 109
- in mixed dementias, 32
- in subcortical dementias, 30
- tau and, 175
- in TBI, 54, *186*

amyloid hypothesis of Alzheimer's Disease (AD), 173–175, 178, 179, 180
amyotrophic lateral sclerosis (ALS), 188
anatomy of white matter, 17–20, 153–155
ANI. *See* asymptomatic neurocognitive impairment

anisotropy/anisotropic (directional) diffusion, 11
Ankney, C. D., 23
antiretroviral therapy (ART), 65, 66–67, 144. *See also* zidovudine
apathy
  in BD, 47, 48, 49
  in gliomatosis cerebri, 74
  in NPH, 70, 71, 123
  in radiation leukoencephalopathy, 52
  in subcortical dementia, 31
  in toxic leukoencephalopathy, *119*
aphasia
  in AD, 29
  in BD, 48
  Broca's/Wernicke's observations on, 156
  conduction aphasia, 6, 105
  in cortical dementia, 30
  intracortical myelin damage and, 109
  in mixed dementias, 32
  neoplasms and, 72–73
  primary progressive aphasia, 153
  tau and, 175
apraxia
  in AD, 29, 59, 175
  in BD, 48
  in cortical dementials, 30
  intracortical myelin damage and, 109
  in NPH, 71
  tau and, 175
Armstrong, C., 53
arousal network, 156
arterial spin labeling PWI, 13
association tracts
  cognition/emotion role, 18
  conduction velocity, 20
  development of, 21
  DTI tractography reconstruction depiction, 12
  LA and, 45
  MS and, 110
  relevance to behavioral neurology, *18*
  TBI and, 189
  WMD resultant from damage to, 36
astrocytomas, 73
asymptomatic neurocognitive impairment (ANI), 65
athletes
  CTE in, 185, 188
  dementia pugilistica in, 187
  diffuse white matter injury in, 189–190
attention deficit-hyperactivity disorder (ADHD)
  NAWM abnormalities in, *119*
  possible white matter derangement in, 38
  sustained attentional disturbances in, 102
autism
  NAWM abnormalities in, *119*
  possible white matter derangement in, 38
autoimmune dementia, *28*, 32
axonal peripheral neuropathy, 96
axo-oligodendroglial synapses, 21, 139

Babikian, V., 48
Balò's concentric sclerosis, 58
bapineuzumab, 174
Bartzokis, G., 105
basal forebrain, 154
basal ganglia, 3
  ADC and, 65, 66, 106
  AD/FTLD and, 29
  arousal network, 156
  gliomatosis cerebri and, 74
  gray matter changes in, 66
  HD/PD and, 3
  HIV infection and, 66, 144
  movement disorders and, 106, 131
  procedural memory and, 107
  subcortical dementia and, 30
  T2 hypointensities in, 50
  white matter tracts in, *18*, 19
BD. *See* Binswanger's Disease
behavioral interventions, in WMD and MCD, 147–148
behavioral neurology. *See also* lesion method
  basic tenet of, 5
  of the cerebellum, 158
  description/focus, 1, 4, 30
  establishment of, 30
  Geschwind's contributions to, 6
  literature review/meta-analysis of, 39
Behçet's disease, *62*
benign senescent forgetfulness, 120–121
Bennett, D. A., *47*
bevacizumab, in recurrent glioblastoma multiforme treatment, 145
Binswanger, Otto, 27, 46
Binswanger's Disease (BD), 46–49
  abnormal NAWM in people with, 48
  AD comparison, 46, 47, 142
  articulation deficits in, 105
  autopsy studies, 142
  CADASIL's similarity to, 75
  cerebrovascular risk factors, 46–47
  characteristics of, 46
  clinical/imaging criteria for antemortem diagnosis, 46–47 *47*
  cognitive dysfunction in, 48–49
  corticospinal dysfunction in, 47
  depression in, 105
  diagnosis, 127
  executive dysfunction in, 101
  hypertension risk factors, 46–47
  leukoaraiosis, relationship to, 43
  medical treatment of, 142
  MRI studies, 46
  neuroradiology of, 48
  NPH comorbidity with, 70
  prognosis, 135, 136
  psychiatric dysfunction in, 47
  questions/controversy about, 46
  relatively preserved language in, 47, 49
  subcortical/frontal-subcortical pathology, 48–49
  sustained attentional disturbances in, 102
bipolar disorder
  cognitive impairment in, 37
  NAWM abnormalities in, *119*
blast injuries, 54, 57, 185
blood-brain barrier, 53, 65, 159
Boone, K. B., 45
Boston Process Approach, 130–131
boxers/boxing. *See* dementia pugilistica
bradyphrenia, 30
brain. *See also* specific structures
  development and aging, 21–22
  neuron count, 20
  19th century view of, 2
  size/intelligence correlation, studies, 23–24
  white matter percentage data, 17
brain-behavior relationships
  corticocentric perspective expansion and, 195, 199
  distributed neural networks and, 155
  Geschwind's interests in, 197
  Gestalt thinking about, 30
  interpretation complications, 63
  leucocentrism and, 198–199
  limitations in understanding, 108
  neuroimaging's role in understanding, 5, 10, 15
  reconsideration of, 1–7
  SLE and, 120
  toluene leukoencephalopathy and, 97
  20th century ignoring of, 2
  white matter tracts implicated in, *18*
brain biopsy, 73, 109, *128*, 131–132
brain connectivity. *See also* brain disconnectivity; connectome

Broca/Wernicke, introduction of, 156
cognition and, 4, 35, 196–197
distributed neural networks, 30, 38, 153, 155–157, *156*, 158, 197
emotion and, 4
foundational association/commissural tracts, 18
in frontal lobes, 21
functional neuroimaging studies, 157, 195
functional/structural, 14
Geschwind on disconnectivity, 6, 197
gray matter microconnectivity, 4, 107
historical background, 197
mapping of, 155, 199–200
musical training benefits, 139
role of myelination, 196
study of Einstein's brain, 198
white matter tracts macroconnectivity, 21, 107

brain disconnectivity. *See also* brain connectivity
disconnection syndrome, 5, 6
DTI studies, 154
frontal/temporal lobe damage and, 76
Geschwind on, 6, 197
leucocentrism and, 197–199
PET studies, 74
schizophrenia, lobotomy and, 146

brain neoplasms, 5, *72*, 72–74. *See also* focal white matter tumors; gliomas; gliomatosis cerebri; lymphomatosis cerebri
CT evaluation of, 9
focal white matter tumors, 72
frontal and temporal lobe, 72
gliomatosis cerebri, 73–74
headaches and, 72–73, 122
with increased intracranial pressure, 32
motor dysfunction and, 73
parenchymal, 72–73
population-based study findings, 72
primary, predilection for white matter, 122
primary central nervous system lymphomas, 72
radiation treatment for, 51
seizures and, 72–73, 122
treatment, 122, 145

brain reserve. *See also* cognitive reserve
concussions and, 191
description, 107, 137–138
onset of dementia and, 110

Brief Repeatable Battery of Neuropsychological Tests for MS, 59
Broca, Paul, 156, 197
Broca's aphasia, 139
Broca's area, 95, 106, 153
Brodmann, Korbinian, *18*, 19, 158
Brodmann areas, cerebral cortex, 17
bromocriptine, in TBI, 143
Brooks, W. M., 64
Brownell, B., 61

CADASIL. *See* cerebral autosomal dominant arteriopathy with subcortical infarcts and leukoencephalopathy
Caenorhabditis elegans, connectome mapping in, 4
Cajal, Santiago Ramon Y, 1
California Verbal Learning Test (CVLT), 131
callosal agenesis, *74*
cancer chemotherapy-induced leukoencephalopathy, 53–54
BCNU (1,3-bis(2-chloroethyl)-1-nitrosourea), 53
causative for leukoencephalopathy, 53
methotrexate, 53
Caplan, L. R., *47*
carbonic anhydrase inhibitors, 145. *See also* acetazolamide
carbon monoxide intoxication, 103, 104
cardiorespiratory fitness in elders, 164
cardiovascular disease
BD risk factors, 48
LA risk factors in, 44, 45
caudate nucleus, involvement in HD, 30
central pontine myelinolysis, *67*, 136
cerebellar-cognitive-affective syndrome (CCAS), 157
cerebellum, 3, 17
behavioral neurology of, 158
distributed neural networks in, 155
FXTAS and, 78
MLD and, 77
movement disorders and, 131
MRI studies, findings, 157–158
neurobehavioral importance of, 153
role in cognition and emotion, 157–158
subcortical dementia and, 30
toluene leukoencephalopathy and, 50, 98
white matter tract connections, *18*, 19
cerebral amyloid angiopathy (CAA), *43*, 173

cerebral autosomal dominant arteriopathy with subcortical infarcts and leukoencephalopathy (CADASIL), 37, 75–76
BD's similarity to, 75
cholinergic projections' vulnerability in, 154
diagnosis, 127
diagnostic challenges, 75–76
memory retrieval deficit in, 103
MRI studies, findings, 76
MS's similarity to, 75
neurobehavioral manifestations of, 76
neuroimaging studies of, 76
relatively preserved language in, 75
cerebral cortex
AD and, 177
Alzheimer's studies of, 2
autopsy study findings, 50
Brodmann areas, 17, 19
cognition association, 2
corticocentric bias and, 23
distributed neural networks in, 156
electroencephalographic studies, 3
Gall's research on, 2
gliomatosis cerebri and, 73, 74
importance/functions, 28
lesion method examination of, 5
Luria's research on, 2
mapping of, *18*
myelinated fascicles in, 154, 155
myelination patterns, 19
neuroimaging studies of, 3, 4, 14, 19
neurotransmitters in, 154
NPH and, 71
Penfield's research on, 2
plasticity in, 138
radiation and, 52
repetitive mTBI and, 191
role of, 2
special place in neuroscientific thinking, 1
subcortical dementia and, 29, 31
varied cellular architecture of, 158
Vogt and Vogt, parcellating of, 19
white matter fascicles in, 61
white matter location relative to, 35
white matter tracts, *18*
WMD and, 100
cerebral disconnection syndrome, 5, 6
cerebral ischemia, 158
cerebrospinal fluid abnormalities, in mixed dementias, 32
cerebrovascular disease. *See also* Binswanger's Disease; leukoaraiosis
BD risk factors, 46–47
as causative for cognitive dysfunction, 38

cerebrovascular disease (cont.)
  classification confusion, 42
  cognitive decline in, 128, 163
  dementia risk factors, 163
  diffusion weighting treatment value for, 11
  global prevalence of, 165
  homocysteine risk factor, 68
  morbidity/mortality in patients, 163
  white matter-behavior relationships in, 49
  young-onset dementia and, 37
Charcot, Jean-Martin, 58, 95
chemotherapy. *See also* cancer chemotherapy-induced leukoencephalopathy
  in brain neoplasia, 145
  "chemobrain" from, 122
  cognitive impairment from, 72, 122
  demyelination in, 53–54
  leukotoxic effects of, 72
  reduction of white matter disease burden, 145
children
  ADHD study, 102
  dementia in, 37
  exercise benefits for, 164
  genetic white matter disorder treatment challenges, 145
  gliomatosis cerebri in, 73
  hydrocephalus in, 104
  learning disabilities in, 52
  MLD in, 76, 77
  MS cognitive decline in, 109
  radiation leukoencephalopathy and, 52
  traumatic brain injury in, 56
cholinesterase inhibitors. *See also* donepezil; rivastigmine
  in TBI, 143
  in vascular cognitive impairment, 142
  in vascular dementia, 142
chronic painters' syndrome, 51. *See also* toluene leukoencephalopathy
chronic traumatic encephalopathy (CTE), 163, 187–190
  in athletes, 185, 188
  clinical phenomenology of, 188
  cognitive reserve and, 189
  in combat veterans, 185, 188
  corticocentric bias and, 190
  dementia pugilistica similarity, 187, 190
  frontotemporal dementia (FTD) similarity, 188
  incidence of, 188
  pathogenesis of, 191
  tau lesions in, 190
  TBI link with, 57, 165
  white matter changes and, 165, 189
clinical evaluation
  HIV infection, 128
  metachromatic leukodystrophy, 127
  mild cognitive dysfunction, 127–129
  multiple sclerosis, 127
  toluene leukoencephalopathy, 127
  white matter dementia, 127–129
Clock Drawing Test (CDT), 129
cobalamin (vitamin B_{12}) deficiency, 67–69
  corticospinal dysfunction in, 47
  mild cognitive impairment and, 145
  MRI studies, findings, 68
  myelination and, 68
  neurobehavioral manifestations of, 68
  neuropathological brain observations in, 68
  reversibility of, 68–69
  treatment, *142*, 145
cognition
  association/commissural tracts and, 18
  brain connectivity and, 4, 35, 196–197
  cerebral cortex and, 3
  early teachings on, xi, 2
  frontal lobe white matter losses and, 22
  gray matter's importance for, 24, 49, 109, 153
  myelinated systems role in, 17, 22
  neural networks mediation of, 1, 14
  subcortical gray matter and, xi
  and white matter, research perspectives, 153–159
  white matter lesions' impact on, 5
  white matter's role in, 5, 6, 17, 37
cognitive behavioral therapy (CBT), 148
cognitive impairment, 30, 32
  in Binswanger's Disease, 48–49
  cancer chemotherapy and, 122
  in cerebrovascular disease, 38
  in cobalamin deficiency, 68
  concussions and, 188
  in depression, bipolar disorder, schizophrenia, 37
  in diffuse axonal injury in TBI, 57
  education's impact on, 45
  HIV cognitive impairment and, 66
  inflammation in, 158
  in leukoaraiosis, 44, 45
  in mixed dementias, 32
  MRI's role in understanding, 5
  in MS, 37, 58–62, 101, 121
  no dementia, 121
  normal aging and, 121
  in normal pressure hydrocephalus, 70, 71, 122–123
  in NPH, 71
  radiation-related, 52
  in subcortical dementia, 30, 101
  in systemic lupus erythematosus, 64
  in toluene leukoencephalopathy, 97–98
  vascular cognitive impairment, 122
  in white matter dementia, 100, 101
  white matter's implication in pathogenesis, 4
cognitive processing speed, 5, 100
cognitive reserve. *See also* brain reserve
  concussions and, 191
  CTE and, 189
  description, 107, 137–138
  epidemiological studies of AD, 137
  onset of dementia and, 110
  role in LA mitigation, 45
Colorado Medical Society Guidelines for the Management of Concussion in Sports, *186*
commissural tracts
  cognition/emotion role, 18
  conduction velocity, 20
  development of, 21
  DTI tractography reconstruction depiction, *13*
  importance for higher functions, 20
  relevance to behavioral neurology, *18*
  role in linking hemispheres, 18
  TBI and, 56
  vascular insults and, 176
  WMD and, 36
computed tomography (CT), *9*
  history of development, 9
  in HIV infection, 65
  inadequacy in white matter disorders, 129
  LA studies, 42
  MLD studies, findings, 77
  MRI comparison with, 9
  review of brain size/GMA studies, 23
  toluene leukoencephalopathy studies, 51, 98
  visuospatial function study, findings, 104
concussions (mTBI)
  amnesia/confusion from, 54, 185
  in athletes, 186, 187
  blast injury similarity, 57
  Colorado Medical Society Guidelines for, *186*

global mTBI prevalence, 186
in military personnel, 186, 187
prognosis, 186
subconcussive injuries, 186–187
tauopathy and, 165
tau's protective role in, 191
TBI and, 185–187
conduction aphasia, 6, 105
confusion, 42
in BD, 48
cancer chemotherapy and, 53
cobalamin deficiency and, 68
in concussions, 185, *186*
in gliomatosis cerebri, 74
in metabolic toxic encephalopathy, 165
in mixed dementias, 32
in radiation leukoencephalopathy, 52
in TBI, *186*
in toluene leucoencephalopathy, 97
in toxic leucoencephalopathy, *119*
connectivity. *See* brain connectivity
connectome
changes during sleep, 21
defined, 4
Human Connectome Project, 4, 195–196
mapping in *Caenorhabditis elegans*, 4
neuroimaging studies of, 4, 17
white matter tracts and, 21
continuous positive airway pressure (CPAP), 164–165
corpus callosotomy, *54*
corpus callosum
CADASIL and, 76
creativity, association tracts, and, 198
DAI and, *55*, 55
dementia pugilistica and, 187
disconnection syndrome and, 5
FXTAS and, 78
gliomatosis cerebri and, 73
HIV infection and, 65, 66
leukodystrophies and, 76
linking role of, 18
memory retrieval and, 104
MS and, 76, *136*
musical training impact on, 139
neuroimaging studies, findings, 66, 71, 136, 144, 147–148, 164
NPH and, 71
role in attentional processing, 102
TBI with DAI and, 189, *189*
cortical atrophy, 36
cortical contusion, 55
cortical dementia, 28–29. *See also* Alzheimer's Disease; frontotemporal lobar degeneration; Pick's Disease
associated symptoms, 30
cortical damage in, 36
distinction from subcortical dementia, 3, 28, 30, 31, 95, 100, 107
encoding deficit in, 62
MS differentiation from, 62
overlap with other dementias, 38
cortical mantle, 1
corticobasal degeneration, *28*, 32
corticocentric bias (view of brain-behavior relationships)
AD diagnosis and, 46
contemporary neuroscientists' belief in, 1, 3, 23, 108–109, 138
CTE and, 190
example of justification for, 96–97
functional neuroimaging and, 14
going beyond, 195–200
Hughlings-Jackson's advancement of, 2
MRI's role in counteracting, 97
problems created by belief in, 35–36
corticospinal dysfunction, 47, 50, 128
corticosteroids
in brain neoplasia treatment, 145
in SLE treatment, 63, *142*, 144
cranial irradiation
DTI studies, findings, 122
self-limited confusional state from, 135
C-reactive protein, 121, 158, 164
Creutzfeldt-Jakob Disease, *28*, 32
Critchley, Macdonald, 188. *See also* chronic traumatic encephalopathy
CT. *See* computed tomography
CTE. *See* chronic traumatic encephalopathy
Cummings, I. L., 48–49

DAI. *See* diffuse axonal injury
Darwin, Charles, 22, 38
DBS. *See* deep brain stimulation
declarative memory
AIDS-dementia complex and, 66
description, 103
distributed network for, 157
TBI and, 56
white matter dementia and, 100
deep brain stimulation (DBS), 149
default mode network (DMN), 14
degenerative dementia, 54. *See also* Alzheimer's Disease; chronic traumatic encephalopathy
delirium
abnormal NAWM in, 119
critical illness/cognitive impairment and, 165
white matter damage in, 163
delusions
in white matter lacunar dementia, 105
dementia. *See also* Alzheimer's Disease; cortical dementia; mixed dementias; strategic infarct dementia; subcortical dementia; white matter dementia
age-related onset data, 37
causes of, 2, 27, 32, 36, 37
circular reasoning on structural basis of, 3
definition, 27
early-onset, 37
epidemiological studies, 38, 39, 162–163
genetic-mediation/genetic mutations and, 162
hypertension control and, 180
modifiable risk factors, 162
Netherlands study of risks in elders, 33
neuritic plaques/neurofibrillary tangles in, 3
neuroanatomic overview of, 27–33
phenomenology/etiopathogenesis of, 2
public health prevention approach, 163
radiation-induced, 52
traditional categories, specific diseases, *28*
white matter's neurorelevance in, 35
dementia pugilistica, 185, 187, 190
demyelination. *See also* demyelinative diseases; myelination; remyelination
in ADC, 65, 67
in BD, 70
in brain tumors, 72
in cancer chemotherapy, 53–54
cobalamin and, 68
CT observations of, 74
dysmyelination distinction, 75
fatal dementia from, 52
gliomas and, 73
in gliomatosis cerebri, 74
in HIV infection, 67
in LA, 44
LA and, 44
in MLD, 76–77
in MS, 20, 44, 59–60, 61–62, 103, 104, 110, 120, 121, 166
myelin repair and, 166–168

demyelination (cont.)
neurobehavioral consequences of, 20
in NPH, 71
in radiation leukoencephalopathy, 52
in SLE, 64, 120
in toluene leukoencephalopathy, 50, 98–99, 108, 110, 136
in toxic leukoencephalopathies, 101, 143
vascular dementia, 43
in white matter lesions, 132, 136
demyelinative diseases, *58*, 58–62. *See also* multiple sclerosis
acute disseminated encephalomyelitis, *58*
Balò's concentric sclerosis, *58*
infectious disease similarities, 64
Marburg's disease, *58*
neuromyelitis optica, *58*
Schilder's disease, *58*
tumefactive multiple sclerosis, *58*
demyelinative peripheral neuropathy, 96
depression
AD risk factors, 162
BD and, 47
CADASIL and, 76
cognitive impairment in, 37
in CTE, 188
deep brain stimulation for, 149
inflammatory mechanisms in, 158
in MS, 105
neoplasms and, 72
The Descent of Man (Darwin), 22
descriptive studies, value of, 38
Deter, Auguste, 2, 37
developmental dyslexia, 38
diabetes mellitus
AD risk factors, 162
dementia risk factors, 163
LA risk factors in, 44
diffuse axonal injury (DAI), in TBI, 165, 176
AD and, 165
autopsied brain findings, 189, *189*
concussions and, 192
CTE and, 165, 190–191, 192
Glasgow Coma Scale assessment, 56
medical therapy treatment, 143
microscopic studies, findings, 55–56
in mild/severe TBI, 55
monkey studies, 108
neurobehavioral impact of, 56–57, 136
neuroimaging studies, findings, 56
phosphorylated tau accumulation in, 190, 191, 192
post-mortem study, *55*
prefrontal leucotomy and, 191
prognosis, 136
static encephalopathy and, 165
tauopathy and, 190–192
widespread damage caused by, 55–57, 166
diffuse necrotizing leukoencephalopathy, 53
diffusion kurtosis imaging (DKI), *9*
crossing fibers phenomenon and, 13
enabling of quantification of non-Gaussian water diffusion, 13
gliomatosis cerebri studies, findings, 74
diffusion spectrum imaging (DSI), *9*, 12
diffusion susceptibility contrast PWI, 13
diffusion tensor imaging (DTI), 6, *9*
CADASIL studies, findings, 76
capturing of Gaussian diffusion by, 13
of cardiorespiratory fitness in elders, 164
children/ADHD studies, findings, 102
cognitive processing observations, 101
connectome mapping by, 17
corpus callosum studies, findings, 66, 144, 147–148, 164
crossing fibers phenomenon issues, 12
delirium assessment, 165
evaluation of strokes, 104
FXTAS studies, findings, 123
glioma/cranial irradiation, studies, findings, 122
gliomatosis cerebri studies, findings, 74
history of development, 11–12
HIV studies, findings, 66
leukoaraiosis studies findings, 45
memory retrieval studies, 104
MS studies, findings, 61
NAWM investigations, 13, 48, 119
NPH studies, findings, 71
SLE studies, findings, 64
studies of non-pharmacologic interventions, 148
TBI studies, 56, 57, 189–190
tract-based spatial statistics, 12
tract identification challenges, 14
of white matter tracts, 12, 57, 74
diffusion weighting amplification, MRI, 11
disconnection syndromes, 5, 6, 154
disconnectivity. *See* brain disconnectivity
distributed neural networks, 30, 38, 153, 155–157, *156*, 158, 197
DMN. *See* default mode network
donepezil
for Binswanger's Disease, 142
in TBI, 143
in vascular dementia, 142
dysmyelination
CT observations of, 74, 77
demyelination distinction, 75
MLD and, 76–77

early-onset Alzheimer's Disease, 33, 178
early-onset autosomal dominant Alzheimer's Disease, 37, 162
early-onset dementia, 37
early-onset familial Alzheimer's Disease, 33, 178
Einstein, Albert, 39, 198
electroconvulsive therapy, 148
electroencephalography (EEG)
epilepsy monitoring, 129
for excluding white matter involvement, 129
of toluene leukoencephalopathy, 98
of white matter, 3
emotion
association/commissural tracts and, 18
myelinated systems role in, 17, 22
neural networks mediation of, 1
white matter lesions' impact on, 5
white matter's role in, 5, 6, 17
encephalitis subcorticalis chronica progressiva, 46
encephalomalacia, 48
ependymoma, 73
epidemiological studies
of cognitive reserve in AD, 137
of dementia, 38, 39, 162–163
epidural hematoma, 55
epilepsy, 2, 129
executive function
ADC and, 66
Binswanger's Disease and, 49, 101
cerebral white matter's role in, 5
cognitive slowing and, 64
cortical structure's role in, 97
distributed network for, 157
fragile X tremor ataxia syndrome and, 102
leukoaraiosis and, 45
metachromatic leukodystrophy and, 77, 102
MS and, 62
neoplasms and, 72
NPH and, 71, 101–102, 123

radiation treatment and, 52
SLE and, 64
TBI and, 56
toluene leukoencephalopathy and, 50–51
toxic leukoencephalopathy and, 101
vitamin B_{12} deficiency and, 68
white matter dementia and, 100, 101–102
exercise
AD prevention and, 180
white matter benefits from, 139, 164
Extended Disability Status Scale (EDSS), 59
extrapyramidal function/dysfunction
Binswanger's Disease and, 47
forms of dysfunction, 106
mixed dementia and, 32
white matter dementia and, 106

florbetapir (amyloid ligand), 174, 179
fluid-attenuated inversion recovery (FLAIR) images, 59
focal cerebral infarctions, 42
focal cerebral lesions, 27
focal damage, 6, 197
focal neurobehavioral syndromes, 7
focal white matter tumors, 72
Folstein, Marshall, 30
fractional anisotropy (FA), 12, 158
fragile X tremor ataxia syndrome, 78
executive dysfunction in, 102
memory retrieval deficit in, 103
MRI studies, findings, 78
NAWM abnormalities in, *119*
neuroimaging studies, findings, 123
relatively preserved language in, 78
white matter hyperintensities and, 78
Franklin, G. M., 59
Freud, Sigmund, 2, 30, 197
frontal aslant tract, 153
Frontal Assessment Battery (FAB), 71, 129
frontal lobe neoplasms, 72
frontal lobotomy, *54*
frontally-predominant leukodystrophy, 77
frontal systems dementia. *See* subcortical dementia
fronto-subcortical dementia. *See* subcortical dementia
frontotemporal dementia (FTD), 188
frontotemporal lobar degeneration (FTLD), *28*
AD's comparison with, 29
comparison with Alzheimer's disease, 29
cortical damage in, 29, 36
HD/PD, distinctions from, 30–31
young-onset dementia and, 37
FTLD. *See* frontotemporal lobar degeneration
fulminant fatal leukoencephalopathy, 65
functional magnetic resonance imaging (fMRI), *9*, 14
cerebellum, studies and findings, 157–158
connectivity studies, 157
neural network identification, 14
functional neuroimaging methods, 14–15. *See also* functional magnetic resonance imaging; positron emission tomography; single photon emission computed tomography
gray matter emphasis of, 14
neural networks identification by, 14
FXTAS. *See* fragile X tremor ataxia syndrome

gait disorder
4-aminopyridine treatment, 144
in BD, 47
in CTE, 188
leukoaraiosis and, 45
in MLD, 76
MRI/DTI studies, findings, 128
in NPH, 70, 71–72
periventricular lesions in, 44
galantamine
in Binswanger's Disease, 142
in vascular cognitive impairment, 142
Gall, Franz Joseph, 2, 95, 156, 197
general mental ability (GMA), 23
gene therapy, 77, 146
genetic diseases, *74*, 74–78. *See also* specific genetic diseases
Gennarelli, T. A., 108
Geschwind, Norman, 154, 197. *See also* disconnection syndromes
on brain disconnectivity, 6, 197
founding of behavioral neurology, 6
NPH and, 70
Glasgow Coma Scale, 54, 56, 57
glatiramer, in MS treatment, 143
gliomas, *72*, 104. *See also* astrocytomas; ependymoma; oligodendroglioma
cranial irradiation studies. findings, 122
description, 73
gliomatosis cerebri comparison, 73
NAWM abnormalities in, *119*, 122
radiation treatment study, 52
gliomatosis cerebri, *72*, 73–74
characteristics, 73
diagnostic challenges, 73
mortality rate, 73
neurobehavioral alterations from, 74
neuroimaging studies, findings, 73–74
predilection for cerebral white matter, 122
prognosis, 135
global brain atrophy, 36, 109
glutamatergic transmission, 21, 147
Golgi, Camillo, 1
gradient echo (GRE) imaging, 56
gray matter
AD and, 100, 107–108
ADC and, 66
aging and trajectory of, 21
association tract interconnectivity, 18
changes in HIV infection, 66
cognitive importance of, 24, 49, 109, 153
conventional emphasis on, 1–4
conventional synapses in, 21
cortical/deep fascicles of white matter, 20, 95
cortical infarcts and, 96
extrapyramidal function and, 106
formation/development, during gestation, 21
gliomatosis cerebri involvement, 66
HD/PD neuropathology and, 30, 96
intelligence and, 1
lesion method examination of, 5
MCI and, *124*, 124
metabolic activity comparison, 17
microconnectivity of, 4, 107
MRI scan, distinction from white matter, *10*
MS and, 59, 61, 62, 100, 138
myelinated tracts within, 36, 106
normal brain perfusion comparison, 13
in NPH, 71
plasticity property of, 138, 139, 147
PWI assessment of, 14
retrieval deficits/procedural memory and, 107
subcortical, 1–4
white matter's parallel functions with, 4
WMD and, 108

Hachinski, V. C., 43
HAD. *See* HIV-associated dementia
hallucinations
mixed dementias and, 32

hallucinations (cont.)
neoplasms and, 72
white matter lacunar dementia and, 105
HAND. *See* HIV-associated neurocognitive disorder
HD. *See* Huntington's Disease
Head, Henry, 197
headaches
mixed dementias and, 32
neoplasms and, 72–73, 122
Heaton, R. K., 58
hematopoietic stem cell transplantation (HSCT), 145–146
hemiparesis, neoplasms and, 72–73
Higher Cortical Functions in Man (Luria), 2
histograms, whole brain, 11
Hitler, Adolf, 22–23
HIV-associated dementia (HAD), 47, 65, 67
HIV-associated mild neurocognitive disorder (MND), 65, 67
HIV-associated neurocognitive disorder (HAND), 65, 67
Hughes, J. T., 61
Hughlings-Jackson, John, 2
Huisa, B. N., *47*
Human Connectome Project (U.S.), 4, 195–196
De Humani Corporis Fabrica (Vesalius), 95
human immunodeficiency virus (HIV) infection, 65–67. *See also* AIDS (acquired immunodeficiency syndrome)
antiretroviral therapy treatment, 65, 66–67, 144
associated terminology, 65
brain/cognitive reserve studies, 137, 138
brain cortex studies, findings, 65, 66
as causative for dementia, 37
clinical evaluation, 128
cognitive profile of brain infection in, 66
DTI studies, findings, 66
fulminant fatal leukoencephalopathy in, 65
gray matter changes in, 66
NAWM abnormalities in, 66, *119*, 122
prognosis, 136
treatment, *142*, 144
Huntington's Disease (HD), 3, *28*
caudate nucleus involvement in, 30
genetic mutations in, 162
impaired procedural memory in, 106–107
memory disturbances in, 102
MS comparison studies, 100
stem cell therapeutics potential, 168
subcortical dementia symptoms in, 30
hydrocephalus, *69*. *See also* normal pressure hydrocephalus
hydrocephalus ex vacuo, *69*
hyperlipidemia, 163
hypertension
AD risk factors, 162, 164
BD risk factors, 46–48
dementia risk factors, 163
LA risk factors in, 44
SYST-EUR study, 164, 180
WHIs and, 164
hypoxic-ischemic encephalopathy, *28*, 32, 55

immunomodulatory drugs, in MS treatment, 143–144
immunosuppressive drugs
in MS treatment, 143
in SLE treatment, 144
infectious diseases of white matter, *64*, 64–67. *See also* specific diseases
inflammation
in Alzheimer's Disease, 121
C-reactive protein and, 121
in MS, 60, 61, 158
radiation leukoencephalopathy and, 53
in SLE, 63, 120, 121, 158
white matter and, 158–159
inflammatory white matter diseases, *64*, 62–64. *See also* acute disseminated encephalomyelitis; Balò's concentric sclerosis; Marburg's disease; multiple sclerosis; neuromyelitis optica; Schilder's disease; tumefactive multiple sclerosis
integrative review process, 38–39
interferon β-1-a, in MS, 143
interferon β-1-b, in MS, 143
intracerebral hemorrhage, 55
intracortical myelin, 20, 21–22, 109–110, 149, 155
IQ, white matter integrity and, 104
ischemic vascular dementia, 103
ischemic white matter hyperintensities, 109

Kaplan, Edith, 130. *See also* Boston Process Approach
knowledge synthesis, 39
Krabbe's Disease, 145

LA. *See* leukoaraiosis
Lafosse, J., 107
language. *See also* relatively preserved language
articulation deficits, 105
cortical structure's role in, 97, 106
frontotemporal lobar degeneration and, 29
gray matter contributions, 4
impairment in AD, 100, 102
networks, neuroimaging identification, 14
radiation treatment and, 52
subcortical dementia and, 30
white matter's role in, 5, 32, 106
Lashley, Karl, 197
left inferior frontal cortical injury, 5
lesion method, in examining white matter, 5, 14, 27–28
leucocentrism, disconnection and, 197–199
leukoaraiosis (LA)
abnormal NAWM in people with, 45
arteriosclerotic changes in, 44
Binswanger's Disease's relationship to, 43
cardiovascular disease risks, 44, 45
as causative for cognitive dysfunction, 38
cholinergic projections' vulnerability in, 154
DTI studies findings, 45
education's impact on, 45
executive function and, 45
gait disorder and, 45
genetic influences, 44
historical background, 43–44
incomplete infarction of, 122
MRI studies, 42, 43, *43*, 44, 45
NAWM abnormalities in, *119*
neurobehavioral significance of, 44–45
neurologic morbidity, mortality and, 45
pathogenesis of, 44
stroke risk factors, 44, 45
treatment, 46
white matter hyperintensities and, 43, 44
leukodystrophies, 37
Lewy bodies, 32
Lewy body dementia, *28*, 32
limbic system, *18*, 18, 157
Luria, Alexander, 2
lymphomatosis cerebri, 122, 145

magnetic resonance imaging (MRI), 5, *9*, 9–11
AD studies, findings, 108
advantage in WMD studies, 36, 38, 97, 129–130, 136

BD studies, 46
CADASIL studies, findings, 76
cobalamin deficiency studies, findings, 68
cognitive processing observations, 101
community-based brain scan studies, 195
CT comparison with, 9
detection of UBOs, 10
detection of WMH, 10–11
diffusion weighting amplification of, 11
FXTAS studies, findings, 78
gliomatosis cerebri studies, findings, 74
history of development, 9, 36
leukoaraiosis studies, 42, 43, 45
macrostructural disruption evaluation, 6
memory retrieval studies, 103–104
MLD studies, findings, 77
MS studies, findings, 5, 10, 15, 58, 59, 60–61
neuropsychological testing combination, 130
NPH studies, findings, 70
post-mortem human neocortex studies, 20
as preferred white matter assessment modality, 10–11
radiation leukoencephalopathy studies, 53
review of brain size/GMA studies, 23
role in detecting/understanding diseases, 5–6
role in toxic drug discoveries, 49
role in understanding MS, 5, 10, 15
SLE studies, findings, 64, 119–120
tau studies, 191
TBI assessment, 56
toluene leukoencephalopathy studies, findings, 50–51, 98
vascular dementia studies, 49
white matter fascicles' studies, 155
WMD studies, findings, 119
WMH recognized by, 10–11, *43*, 43, 51, 98
magnetic resonance spectroscopy (MRS), 6, *9*
early abnormalities detected with, 11
FXTAS studies, findings, 123
gliomatosis cerebri studies, findings, 74
NAWM investigations, 13, 119
SLE studies, findings, 64, 120
vascular dementia studies, findings, 48
magnetization transfer imaging (MTI)
advanced neuroimaging capabilities, 6, *9*
description/usefulness, 11
NAWM investigations, 13, 119
vascular dementia studies, 48
magnetization transfer ratio (MTR), 11
Marburg's disease, *58*
Markowitsch, H. J., 103
MCD. *See* mild cognitive dysfunction
McHugh, Paul, 30
medulloblastoma, 53
memory retrieval deficit, 102–104
Mendez, M. F., 108
meningismus, mixed dementias and, 32
metabolic disorders of white matter, *67*, 67–69. *See also* specific disorders
metabolic-toxic encephalopathy. *See* delirium
metachromatic leukodystrophy (MLD), 76–78
adult-onset, 105
in children, 76, 77
clinical evaluation, 127
diagnosis, 77, 127
executive dysfunction in, 102
HSCT treatment, 145–146
NAWM abnormalities in, *119*
neuroimaging studies, findings, 77
neuropathology of, 76–77
neuropsychological testing, findings, 77
relatively preserved language in, 77
treatment, 77–78, *142*
methylphenidate, in TBI, 143
mild cognitive dysfunction (MCD), 118–124
ADC and, 65
background research, 118–120
characteristics, 120
definition, 120
diagnosis, 100, 127–132, *128*
brain biopsy, 131–132
clinical evaluation, 127–129
laboratory testing, 129
neuroimaging, 129–130
neuropsychology, 130–131
increasing legitimacy of, 195–196
inflammatory processes, 121
leucocentrism and, 198
mild cognitive impairment comparison, 123–124, *124*
MND similarities, 120, 122
in MS, 120
neurobiological advantage of, 123
as precursor syndrome, 38
preventive measures, potential, 154
prognosis
brain/cognitive reserve, 137–138
influential factors, *135*
natural history, 135–137
plasticity, 138–139
in SLE, 64, 120
treatment, *142*, 142–149
behavioral, *147*, 147–148
cholinergic augmentation, 154
medical, 142–146
psychiatric, 148–149
rehabilitative, 147–148
surgical, 146–147
vitamin B_{12} and, 69
white matter tracts and, 124
mild cognitive impairment (MCI)
MCD comparison, 123–124, *124*
as pre-dementia state, 118, 178, 180
vitamin B_{12} supplementation and, 145
WMH in, 177
mild neurocognitive disorder (MND)
in HIV infection, 65, 67
MCD similarities, 120, 122
mild traumatic brain injury (mTBI). *See* concussions
military personnel
blast injuries in, 54, 57, 185
chronic traumatic encephalopathy in, 185
concussions in, 186
Luria's study of Russian soldiers, 2
tauopathy in, 190
VA TBI assessment, *186*, 186
mindfulness meditation, DTI study, 148
Minimal Assessment of Cognitive Function in MS (MACFIMS), 59
Mini-Mental State Examination (MMSE), 128–129
mixed dementias, *28*, 32–33. *See also* autoimmune dementia; corticobasal degeneration; Creutzfeldt-Jakob Disease; hypoxic-ischemic encephalopathy; Lewy body dementia; multi-infarct dementia; neurosyphilis; subdural hematoma
MLD. *See* metachromatic leukodystrophy
MND. *See* mild neurocognitive disorder
Montreal Cognitive Assessment (MoCA), 129
morbidity/mortality, 147
APP knockout mice studies, 176
cerebrovascular disease and, 163
inflammation and, 158

morbidity/mortality (cont.)
leukoaraiosis and, 45
TBI and, 163
movement disorders. *See also* gait disorder; Parkinson's Disease
causes of, 106
in dementia in BD, 48
extrapyramidal dysfunction and, 106
in MS, 106
myoclonus in ADC, 106
uncommon in white matter disorders, 128
MRI. *See* magnetic resonance imaging
MRS. *See* magnetic resonance spectroscopy
MTI. *See* magnetization transfer imaging
MTR. *See* magnetization transfer ratio
mucopolysaccharidoses, *74*
multi-infarct dementia, *28*, 32
multiple sclerosis (MS)
AD comparison, 100, 102, 105, 138, 167
assessment screening tools, 59
brain atrophy in, 60, 61
brain/cognitive reserve and, 137, 138
brain inflammation in, 60, 61, 121
CADASIL's similarity to, 75
Charcot's initial insights about, 58
clinical evaluation, 127
cognitive impairment in, 37, 58–62, 101, 121
cortical demyelination in, 20, 59–60, 61–62, 103, 104, 110, 120, 121
corticospinal dysfunction in, 47
depression in, 105
differentiation from cortical dementias, 62
DTI studies, findings, 61
FLAIR studies, 59
gray matter lesions in, 62
HD comparison studies, 100
inflammation in, 60, 61, 158
intracortical myelin in, 109–110
MCD in, 120
memory retrieval deficit in, 103, 104
MRI studies, 5, 10, 15, 58, 59, 60–61
MRS studies, 11
NAWM findings in, 58, 61, *119*, 121
neuropathology of, 59–60, 61
neuropsychological deficits in, 61–62
normal procedural memory in, 106
prognosis, 135
relatively preserved language in, 59, 62
remyelination process in, 166–167, 168
sustained attentional disturbances in, 102
treatment, *142*, 143–144
Multiple Sclerosis Functional Composite (MSFC), 59
muscular dystrophy, *74*
myelin. *See also* demyelination; demyelinative diseases; dysmyelination; myelination; remyelination; white matter tracts
altered formation of, 22
BD and, 48
cancer chemotherapy and, 53–54
cobalamin and, 67
cognitive processing speed and, 100
core neurophysiological function, 101
DAI and, 55, 165
intracortical myelin, 20, 21–22, 109–110, 149, 155
language processing and, 106
movement disorders and, 106
MRI studies, 119
MTI imaging, 11
NAA as injury marker, 11
repair of, 166–168
role in white matter, 21
role in white matter disorders, 36
SLE and, 136, 144
white matter anatomy and, 17, 19–20, 153–155
white matter neuropathology and, 135
myelination. *See also* demyelination
in adolescents, young adults, 105
of cerebral axons, 23, 36
connectivity role, 196
connectome role, 21
evolution in the brain, 21, 22, 24
MLD and, 76, 77
plasticity of, 21, 139, 147
psychiatric disturbance and, 105
retardation in schizophrenia, 149
role in cognition/emotion, 17, 22
role in electrical conduction, 20
schizophrenia treatment and, 149
thyroid hormones and, 129
treatments for enhancement of, 167
Vogts' studies, findings, 19, 155
myelin model of Alzheimer's Disease (AD), 175–179, 180, 181, 191
myoclonus, 32, 106

N-acetyl aspartate (NAA), 11, 120, 136, 146
natalizumab, in MS treatment, 143
Naville, F., 30
NAWM. *See* normal-appearing white matter
neoplasms. *See* brain neoplasms
neuritic plaques/neurofibrillary tangles, in Alzheimer's Disease, 2, 3
Alzheimer's discovery of, 28
autopsy study findings, 173
as cortical hallmarks in AD, 29, 172
counteractive mechanisms, 108
sequence in neuropathological appearance, 173
white matter changes and, 33
neuroanatomic overview of dementia, 27–33
cortical dementia, 28–29
mixed dementia, 32–33
subcortical dementia, 29–32
traditional categories, diseases, *28*
neurobehavioral domains, 5
neurobiology of white matter, 17–24
anatomy, 17–20
brain development and aging, 21–22
physiology, 20–21
neuroimaging technologies. *See also* specific technologies
in AD research, 174
essential contributions of, *9*, 9–15
functional neuroimaging, 14–15, 17, 103
growing advantages of, 5
historical background, 5, 35, 100
neuroanatomy combination, 18, 153–154
role in observing white matter, 4, 5, 42
structural neuroimaging, 11–14, 17, 23
of tau, in the brain, 191
neuromyelitis optica, 58
neuron doctrine, 1, 36
neuropsychiatric syndromes, 7, 63
neuropsychological testing, 30
of attention, 102
in BD, *47*
Boston Process Approach, 130–131
cognitive slowing and, 101
forms of, 130–131
MRI combination, 130
of procedural memory, 106
role in WMD/MCD diagnosis, 130–131
neurosyphilis, *28*, 32, 46
neurotransmitter systems in white matter, *154*
Nevin, S., 55
Niemann-Pick Disease, 77
nitrendipine, 164
non-fluent aphasia, 5

non-paraneoplastic autoimmune dementia, 32
normal-appearing white matter (NAWM)
abnormal appearance of, *119*, 119
appearance in non-demented patients, 122
BD studies, 48
CADASIL studies, findings, 76
cognition and, *123*
C-reactive protein and, 121
HIV findings, 66, *119*, 122
LA studies, 45
microstructural changes in, 111
MS studies, 58, 61, *119*, 121
neuroimaging studies, findings, 13, 48, 58, 66, 110, 119, 120
NPH studies, 70
radiation therapy and, 122
TBI studies, 56
white matter inflammation and, 119
normal pressure hydrocephalus (NPH), 37, *69*, 69–72
AD comparison, 101–102
BD comorbidity with, 70
clinical presentation, 70
cognitive impairment in, 70, 71, 122–123
CT evaluation, 9
diagnosis of, 70
DTI studies, findings, 71
executive dysfunction in, 71, 101–102, 123
Frontal Assessment Battery in, 71
gait disorder in, 71–72
gray matter in, 71
MRI studies, findings, 70
NAWM abnormalities in, *119*
neurobehavioral profile of, 71
pathophysiology of, 70–71
prognosis, 136
treatment of, *142*
pharmacologic, 72, 145
surgical, 69, 71, 146
white matter hyperintensities and, 72
NPH. *See* normal pressure hydrocephalus

obesity, 44, 162, 180, 181
obstructive sleep apnea (OSA), 164–165
oligodendroglioma, 73
Olszewski, J., 46
Osimani, A., 68

Paced Auditory Serial Addition Test (PASAT), 101, 131
painted brain syndrome, 97. *See also* toluene leukoencephalopathy
panic attacks, 72
papilledema, 32
paraneoplastic autoimmune dementia, 32
parenchymal brain neoplasms, 72–73
parkinsonism
from carbon monoxide poisoning, 106
in CTE, 188
in dementia pugilistica, 187
lower body (cerebrovascular gait disorder), 128
mixed dementias and, 32
postencephalitic, 30
Parkinson's Disease (PD), 3, *28*
AD distinctions from, 30–31, 96
brain reserve and, 137
concussions and, 188
dementia in, 30
stem cell therapeutics potential, 168
substantia nigra involvement, 30
Penfield, Wilder, 2
perfusion-weighted imaging (PWI), *9*, 13–14. *See also* arterial spin labeling PWI; diffusion susceptibility contrast PWI
periventricular lesions, 44, 145
Peyser, J. M., 58
phakomatoses, *74*
physiology of white matter, 20–21
Pick, Arnold, 27, 29
Pick bodies, 32
Pick's Disease, 28, 29. *See also* frontotemporal lobar degeneration
plasticity
benefits for WMD/MCD, 70, 139, 147
bilingualism benefits, 139
in the cerebral cortex, 138
definition, 138
of gray matter, 138, 139, 147
musical training benefits, 138–139
therapeutics for, 148
white matter tracts and, 139
polyarteritis nodosa, *62*
positron emission tomography (PET), *9*
amyloid studies, 174
cerebral cortex studies, 3, 74
connectivity studies, 157
gliomatosis cerebri studies, findings, 74
mechanics of, 14
subcortical dementia study, findings, 109
tau studies, 191
post-concussion syndrome, 186
postencephalitic parkinsonism, 30
post-traumatic stress disorder, 185
prefrontal leucotomy, 191
primary angiitis of the central nervous system, *62*
primary progressive aphasia, 153
procedural memory
AIDS-dementia complex and, 66
description, 103
preservation in AD, 106
TBI and, 56
white matter dementia and, 100, 106–107
progressive multifocal leukoencephalopathy, 37
progressive supranuclear palsy, *28*
projection tracts, 17, 156
psychosis, in adult-onset MLD, 105
PWI. *See* perfusion-weighted imaging

radiation, 51–53
causative for dementia, 37, 52
children's learning disabilities and, 52
cognitive impairment from, 52, 72
executive dysfunction from, 51–52
leukotoxic effects of, 52, 72
MRI studies, findings, 53
neurotoxic effects of, 51–52
radiation leukoencephalopathy
cancer chemotherapy comparison, 53
clinical sequelae of, 52
cranial irradiation and, 52
dosages causing, 52
focal *vs.* whole brain, 52
hypothesized causes of, 53
memory retrieval deficit in, 103
neuropathological abnormalities in, 52
Rao, S. M., 58
recognition memory, 103, 108, 131
relatively preserved language
in ADC, 66
in Binswanger's Disease, 47, 49
in CADASIL, 75
in FXTAS, 78
in MLD, 77
in MS, 59, 62
in SLE, 64
in TBI, 57
in vitamin B_{12} deficiency, 68
in WMD, 105–106
remyelination
in MLD, 77
in MS, 166–167, 168
in normal aging, 166
repetitive transcranial magnetic stimulation (rTMS), 148
reticular theory, Golgi's defense of, 1

rivastigmine, in TBI, 143
Roberts, A. H., 187
rodent studies, 2–3
Román, G. C., 48
Ropper, A. H., 48
Rosenberg, N. L., *47*
rTMS. *See* repetitive transcranial magnetic stimulation
Rushton, J. P., 23

sarcoidosis, *62*
Schilder's disease, *58*
schizophrenia
  brain reserve and, 137
  cognitive impairment in, 37
  medication treatment, 146, 149
  myelination and 37, 105
  NAWM abnormalities in, *119*
  surgical treatment, 146, 191
  tau and, 191
scleroderma, *62*
seizures
  gliomatosis cerebri and, 73
  in mixed dementias, 32
  neoplasms and, 72–73, 122
  uncommon in white matter disorders, 128
shaken baby syndrome, *54*
Sheline, G. E., 52
single photon emission computed tomography (SPECT), *9*, 14
Sjögren's syndrome, 62
SLE. *See* systemic lupus erythematosus
sleep medicine, 164–165
smoking
  AD risk factors, 162
  LA risk factors in, 44
solanezumab, 174
somatic therapies, 148
somnolence syndrome, 52
spatial attention network, 157
Spurzheim, Johann Kaspar, 2, 95, 156
static encephalopathy, 54, 57, 165
stem cell therapeutics, 77, 146, 168–169
strategic infarct dementia, 27
strokes
  BD and, 49
  brain inflammation in, 121
  CT evaluation of, 9
  DTI evaluation of, 104
  focal cerebral lesions from, 27
  LA risk factors in, 44, 45
  mixed dementias and, 32
  rehabilitation treatment, 147
structural neuroimaging methods. *See* diffusion kurtosis imaging; diffusion spectrum imaging; diffusion tensor imaging; magnetic resonance imaging; magnetic resonance spectroscopy; magnetization transfer imaging; perfusion-weighted imaging
Stuss, D. T., 48–49
subacute HIV encephalitis, 65
subcortical arteriosclerotic encephalopathy, 46
subcortical dementia, 3, 28, 29–32. *See also* Huntington's Disease; Parkinson's Disease; progressive supranuclear palsy; white matter disorders; Wilson's Disease
  ADC characterization as, 66
  alternate descriptors, 30
  BD classification as, 48
  cobalamin deficiency and, 68
  cognitive impairment in, 30, 101
  contributions of concept of, 32
  cortical dementia distinction from, 3, 28, 30, 31, 95, 100, 107
  defense of concept of, 31
  historical background, 30, 35, 96
  MS qualification as, 62
  NPH's features of, 71
  opposition to concept of, 31
  overlap with other dementias, 38
  in SLE patients, 64
  toluene abuse and, 50
  WMD distinction from, 100
subcortical ischemic vascular dementia (SIVD), 43, 46
subcortical lesions, 44, 75, 167
subdural hematoma, *28*, 32, 55
substantia nigra, in PD, 30
supranuclear palsy, 30
susceptibility-weighted images (SWI), 56
Symonds, Sir Charles, 70, 137
systemic lupus erythematosus (SLE), 63–64
  cognitive slowing in, 64
  immune-related myelinopathy in, 120
  inflammation in, 63, 120, 121, 158
  MCD in, 64, 120
  MMSE assessment, 144
  MRI studies, findings, 119–120
  MRS studies, findings, 64, 120
  NAWM abnormalities in, *119*
  neuroimaging studies, 64
  neuropsychological study of cognitive dysfunction, 63–64
  pathogenesis of neuropsychiatric dysfunction, 63
  pathology of, 63
  prognosis, 136
  relatively preserved language in, 64
  treatment, 63, *142*, 144
  white matter hyperintensities and, 64
Systolic Hypertension in Europe (SYST-EUR) study, 164, 180

Takeuchi, H., 147
TAR DNA-binding protein 43 (TDP-43), 29
tau
  as hallmark CTE lesion, 190
  mechanisms of spreading in the brain, 192
  neuroimaging of, 191
  protective role in concussions, 191
  vulnerability to injury, 190
tauopathy
  in athletes, military personnel, 190
  CTE and, 165, 188
  diffuse axonal injury and, 190–192
  prefrontal leucotomy study, 191
tau-positive (FTLD-TAU) protein, 29
Tay-Sachs Disease, 77
tCDS. *See* transcranial direct current stimulation
temporal arteritis, *62*
temporal lobe neoplasms, 72
thalamus, 3
  AD/FTLD and, 29
  arousal network, 156
  gliomatosis cerebri and, 74
  gray matter changes in, 66
  isolated vascular lesions of, 27
  subcortical dementia and, 30
  T2 hypointensities in, 50
  white matter tracts in, *18*, 19
therapeutic innovations in treatment, 162–169
  damage prevention, 162–165
  hypertension control, 164
  lifestyle modifications, 164
  myelin repair, 166–168
  sleep medicine, 164–165
  stem cell therapeutics, 168–169
  TBI control, 165
toluene-induced cardiac arrhythmia, 98
toluene leukoencephalopathy, 49–51
  alternate names for, 51, 97
  articulation deficits in, 105
  autopsy findings, 50, 97
  brain-behavior relationships and, 97
  causes of, 97, 98–99
  clinical evaluation, 127
  cognitive impairment in, 97–98
  corticospinal dysfunction in, 50
  CT studies/findings, 51, 98
  MRI studies/findings, 50–51, 98

neurobehavioral sequelae of toluene abuse, 51
neuropathological investigations, 51
nonverbal ability impairment in, 104
pathogenesis of dementia in, 50–51
prognosis, 135, 136
white matter dementia and, 96–99
toxic leukoencephalopathy, 49, *50*
drug abuse and, 148
executive dysfunction in, 101
MRI studies, 53, 143
stages of severity, *119*, 119
treatment of, 143, 148–149
Tozzi, V., 144
tracts. *See* white matter tracts
Trail Making Test, Form A, 146
transcranial direct current stimulation (tCDS), 148
traumatic axonal injury (TAI). *See* diffuse axonal injury
traumatic brain injury (TBI), 54–58. *See also* diffuse axonal injury (DAI), in TBI
AD association, 57
from blast injuries, in military conflicts, 54, 57, 185
brain/cognitive reserve studies, 137, 138
clinical presentation, 54–55
concussion and, 185–187 (*See also* concussions)
CTE link, with, 57
CT evaluation of, 9
diagnostic challenges, 55
diffuse axonal injury in, 55–57, 165
disinhibition/impaired impulse behavior in, 57
DTI studies, 56, 57, 189–190
executive function impacted by, 56
Glasgow Coma Scale assessment, 54, 56, 57
global prevalence of, 165
lesions produced by, 55
long-term outcomes, 57–58
monkey research, 108
morbidity/mortality of patients, 163
mortality rate, U.S., 54
MRI assessment, 56
NAWM abnormalities in, *119*
NAWM studies in, 56
neurobehavioral sequelae, 55
neuropathology of, 57
Nevin's research on, 55
phosphorylated tau accumulation in, 190, 191
prognosis, 135, 136
recovery potential, 57
relatively preserved language in, 57
severity classification, *186*, 186
static encephalopathy and, 54, 57, 165
tauopathy and, 188
terminology related to, 54
therapeutic innovations, 165
treatment
challenges, 57
medical therapy, 143
rehabilitation, 147
therapeutic innovations, 165
WAIS scores, 57
in young adulthood, 54
young-onset dementia and, 37
treatment of WMD and MCD, *142*, 142–149. *See also under* specific disorders
medical, 142–146
psychiatric, 148–149
rehabilitative, *147*, 147–148
surgical, 146–147
therapeutic innovations, 162–169
tumefactive multiple sclerosis, 58

unidentified bright objects (UBOs), 10
unspecified leukoencephalopathy, 37
urinary incontinence
in frontal white matter dysfunction, 128
in NPH, 70

van Bogaert, L., 75. *See also* cerebral autosomal dominant arteriopathy with subcortical infarcts and leukoencephalopathy
vascular cognitive impairment (VCI), 122, 142
vascular cognitive impairment (VCI), no dementia (VCI-no dementia), 122
vascular dementia. *See also* Binswanger's Disease; cerebral autosomal dominant arteriopathy with subcortical infarcts and leukoencephalopathy
AD combination, 32
BD as causative for, 42–43
hypertension control and, 180
ischemic vascular dementia, 103
medical treatment of, 142
MRS studies, findings, 48
MTI studies, findings, 48
reversibility of, 122
rTMS treatment for, 148
strokes and, 42
subcortical, 109
subcortical ischemic vascular dementia, 43, 46
subcortical vascular dementia, 109
SYST-EUR treatment study, 164
vascular diseases of white matter, 42–49, *43*
Binswanger's Disease, 46–49 (*See also* Binswanger's Disease)
cerebral amyloid angiopathy, *43*, 173
leukoaraiosis, 43–46 (*See also* leukoaraiosis)
migraine, *43*, 75
MRI studies, 42, *43*, 44, 45, 49
MTI studies, 48
subcortical ischemic vascular dementia, 43, 46
ventricular enlargement, 36
Vesalius, Andreas, 95
visual recognition network, 157
visuospatial function/dysfunction
AIDS-dementia complex and, 66
BD and, 47, 49
cerebral white matter's role in, 5
cortical structure's role in, 97
CT study of, 104
metachromatic leukodystrophy and, 77
radiation treatment and, 52
SLE and, 63
vitamin B_{12} deficiency and, 68
white matter dementia and, 104
visuospatial network, 157
vitamin B_{12} deficiency, 68. *See also* cobalamin (vitamin B_{12}) deficiency
Vogt, Cecile and Oskar, *18*, 19, 155

WAIS. *See* Wechsler Adult Intelligence Scale
Wechsler Adult Intelligence Scale (WAIS), 57
Wegener's granulomatosis, *62*
Wernicke, Karl, 95, 156
white matter
Alzheimer's Disease and, 172–181
anatomy, normal, of, 153–155
anisotropic (directional) diffusion in, 11
axo-oligodendroglial synapses in, 21, 139
behavioral neurology of, 5–7
cognition and
reflections on the study of, 199–200
research perspectives, 153–159
CTE and, 165
defined, 155
in distributed neural networks, 155–157, *156*
electroencephalographic studies, 3
enhanced electrical conduction by, 20–21

white matter (cont.)
evolution of, 4, 22–24
formation/development, at birth, 21
frontal lobes, losses in late life, 22
gray matter's parallel functions with, 4
historical background, 95–96
inflammation and, 158–159
lesion method examination of, 5
myelin's special role in, 21
neurobiology of, 17–24
anatomy, 17–20
physiology, 20–21
neurorelevance in dementia pathogenesis, 35
neurotransmitter systems within, 154
pathology spectrum, 121–123
percentage in non-human animals, 2
role in language, 5, 32, 106
role in lifespan, 5
significance of, 4–5
white matter dementia (WMD), 95–111
AD similarities, 172
categories, 118
clinical profile, *99*
cognitive slowing, 100, 101
executive dysfunction, 101–102
memory retrieval deficit, 102–104
normal extrapyramidal function, 106
normal procedural memory, 100, 106–107
psychiatric disturbance, 105
relatively preserved language, 105–106
sustained attention deficit, 102
visuospatial impairment, 104
cortical/subcortical dementia distinctions, 99–101, *100*
definition, 99, 118
diagnosis, 100, 127–132, *128*
brain biopsy, 131–132
clinical evaluation, 127–129
laboratory testing, 129
neuroimaging, 129–130
neuropsychology, 130–131
historical background, 95–96
increasing legitimacy of, 195–196
integrative review process in studying, 38–39
introduction of, xi
leucocentrism and, 198
neuroimaging studies, findings, 118–119
overlapping dementia disorders, 36, 38
preventive measures, potential, 154
Pub Med search citations for, 195
subcortical dementia as precursor, 32
toluene leukoencephalopathy turning point, 96–99
treatment, *142*, 142–149
behavioral, *147*, 147–148
cholinergic augmentation, 154
medical, 142–146
psychiatric, 148–149
rehabilitative, 147–148
surgical, 146–147
unresolved issues, 107–111
co-existent gray matter neuropathology, 108
corticocentric bias, 108–109
intracortical myelin pathology, 109–110
lack of suitable animal models, 108
threshold effect, 110
WMH/absence of cognitive correlates, 107–108
white matter disease of immaturity, *43*
white matter disorders, 3–4, 42–78. *See also* specific disorders
acquired factors, *163*, 163
in adolescence, young adulthood, 37
cancer chemotherapy-induced leukoencephalopathy, 53–54
cognitive slowing in, 101
declarative memory impairment in, 103
demyelinative diseases, *58*, 58–62
executive dysfunction in, 101
genetic diseases, *74*, 74–78
hydrocephalus, *69*, 69–72
infectious diseases, *64*, 64–67
inflammatory diseases, *62*, 62–64
integrative review of, 39
memory retrieval deficit in, 104
metabolic disorders, *67*, 67–69
methods of studying, 6, 10, 15
MRI's advantages in, 97
neoplasms, 72–74
neuropathology of, 6
pathophysiology of, 21
prognosis, 135–139
brain/cognitive reserve, 137–138
influential factors, *135*
natural history, 135–137
plasticity, 138–139
radiation, 51–53
relatively preserved language in, 105–106
sustained attentional disturbances in, 102
symptoms, 128
therapeutic innovations, 162–169
damage prevention, 162–165
hypertension control, 164
myelin repair, 166–168
sleep medicine, 164–165
stem cell therapeutics, 168–169
vascular diseases of white matter, 42–49, *43*
Binswanger's Disease, 46–49
cerebral amyloid angiopathy, *43*, 173
leukoaraiosis, 43–46
migraine, *43*, 75
subcortical ischemic vascular dementia, 43, 46
white matter disease of immaturity, *43*
white matter hyperintensities (WMH)
absence of cognitive correlates, 49, 107–108
age-related, 10
in Alzheimer's Disease, 177
FXTAS and, 78
gray matter disease and, 49
hypertension and, 164
leukoaraiosis and, 43, 44
in MCI, 177
MRI recognition of, 10–11, *43*, 43, 51, 98
MS white matter lesions and, 59–60
NPH and, 72
perceptual/constructional deficits with, 104
SLE and, 64
solvent exposure and, 51
vitamin B_{12} deficiency and, 68
white matter lacunar dementia, 105
white matter lesions. *See also* white matter hyperintensities
assumptions made about, 4
cognition-related neurochemical systems and, 154
in the frontal lobes, 4
impact on cognition, emotion, 5
investigational challenges, 10, 36
ischemic and global brain atrophy, 36
neuroimaging studies of, 3, 6, 11, 36
syndromes occurring with, 7
in traumatic brain injury, 55
white matter toxins, *50*
white matter tracts. *See also* association tracts; commissural tracts
connecting peduncles of, 19
connectome and, 21
DKI visualization of, 13
DTI studies, 12, 57, 74, 101
frontal aslant tract, 153
language-related, 106
macroconnectivity of, 21
MCD and, 124

MRI observations, 101
musical training impact on, 139
neural networks in, 14
neurobehavioral impairment and, 35–36
neuroimaging visualization of, *9*, 9
physiology of, 20
plasticity and, 139
projection tracts, 17, 156
relevance to behavioral neurology, *18*
restoration of, 147
rTMS and, 148
size variances, 17
subcortical dementia and, 30
tracts relevant to behavioral neurology, *18*
unanswered questions about, 153
Wallerian degeneration in DAI, 55

Williams, M. A., 71
Wilson, R. K., 71
Wilson's Disease, *28*
Wisconsin Card Sorting Test, 144
WMH. *See* white matter hyperintensities

young-onset dementia, 37

zidovudine (AZT), 67, 144